Pediatric Facial Plastic and Reconstructive Surgery

Editor

SHERARD A. TATUM

FACIAL PLASTIC SURGERY CLINICS OF NORTH AMERICA

www.facialplastic.theclinics.com

Consulting Editor
J. REGAN THOMAS

November 2014 • Volume 22 • Number 4

ELSEVIER

1600 John F. Kennedy Boulevard • Suite 1800 • Philadelphia, Pennsylvania, 19103-2899

http://www.theclinics.com

FACIAL PLASTIC SURGERY CLINICS OF NORTH AMERICA Volume 22, Number 4
November 2014 ISSN 1064-7406, ISBN-13: 978-0-323-32371-0

Editor: Joanne Husovski
Developmental Editor: Susan Showalter

Facial Plastic Surgery Clinics of North America (ISSN 1064-7406) is published quarterly by Elsevier Inc., 360 Park Avenue South, New York, NY 10010-1710. Months of issue are February, May, August, and November. Business and Editorial Offices: 1600 John F. Kennedy Blvd., Suite 1800, Philadelphia, PA 19103-2899. Periodicals postage paid at New York, NY, and additional mailing offices. Subscription prices are $390.00 per year (US individuals), $525.00 per year (US institutions), $445.00 per year (Canadian individuals), $653.00 per year (Canadian institutions), $535.00 per year (foreign individuals), $653.00 per year (foreign institutions), $185.00 per year (US students), and $255.00 per year (foreign students). Foreign air speed delivery is included in all *Clinics* subscription prices. All prices are subject to change without notice. POSTMASTER: Send address changes to *Facial Plastic Surgery Clinics*, Elsevier Health Sciences Division, Subscription Customer Service, 3251 Riverport Lane, Maryland Heights, MO 63043. **Customer service: 1-800-654-2452 (US and Canada); 1-314-447-8871 (outside US and Canada); Fax: 314-447-8029; E-mail:journalscustomerservice-usa@elsevier.com (for print support); journalsonlinesupport-usa@elsevier.com (for online support).**

Reprints. For copies of 100 or more of articles in this publication, please contact the Commercial Reprints Department, Elsevier Inc., 360 Park Avenue South, New York, NY 10010-1710. Tel.: 212-633-3874; Fax: 212-633-3820; E-mail: reprints@elsevier.com.

Facial Plastic Surgery Clinics of North America is covered in *MEDLINE/PubMed* (*Index Medicus*).

Contributors

CONSULTING EDITOR

J. REGAN THOMAS, MD
Mansueto Professor and Chairman,
Department of Otolaryngology–Head and Neck
Surgery, University of Illinois at Chicago,
Chicago, Illinois

EDITOR

SHERARD A. TATUM, MD, FACS, FAAP
Professor of Otolaryngology and Pediatrics,
Division of Facial Plastic and Reconstructive
Surgery, Department of Otolaryngology and
Communication Sciences, Upstate Medical
University, SUNY Upstate Medical University,
Syracuse, New York

AUTHORS

PETER A. ADAMSON, MD, FACS, FRCSC
Professor and Head, Division of Facial Plastic
and Reconstructive Surgery, Department of
Otolaryngology–Head and Neck Surgery,
University of Toronto; Adamson Associates
Cosmetic Facial Surgery, Toronto, Ontario,
Canada

CAROLINE A. BANKS, MD
Facial Plastic and Reconstructive Surgery
Fellow, Department of Otology and
Laryngology, Massachusetts Eye and Ear
Infirmary, Harvard Medical School, Boston,
Massachusetts

MICHAEL BASSIRI-TEHRANI, MD
Otolaryngology–Head and Neck Surgery,
New York Eye and Ear Infirmary of Mount Sinai,
New York, New York

SYDNEY C. BUTTS, MD
Chief of the Division of Facial Plastic and
Reconstructive Surgery, Assistant Professor,
The Department of Otolaryngology–Head and
Neck Surgery, Director of the Greater Brooklyn
Cleft and Craniofacial Team, The State

University of New York, Downstate Medical
Center, Brooklyn, New York

JONATHAN A. CABIN, MD
Otolaryngology–Head and Neck Surgery,
New York Eye and Ear Infirmary of Mount Sinai,
New York, New York

RANDOLPH B. CAPONE, MD, FACS
Assistant Professor, The Department of
Otolaryngology–Head and Neck Surgery,
Co-Director of the Greater Baltimore Cleft Lip
and Palate Team, The Johns Hopkins University
School of Medicine, Baltimore, Maryland

DAVID J. CROCKETT, MD
Department of Otolaryngology–Head and Neck
Surgery, Vanderbilt University Medical Center,
Nashville, Tennessee

JOSHUA C. DEMKE, MD
Assistant Professor, Facial Plastic and
Reconstructive Surgery, Department of
Surgery, Co-director, West Texas Craniofacial
Center of Excellence, Texas Tech Health
Sciences Center, Lubbock, Texas

NICOLE M. FOWLER, MD
Department of Otolaryngology–Head and Neck Surgery, University of Washington, Seattle, Washington

JAMIE L. FUNAMURA, MD
Resident Physician, Department of Otolaryngology–Head and Neck Surgery, University of California, Davis Medical Center, Sacramento, California

NEAL D. FUTRAN, MD, DMD
Allison T. Wanamaker Professor and Chair, Department of Otolaryngology–Head and Neck Surgery, University of Washington, Seattle, Washington

STEVEN L. GOUDY, MD
Associate Professor, Department of Otolaryngology–Head and Neck Surgery, Vanderbilt University Medical Center, Vanderbilt University, Nashville, Tennessee

TESSA A. HADLOCK, MD
Director, Division of Facial Plastic and Reconstructive Surgery and Facial Nerve Center, Department of Otology and Laryngology, Massachusetts Eye and Ear Infirmary, Harvard Medical School, Boston, Massachusetts

MARCELO HOCHMAN, MD
Hemangioma and Malformation Treatment Center, Charleston, South Carolina

LAMONT R. JONES, MD
Vice Chairman, The Department of Otolaryngology–Head and Neck Surgery, Director of the Cleft and Craniofacial Clinic, Senior Staff, The Henry Ford Health System, Detroit, Michigan

ROBERT M. KELLMAN, MD, FACS
Professor and Chairman, Department of Otolaryngology, Upstate Medical University, State University of New York, Syracuse, New York

STEVEN R. MOBLEY, MD
Adjunct Associate Professor, Adjunct Track, Division of Otolaryngology–Head and Neck Surgery, University of Utah, Salt Lake City, Utah

LASZLO NAGY, MD
Covenant Health Robert Moore, M.D., Endowed Chair in Pediatrics, Assistant Professor, Pediatric Neurosurgery, Department of Pediatrics, Co-director, West Texas Craniofacial Center of Excellence, Texas Tech Health Sciences Center, Lubbock, Texas

THOMAS ROMO III, MD
Division of Facial Plastic and Reconstructive Surgery, Lenox Hill Hospital, New York, New York

NOAH BENJAMIN SANDS, MD, FRCSC
Clinical Fellow, Division of Facial Plastic and Reconstructive Surgery, Department of Otolaryngology–Head and Neck Surgery, University of Toronto; Adamson Associates Cosmetic Facial Surgery, Toronto, Ontario, Canada

ANTHONY P. SCLAFANI, MD, FACS
Director, Division of Facial Plastic and Reconstructive Surgery, Otolaryngology–Head and Neck Surgery, New York Eye and Ear Infirmary of Mount Sinai, Professor of Otolaryngology, Icahn School of Medicine at Mount Sinai, New York, New York

TIANJIE SHEN, MD
Department of Otolaryngology–Head and Neck Surgery, Kaiser San Francisco, San Francisco, California

KATHLEEN C.Y. SIE, MD
Department of Otolaryngology–Head and Neck Surgery, University of Washington; Division of Pediatric Otolaryngology, Childhood Communication Center, Seattle Children's Hospital, Seattle, Washington

PHAYVANH P. SJOGREN, MD
Resident in Otolaryngology, Division of Otolaryngology–Head and Neck Surgery, University of Utah, Salt Lake City, Utah

JONATHAN M. SYKES, MD, FACS
Professor and Director of Facial Plastic and Reconstructive Surgery, Department of Otolaryngology–Head and Neck Surgery, University of California, Davis Medical Center, University of California, Davis Health System, Sacramento, California

SHERARD A. TATUM, MD, FACS, FAAP
Professor of Otolaryngology and Pediatrics,
Division of Facial Plastic and Reconstructive
Surgery, Department of Otolaryngology and
Communication Sciences, SUNY Upstate
Medical University, Syracuse, New York

RYAN WINTERS, MD
Division of Facial Plastic and Reconstructive
Surgery, Department of Otolaryngology
and Communication Sciences, SUNY
Upstate Medical University, Syracuse,
New York

Contents

Pediatric Facial Nerve Rehabilitation   487

Caroline A. Banks and Tessa A. Hadlock

> Facial paralysis is a rare but severe condition in the pediatric population. Impaired facial movement has multiple causes and varied presentations, therefore individualized treatment plans are essential for optimal results. Advances in facial reanimation over the past 4 decades have given rise to new treatments designed to restore balance and function in pediatric patients with facial paralysis. This article provides a comprehensive review of pediatric facial rehabilitation and describes a zone-based approach to assessment and treatment of impaired facial movement.

Pediatric Septorhinoplasty   503

Jamie L. Funamura and Jonathan M. Sykes

> In the appropriately selected patient, septorhinoplasty can benefit a pediatric patient presenting with significant nasal trauma, abscess, or mass that will likely result in a progressive deformity in the growing nose or with negative functional or psychosocial effect. Clinical and experimental observations support a conservative approach to cartilage scoring and resection in pediatric patients in which septorhinoplasty is deemed necessary.

Infantile Hemangiomas: Current Management   509

Marcelo Hochman

> Management of infantile hemangiomas includes a combination of observation, medical therapy, laser treatments, and surgery. The nomenclature to describe these lesions has been standardized and should be adhered to. The goal of treatment is to obtain the best possible result commensurate with known developmental milestones. Current knowledge of the biology of these tumors as well as experience allows obtaining this goal. "Leave it alone, it will go away" is no longer universally acceptable advice for treatment of infantile hemangiomas.

Craniofacial Anomalies   523

Laszlo Nagy and Joshua C. Demke

 Videos related to pediatric craniofacial surgical procedures (Video 1: Open approach for sagittal synostosis subtotal cranial vault recon without bone grafting and Video 2: Depicts endoscopic-assisted strip craniectomy with wedge craniectomy) accompany this article

> Craniosynostosis, in which 1 or more cranial sutures prematurely fuse, is associated with diverse environmental and genetic factors. Whereas isolated single-suture synostosis is usually sporadic and nonfamilial, FGFR mutations account for most cases of syndromic craniosynostosis. This article reviews the etiology and various clinical manifestations of the most common isolated and syndromic forms of craniosynostosis, and provides a brief overview of genetics. Past and present surgical management approaches and techniques are examined in depth. Outcomes data in the

recent literature are reviewed, and controversies in the field and promising trends in craniofacial surgery discussed.

Head and neck tumors requiring large composite resections are rare in pediatrics. Large soft tissue and/or bony resections are usually the result of a neoplastic, traumatic, or infectious process. Sarcomas are the most common malignancy. Surgical resection is usually recommended after chemotherapy and/or radiation therapy. Free tissue transfer is safe and effective in this population, which has continued craniofacial growth and development. The surgeon must know the anatomic location of the growth centers and facial skeletal relationships because disruption results in abnormal development. Free tissue transfer can restore normal maxillomandibular occlusion and condylar-cranial articulation.

Trauma is a leading cause of death in children. The pediatric facial skeleton goes through progressive development and major changes, including change in the size ratio of the cranium to the face; change in the ratio of facial soft tissue to bone, and pneumatization of the sinuses. The main goal of maxillofacial fracture repair is to reestablish normal or preinjury structure and function. Follow-up is typically recommended until children reach skeletal maturity as trauma may affect growth of the facial skeleton. Problems not obvious immediately after the injury may become an issue later, and secondary surgery might be needed to address such issues.

Cleft lip with or without cleft palate is the most common congenital malformation of the head and neck. Orofacial clefting could significantly affect the quality of life of the child and requires multiple steps of care to obtain an optimal outcome. Each patient should be evaluated for congenital anomalies, developmental delay, neurologic disorders, and psychosocial concerns. A multidisciplinary team is necessary to ensure that every aspect of the child's care is appropriately treated and coordination between providers is achieved. This article discusses the assessment and treatment recommendations for children born with cleft lip and/or cleft palate.

Facial plastic surgeons have a comprehensive understanding of the challenges that patients with cleft lip and palate encounter in form and function. Because there are areas in the United States where access to cleft care is limited, opportunities exist for facial plastic surgeons to develop cleft teams to provide greater availability of services to patients. A consensus statement has been developed by the Cleft and Craniofacial Subcommittee of the Specialty Surgery Committee of the American Academy of Facial Plastic and Reconstructive Surgery that outlines strategies for facial plastic surgeons who are prepared to assume leadership roles in domestic multidisciplinary cleft team initiatives.

Most speech disorders of childhood are treated with speech therapy. However, two conditions, ankyloglossia and velopharyngeal dysfunction, may be amenable to surgical intervention. It is important for surgeons to work with experienced speech language pathologists to diagnose the speech disorder. Children with articulation disorders related to ankyloglossia may benefit from frenuloplasty. Children with velopharyngeal dysfunction should have standardized clinical evaluation and instrumental asseessment of velopharyngeal function. Surgeons should develop a treatment protocol to optimize speechoutcomes while mnimizing morbidity.

Pediatric otoplasty is generally considered to be a "simple" procedure, but an astute surgeon recognizes the challenges of this operation and is mindful of the degree of detail involved in its planning and execution. The vast number of described otoplasty methods, which are ever evolving, is a testament to the complexity of this procedure. In this article, the authors' methodology with respect to preoperative analysis and planning, surgical technique, and postoperative care, including management of complications and potential pitfalls, are highlighted.

 Videos of microtia reconstruction accompany this article

Microtia represents a spectrum of maldevelopment of the external ear. Reconstructive techniques may utilize an autogenous rib cartilage framework and require 2–4 stages; alternatively, an alloplastic framework can be used and typically requires 1–2 stages. Successful reconstruction of microtia with either technique can provide a significant quality of life improvement, and both techniques are described in this article.

Numerous techniques and treatments have been described for scar revision, with most studies focusing on the adult population. A comprehensive review of the literature reveals a paucity of references related specifically to scar revision in children. This review describes the available modalities in pediatric facial scar revision. The authors have integrated current practices in soft tissue trauma and scar revision, including closure techniques and materials, topical therapy, steroid injection, cutaneous laser therapy, and tissue expanders.

Distraction osteogenesis (DO) may be the most versatile tool to become available to the craniofacial surgeon in recent years. It can be used in an ever-expanding register of clinical scenarios and offers major advantages over conventional craniofacial techniques in some circumstances. Craniofacial surgery has significant complications, some of which can be mitigated but not eliminated by choosing DO over conventional approaches. Although some DO applications are in their infancy with limited data, this article provides an overview of current uses of this versatile technology.

FACIAL PLASTIC SURGERY CLINICS OF NORTH AMERICA

DOWNLOAD Free App!

Review Articles THE CLINICS

NOW AVAILABLE FOR YOUR iPhone and iPad

Preface
Pediatric Facial Plastic and Reconstructive Surgery

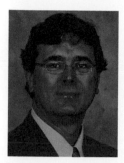

Sherard A. Tatum, MD, FACS, FAAP
Editor

It is indeed an honor to have been asked to guest edit the "Pediatric Facial Plastic and Reconstructive Surgery" issue of *Facial Plastic Surgery Clinics of North America*. I must begin by expressing my deepest gratitude to the *Facial Plastic Surgery Clinics of North America* editors and editorial staff and especially the authors of these excellent articles. Without them, this issue of outstanding articles would not have happened.

Facial plastic and reconstructive surgery has a storied history as was recently emphasized at the 50th anniversary celebration of the American Academy of Facial Plastic and Reconstructive Surgery. For over 100 years, the discipline has been nurtured by great surgeons such as Jacques Joseph, Sir Harold Gilles, John Orlando Roe, Gustave Aufricht, Johann Friedrich Dieffenbach, and Robert Weir. Later, there were John Conley, Samuel Foman, Maurice Cottle, Irving Goldman, Richard Webster, Jack Anderson, and Richard Farrior, to name a few. We have made great strides in furthering the field subsequently, and pediatric facial plastic and reconstructive surgery subspecialization is a logical next step to consider as has been done by so many other medical specialties.

This array of pediatric topics speaks volumes about our growth as a specialty. And there were numerous other topics not included because of size constraints. From scar revision and otoplasty to free tissue transfer and synostosis repair, this issue covers most of the broad field of facial plastic and reconstructive surgery as applied to children. As you read these articles, take note of the quality of our colleagues' work. Their dedication to the welfare of children with facial plastic surgery issues is exemplary. I hope you will find these articles as enjoyable and informative as I have.

Sherard A. Tatum, MD, FACS, FAAP
Division of Facial Plastic and
Reconstructive Surgery
Upstate Medical University State
University of New York
750 East Adams Street, CWB
Syracuse, NY 13210, USA

E-mail address:
tatums@upstate.edu

Facial Plast Surg Clin N Am 22 (2014) xiii
http://dx.doi.org/10.1016/j.fsc.2014.08.004

Pediatric Facial Nerve Rehabilitation

Caroline A. Banks, MD[a], Tessa A. Hadlock, MD[b],*

KEYWORDS

- Facial paralysis • Facial nerve palsy • Pediatric • Gracilis • Synkinesis • Bell palsy

KEY POINTS

- The main goals of facial reanimation are to restore symmetry, balance, resting tone, and movement to the face, and to decrease hyperfunction from aberrant regeneration.
- Special considerations in the pediatric population include the ability to understand and participate in rehabilitation, small-caliber vessels and nerves, and concerns about long-term outcomes with continued craniofacial growth.
- An individualized treatment plan is developed for each patient. The paralyzed face is assessed and treated by zone.
- Free muscle transfer for smile reanimation in children is safe and has superior results compared with adults. It should be considered as first-line therapy for children with lack of meaningful smile.
- Treatments directed at decreasing synkinesis, including botulinum toxin, physical therapy, and surgery, are critical in the overall treatment of children with facial paralysis.

HISTORICAL PERSPECTIVE

Harii and colleagues[1] first described gracilis free muscle transfer with microvascular anastomosis for facial rehabilitation in 1976. Free muscle transfer has since become the gold standard for dynamic smile restoration in the adult population. The treatment of impaired facial movement in children is less defined. Investigators Including Ueda and colleagues,[2] Terzis and colleagues,[3–7] Zuker and colleagues,[8,9] and Hadlock and colleagues[10] have focused specifically on the pediatric population to provide treatment algorithms for children. Advances in facial reanimation over the past 4 decades have given rise to new treatments designed to restore balance and function in pediatric patients with facial paralysis.

INTRODUCTION

Facial palsy in the pediatric population is a rare condition, with an incidence of 21.1 per 100,000 per year for children less than 15 years old.[11] Facial paralysis has variable presentations, ranging from complete hypofunction to hyperfuction and mixed presentations. Injury to the facial nerve can have severe consequences, including physical deformity, ocular complications, nasal valve collapse, inability to express emotion, oral incompetence, and speech difficulty. The treatment of pediatric facial paralysis is especially challenging because of additional psychosocial concerns, the impact of future growth and potential disfigurement, anatomic considerations, and complex parent decision making.

Pediatric facial paralysis is classified as congenital or acquired. Congenital facial paralysis is uncommon and has multiple causes including birth trauma, Moebius syndrome, unilateral lower lip paralysis, hemifacial microsomia, Goldenhar-Gorlin syndrome, CHARGE (Coloboma, Heart defects, Atresia choanae, Retardation of growth and/or development, Genital and/or urinary

Disclosure: The authors have no conflict of interest in relation to this article.
[a] Department of Otology and Laryngology, Massachusetts Eye and Ear Infirmary, Harvard Medical School, 243 Charles Street, Boston, MA 02114, USA; [b] Division of Facial Plastic and Reconstructive Surgery and Facial Nerve Center, Department of Otology and Laryngology, Massachusetts Eye and Ear Infirmary, Harvard Medical School, 243 Charles Street, Boston, MA 02114, USA
* Corresponding author.
E-mail address: tessa_hadlock@meei.harvard.edu

abnormalities, and Ear abnormalities and/or hearing loss) association, Arnold-Chiari malformation, and syringobulbia.[12,13] Physical examination and the presence of synkinesis can help distinguish between traumatic and developmental deficits. Acquired facial paralysis in the pediatric population may be caused by infection, Bell's palsy, neoplasm, or trauma. The most common cause of pediatric facial paralysis is debated in the literature. Although Bell's palsy occurs less frequently in children compared with adults, multiple studies have found that Bell's palsy accounts for most pediatric facial paralysis, occurring in 40% to 50% of cases.[14–17] Other studies have found an identifiable cause in most patients, citing that fewer than 20% of children were diagnosed with Bell's palsy.[18,19] Both Grundfast and colleagues[18] and Evans and colleagues[19] found that infectious causes, most frequently otitis media, and trauma were the most common causes of facial nerve paralysis in children.

TREATMENT GOALS

When facial nerve injury occurs, the primary goal is to reestablish continuity of the facial nerve via direct neurorrhaphy or cable graft. Facial reanimation procedures are performed when reestablishing the nerve is not possible or when reestablishment of the nerve leads to unacceptable results. The main goals of facial reanimation procedures and adjuvant therapies are to restore symmetry, balance, resting tone, and movement to the face, and to decrease hyperfunction from aberrant regeneration. The specific treatment goals vary with each patient.

PREOPERATIVE PLANNING AND PREPARATION

Preoperative planning begins with a thorough history to determine the cause of facial paralysis and the likelihood of spontaneous recovery. Cognitive evaluation is also important in children, because physical therapy and muscle training are often components of facial reanimation. All patients undergo zonal facial assessment, including documentation of resting position and movement on eFACE (Fig. 1), photography of 7 standard facial expressions, videography, and spontaneous smile assay. The clinician then develops an individualized treatment plan. If the treatment algorithm includes surgery, medical clearance is required.

There are special considerations in the pediatric population. Although children as young as 2 years old have successfully undergone free tissue transfer for smile restoration,[6] waiting until at least 5 or

6 years of age, around the time the child is school aged and becomes self-aware, is preferred.[6,20] Delaying major procedures until this age provides time for growth of nerves and vessels, whose small caliber may lead to free flap failure, and allows children to be mature enough to understand and participate in their own care. There is a theoretic concern that surgery may disrupt continued craniofacial growth and lead to disfigurement; however, this has not been established in human studies.[6] In addition, some investigators have found poorer results after long-term follow-up of free flaps for facial reanimation,[21] raising the concern that free flaps in childhood might not function adequately into adulthood. Multiple investigators have refuted these results, reporting excellent aesthetic and functional long-term outcomes following free flap smile reanimation.[2,6,20,22,23]

PROCEDURAL APPROACH TO ZONE-BASED FACIAL REANIMATION SURGERY
Ocular Rehabilitation

After facial nerve injury, ocular protection to prevent dryness, corneal abrasion, and irreversible blindness is paramount.[24] In all children with incomplete eye closure, an aggressive eye care regimen, including artificial tears during the day and ophthalmic ointment with eyelid patching at night, should be established immediately.

Static procedures

Ocular reanimation may involve static and/or dynamic techniques. Pediatric patients with lagophthalmos are candidates for static eyelid procedures to passively assist in upper eyelid closure, including eyelid weights or palpebral springs. Platinum weights are preferred in adults and children because of their thinner profile, decreased tendency for capsule formation, and lower rates of extrusion.[25] In cooperative children, the procedure may be performed under local anesthesia. For younger children or those who require multiple procedures for facial reanimation, the eyelid weight is placed under general anesthesia. The supratarsal crease is marked before surgery. The patient is placed in a supine position. An incision is made in the crease, and dissection is performed through the orbicularis oculi to the tarsal plate. The implant is centered between the midpupillary line and the medial limbus and sutured in 3 places to the tarsal plate with 6-0 clear nylon sutures (Fig. 2). Eyelid weights can easily be removed during a brief office procedure if facial paralysis resolves.

Lower lid malposition occurs less commonly in the pediatric population. In children with lower lid

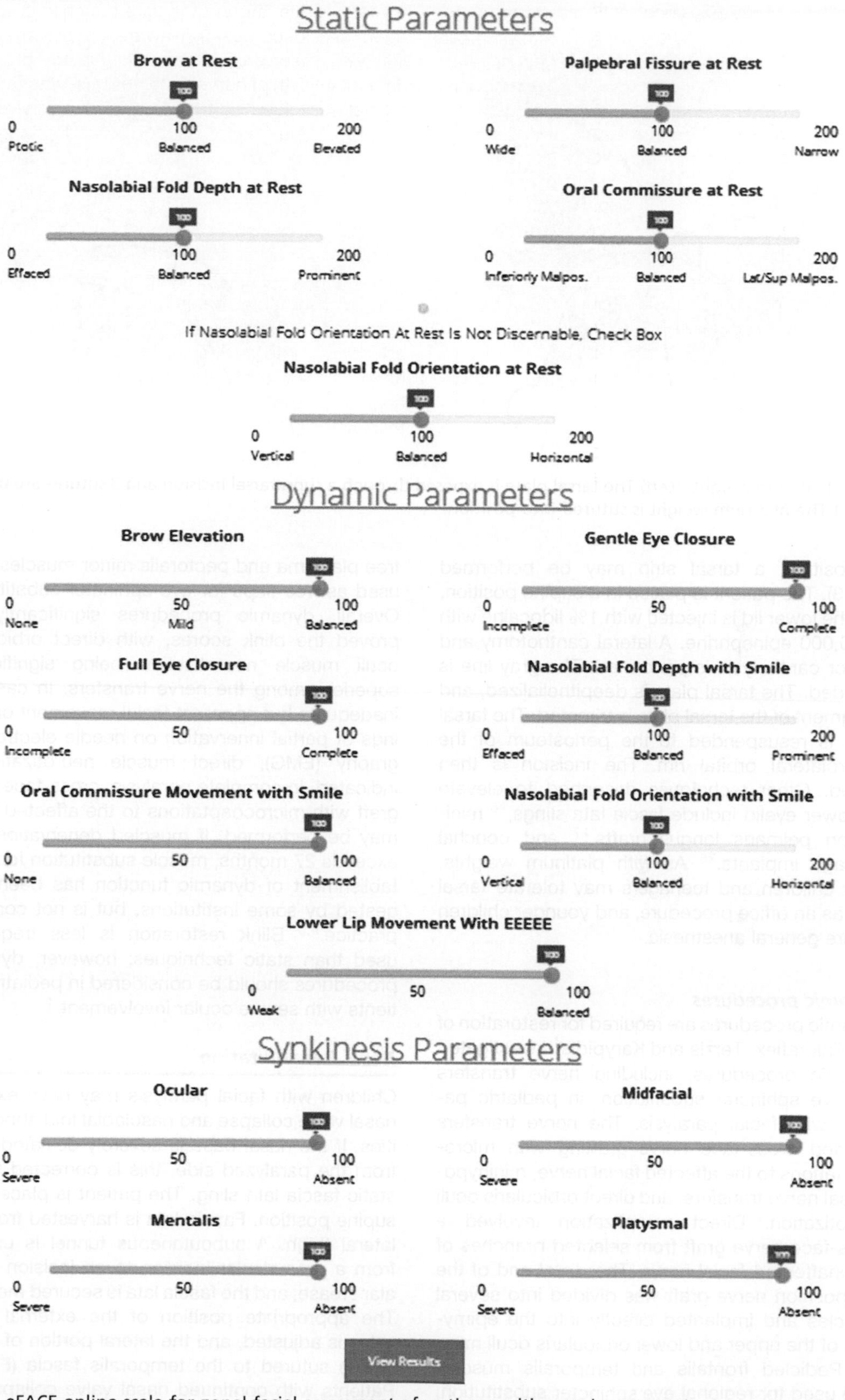

Static Parameters

Brow at Rest

0 — Ptotic
100 — Balanced
200 — Elevated

Palpebral Fissure at Rest

0 — Wide
100 — Balanced
200 — Narrow

Nasolabial Fold Depth at Rest

0 — Effaced
100 — Balanced
200 — Prominent

Oral Commissure at Rest

0 — Inferiorly Malpos.
100 — Balanced
200 — Lat/Sup Malpos.

If Nasolabial Fold Orientation At Rest Is Not Discernable, Check Box

Nasolabial Fold Orientation at Rest

0 — Vertical
100 — Balanced
200 — Horizontal

Dynamic Parameters

Brow Elevation

0 — None
50 — Mild
100 — Balanced

Gentle Eye Closure

0 — Incomplete
50
100 — Complete

Full Eye Closure

0 — Incomplete
50
100 — Complete

Nasolabial Fold Depth with Smile

0 — Effaced
100 — Balanced
200 — Prominent

Oral Commissure Movement with Smile

0 — None
50
100 — Balanced

Nasolabial Fold Orientation with Smile

0 — Vertical
100 — Balanced
200 — Horizontal

Lower Lip Movement With EEEEE

0 — Weak
50
100 — Balanced

Synkinesis Parameters

Ocular

0 — Severe
50
100 — Absent

Midfacial

0 — Severe
50
100 — Absent

Mentalis

0 — Severe
50
100 — Absent

Platysmal

0 — Severe
50
100 — Absent

View Results

Fig. 1. eFACE online scale for zonal facial assessment of resting position and movement.

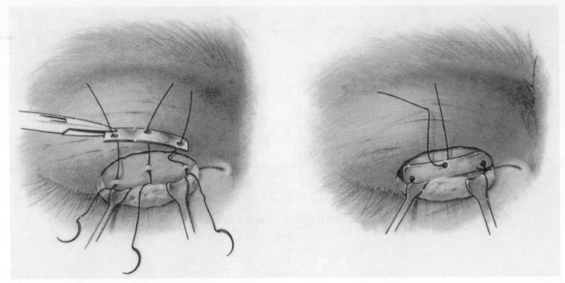

Fig. 2. Platinum weight. (*Left*) The tarsal plate is exposed through a supratarsal incision and 3 sutures are placed. (*Right*) The platinum weight is sutured into position.

malposition, a tarsal strip may be performed (**Fig. 3**). The patient is placed in a supine position, and the lower lid is injected with 1% lidocaine with 1:100,000 epinephrine. A lateral canthotomy and inferior cantholysis is performed. The gray line is denuded. The tarsal plate is deepithelialized, and a segment of the tarsal plate is trimmed. The tarsal plate is resuspended to the periosteum of the superolateral orbital rim. The incision is then closed. Other techniques described to elevate the lower eyelid include fascia lata slings,[26] minitendon palmaris longus grafts,[27] and conchal cartilage implants.[28] As with platinum weights, older children and teenagers may tolerate tarsal strip as an office procedure, and younger children require general anesthesia.

Dynamic procedures

Dynamic procedures are required for restoration of the blink reflex. Terzis and Karypidis[4] investigated dynamic procedures, including nerve transfers and eye sphincter substitution, in pediatric patients with facial paralysis. The nerve transfers included cross-face nerve grafting with microcoaptations to the affected facial nerve, minihypoglossal nerve transfers, and direct orbicularis oculi neurotization. Direct neurotization involved a cross-face nerve graft from selected branches of the unaffected facial nerve. The distal end of the interposition nerve graft was divided into several fascicles and implanted directly into the epimysium of the upper and lower orbicularis oculi muscle. Pedicled frontalis and temporalis muscles were used for regional eye sphincter substitution;

free platysma and pectoralis minor muscles were used as free flaps for eye sphincter substitution. Overall, dynamic procedures significantly improved the blink scores, with direct orbicularis oculi muscle neurotization being significantly superior among the nerve transfers. In cases of inadequate but apparent facial movement or findings of partial innervation on needle electromyography (EMG), direct muscle neurotization is indicated. In complete paralysis, cross-face nerve graft with microcoaptations to the affected nerve may be performed. If muscled denervation time exceeds 27 months, muscle substitution for reestablishment of dynamic function has been suggested by some institutions, but is not common practice.[4,5] Blink restoration is less frequently used than static techniques; however, dynamic procedures should be considered in pediatric patients with severe ocular involvement.[4]

Nasal Rehabilitation

Children with facial paralysis may have external nasal valve collapse and nasolabial fold abnormalities. If the nasal base is severely deviated away from the paralyzed side, this is corrected with a static fascia lata sling. The patient is placed in a supine position. Fascia lata is harvested from the lateral thigh. A subcutaneous tunnel is created from a preauricular incision to an incision in the alar crease, and the fascia lata is secured medially. The appropriate position of the external nasal valve is adjusted, and the lateral portion of fascia lata is sutured to the temporalis fascia (**Fig. 4**). Patients with continued nasal valve collapse are

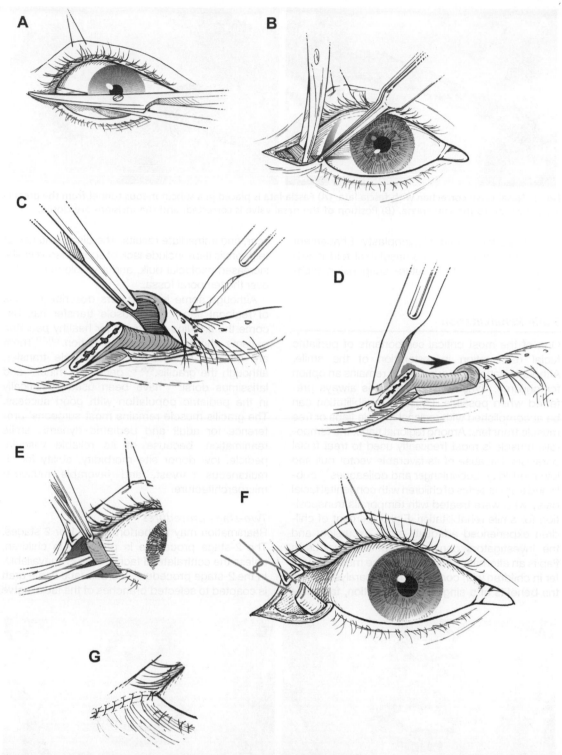

Fig. 3. Lower lid elevation in the paralyzed eye. (*A*) Canthotomy. (*B*) Inferior cantholysis. (*C*) Denuding the gray line. (*D*) Sharp deepithelialization of the conjunctival covering of the tarsal plate. (*E*) Amputation of segment of the tarsal plate. (*F*) Suture resuspension of tarsal plate to periosteum of superolateral orbital rim. (*G*) Final closure.

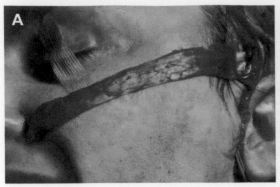
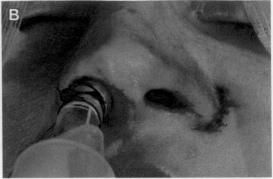

Fig. 4. Nasal valve correction with fascia lata. (*A*) Fascia lata is placed in a subcutaneous tunnel from the preauricular incision to the alar crease. (*B*) Position of the nasal valve is corrected, and the incisions are closed.

candidates for functional rhinoplasty. Effacement or hyperprominence of the nasolabial fold is addressed through static suture suspension techniques (**Fig. 5**).[29,30]

Smile Rehabilitation

One of the most critical components of pediatric facial reanimation is restoration of the smile. Although static facial suspension remains an option for children, dynamic reanimation is always preferred when possible. Dynamic rehabilitation can be accomplished with regional muscle flaps or free muscle transfers. Among regional flaps, the temporalis muscle is most frequently used to treat facial paralysis, because of its favorable vector pull and low morbidity. Leboulanger and colleagues[12] published a small series of children with congenital facial palsy who were treated with temporalis transposition for smile rehabilitation. Eighty percent of children experienced adequate smile excursion, and the investigators concluded that the temporalis flap is an alternative treatment to free muscle transfer in children with congenital facial paralysis, citing the benefits of a single-stage operation, favorable

scar, and immediate results. The disadvantages of temporalis flaps include lack of spontaneous smile, increased midfacial bulk, and a visible depression over the temporal fossa.

Although some investigators describe the use of regional flaps, free muscle transfer has become the first-line treatment for healthy pediatric patients who desire smile reanimation.[2,6,10] There are multiple options for free muscle transfer, although the gracilis,[2,6,10] pectoralis minor,[6] and latissimus dorsi[2,6] have been used specifically in the pediatric population with good success. The gracilis muscle remains most surgeons' preference for adult and pediatric dynamic smile reanimation, because of its reliable vascular pedicle, low donor site morbidity, ability for simultaneous harvest, and favorable muscular microarchitecture.

Two-stage procedures
Reanimation may be performed in 1 or 2 stages. The 2-stage procedure is preferred in children, unless the contralateral facial nerve is unavailable. In the 2-stage procedure, a cross-face nerve graft is coapted to selected branches of the facial nerve

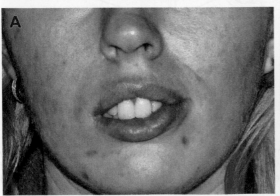
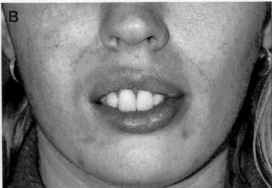

Fig. 5. Nasolabial fold correction. (*A*) Before surgery, with effacement of the right nasolabial fold. (*B*) After suture suspension of the right nasolabial fold.

on the unaffected side and buried in the lip for 6 to 12 months. The sural nerve is the most frequently used nerve for the cross-face nerve graft.[31] The gracilis muscle is then harvested, transferred to the paralyzed side, and driven by the cross-face nerve graft. The greatest benefit of the 2-stage procedure is the ability to restore spontaneous, emotive facial expression, which is the main goal of pediatric smile restoration (**Fig. 6**). The major disadvantage is the higher failure rate compared with 1-stage procedures, resulting from inadequate penetration across the 2 neurorrhaphies, which occurs in approximately 20% of adults and children.[32]

One-stage procedures

The 1-stage procedure is reserved for children who have bilateral facial paralysis (ie, Moebius syndrome), those whose contralateral facial nerve is at risk for paralysis (ie, neurofibromatosis 2), or for children who have failed a 2-stage gracilis. One-stage procedures are classically innervated by the masseteric nerve and provide earlier results, because of the single neurorrhaphy and close proximity of the donor nerve. Flaps innervated by the masseteric nerve have reliably strong voluntary contraction; however, they do not deliver a spontaneous smile (**Fig. 7**). One-stage free flaps have higher success rates, approximately 92%, compared with flaps innervated by cross-face nerve grafts.[32]

First stage cross-face nerve grafting

Patient positioning The patient is placed in a supine position and general nasotracheal intubation is achieved.

Procedural approach A preauricular incision, extending from the temporal region to 2 to 3 cm inferior to the angle of the mandible, is made with a #15 blade. The parotidomasseteric fascia (PMF) is identified, and a skin flap is raised and brought forward to the masseteric fascia. At the anterior border of the parotid gland, facial nerve branches are identified. Donor branches of the facial nerve that produce isolated smile movement are selected using a Montgomery nerve stimulator (Boston Medical Products, Worcester, MA) and isolated with vessel loops.

Harvest of the sural nerve is performed endoscopically through a 2-cm incision lateral to the lateral malleolus (**Fig. 8**). The nerve is transferred to the face and tunneled subcutaneously from the nonparalyzed side, across the upper lip, to the gingivobuccal sulcus on the paralyzed side, using a Wright needle (**Fig. 9**). The previously selected branches of the unaffected facial nerve are transected, and the sural nerve is sutured to

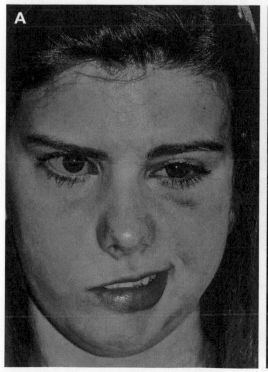 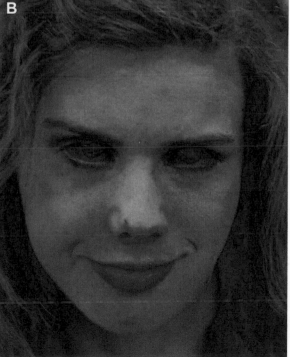

Fig. 6. (*A*) Right facial paralysis and poor smile excursion before surgery. (*B*) After 2-stage free gracilis transfer. Note the balanced, spontaneous smile.

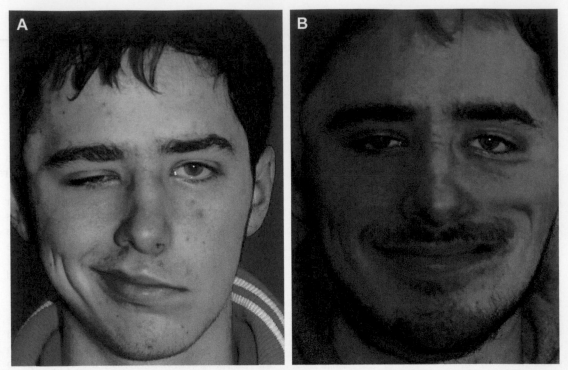

Fig. 7. (*A*) Left facial paralysis before surgery in a patient with neurofibromatosis. (*B*) After 1-stage free gracilis transfer. Note the strong, voluntary smile.

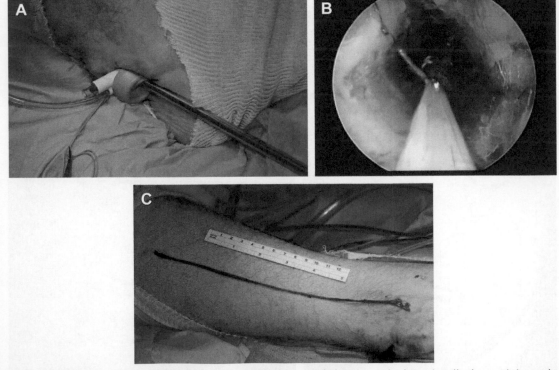

Fig. 8. Endoscopic sural nerve harvest. (*A*) A 2-cm incision is made lateral to the lateral malleolus, and the endoscope is inserted into the leg. (*B*) Endoscopic view of the sural nerve. (*C*) The sural nerve is harvested through a single incision.

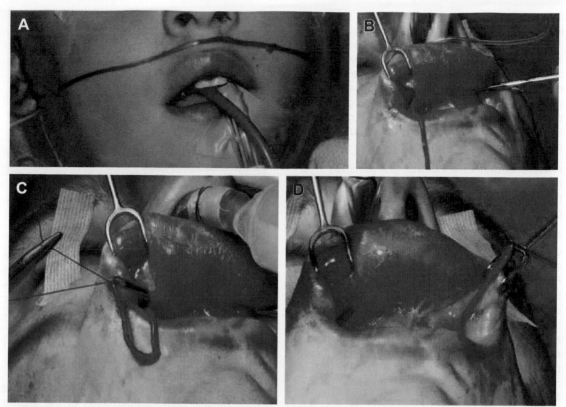

Fig. 9. Cross-face nerve graft. (*A*) The sural nerve is transferred to the face. (*B*) The nerve is tunneled subcutaneously from the nonparalyzed side. (*C*) A Wright tissue needle is passed across the upper lip from the paralyzed side to the nonparalyzed side. (*D*) The tip of the nerve graft is brought to the gingivobuccal sulcus on the paralyzed side.

facial nerve branches with 10-0 nylon and fibrin glue (**Fig. 10**). The tip of the nerve graft is marked with a 4-0 nylon suture and banked in the gingivobuccal sulcus of the paralyzed side for coaptation during the second-stage procedure. A figure-of-

eight, 4-0 chromic suture is used to close the lip. A Penrose drain is placed in the face, and the incision is closed using 4-0 monofilament absorbable suture for the deep dermal layer and running 5-0 nylon suture for the skin. An Ace wrap and ice glove are placed around the head to encourage hemostasis.

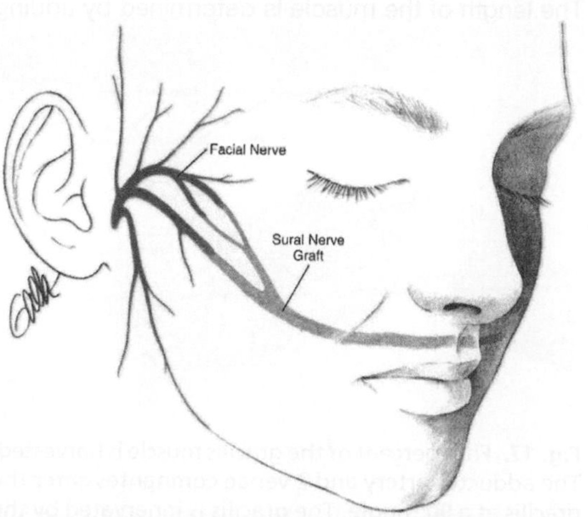

Potential complications and management Hematoma in the face can occur after cross-face nerve graft, and this can lead to disruption of the neurorrhaphy. Most hematomas are evacuated at the bedside with a small Frasier tip suction. The pressure wrap and ice glove are reapplied. The nonparalyzed side of the face may be slightly weak after cross-face nerve grafting. In general, this leads to improved facial balance and symmetry, and the weakness gradually resolves over time. Disfiguring paresis after cross-face nerve graft is rarely encountered because of the rich arborization of the facial nerve. All patients have numbness over a patch of skin on the lateral aspect of the foot from sural nerve harvest. Minor wound dehiscence at the leg incision may occur, and is treated with primary closure in a clean wound. As an

Fig. 10. Cross-face nerve graft connected to isolated smile branches of the nonparalyzed side.

alternative, the leg incision can heal by secondary intention.

Long-term complications include absence of the Tinel sign. In such cases, second-stage gracilis is delayed for several more months. The tip of the nerve graft is sent for an axon count at the time of the second stage, and the surgeon may consider dual innervation with the masseteric nerve if there is concern for the adequacy of the cross-face nerve graft.

Postprocedural care Patients are admitted overnight for observation. On postoperative day 1, the Penrose drain is removed, and the patient is discharged home.

Rehabilitation, recovery, and follow-up Patients can ambulate after surgery. They return for a postoperative check and suture removal in 2 weeks. Patients are asked to check the Tinel sign intermittently by tapping on the graft. This tapping produces tingling in the zygomaticus muscle groups of the unaffected side and represents regenerating axons. The second-stage gracilis muscle transfer is scheduled for 6 to 9 months after the cross-face nerve graft.

Free muscle transfer

Patient positioning The patient is placed in a supine position, and nasotracheal intubation is achieved on the nonparalyzed side. The patient's leg is placed in a frog-leg position by adducting and flexing the leg at the knee. This position aids in harvesting the gracilis muscle and dissection of the pedicle.

Procedural approach The procedure begins with preparation of the face and neck for free muscle transfer. An extended Blair incision is made from the temporal region to 2 to 3 cm below the angle of the mandible. The PMF is identified, and dissection is carried along the PMF to the anterior border of the parotid gland. In patients with functioning facial nerves on the affected side, a Montgomery nerve stimulator is used to identify and protect the branches.

The modiolus, or the chiasm of facial muscles involved in oral commissure movement, is identified using the zygomaticus major and the facial vessels (**Fig. 11**). The facial artery and vein are isolated in preparation for anastomosis with the free flap vessels. Inset sutures are placed in the muscles of the oral commissure taking care to avoid tethering the oral commissure mucosa or overlying dermis.

In 1-stage procedures, the masseteric branch of the trigeminal nerve is exposed through a vertical incision located 3 cm anterior to the free edge of the tragus and 1 cm inferior to the zygoma.[33–35]

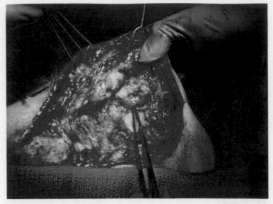

Fig. 11. Intraoperative identification of the oral commissure.

The masseteric nerve, running on the undersurface of the masseter muscle, is identified and isolated with a vessel loop. For 2-stage gracilis muscle transfers, the tip of the cross-face nerve graft is located in the gingivobuccal sulcus of the paralyzed side.

Gracilis harvest begins with an incision 1.5 cm medial and parallel to a line connecting the pubic tubercle to the medial condyle of the tibia. Dissection is carried down through subcutaneous tissue to the muscle belly. Confirmation of the gracilis muscle is achieved by identification of the pedicle entering the deep surface of the muscle. The vascular pedicle, consisting of the adductor artery and 2 venae comitantes, enters the gracilis at a 90° angle. In adults, the vascular pedicle lies 8 to 10 cm inferior to the pubic tubercle; however, this distance is variable in children. The obturator nerve innervates the muscle obliquely, running superior to the vascular pedicle. The muscle is freed superior and inferior to the pedicle.

Fifty percent of the muscle is harvested (**Fig. 12**). The length of the muscle is determined by adding

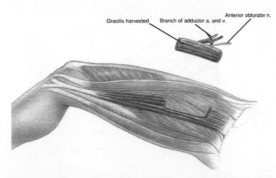

Fig. 12. Fifty percent of the gracilis muscle is harvested. The adductor artery and 2 venae comitantes enter the gracilis at a 90° angle. The gracilis is innervated by the anterior obturator nerve, which enters the muscle obliquely and superior to the vascular pedicle.

2.5 cm to the length from the tragus to the oral commissure. For contralateral muscle transfer, one-third of the muscle length is taken superior to the pedicle; for ipsilateral muscle transfer, two-thirds of the muscle length is taken superior to the pedicle, making dissection more challenging. The obturator nerve is dissected superiorly and divided distal to the branching of the nerve. The pedicle is then dissected and divided, ligating perforators to adductor longus to achieve adequate length.

In children, the gracilis muscle is thinned to 12 g or less to avoid excess bulk in the face (**Fig. 13**). A running, interlocking 2-0 polyglactin suture is placed along the end of the flap to create a neo-tendon to reduce muscle shearing during inset. The muscle is placed parallel to the zygomaticus major (**Fig. 14**). In 2-stage procedures, a Wright needle is used to pass the obturator nerve into the gingivobuccal sulcus near the cross-face nerve graft. The gracilis is then inset to the oral commissure using the previously placed polyglactin sutures. Microvascular anastomosis is accomplished. A neotendon is placed on the superior edge of the flap, and the flap is inset into the deep temporalis fascia (**Fig. 15**). The commissure is slightly overcorrected (**Fig. 16**). Neurorrhaphy is performed. The face is irrigated with antibiotic-impregnated solution, and hemostasis is achieved. The wound is closed over a Penrose drain; a suction drain is used if there is increased concern for postoperative hematoma. The incision is closed using 4-0 monofilament absorbable suture for the deep dermal layer and running 5-0 nylon suture for the skin.

Potential complications and management The most common complication after gracilis free muscle transfer is hematoma in the face. Prompt identification and drainage is critical to avoid

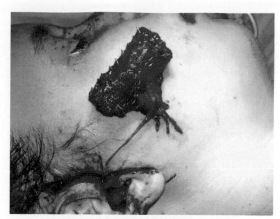

Fig. 14. The gracilis muscle is oriented along the direction of the zygomaticus major with the pedicle positioned along the inferior edge of the muscle belly.

vascular compromise of the flap or disruption of the neurorrhaphy. Hematomas may also occur at the gracilis or fascia lata harvest site, and require rapid detection and evacuation.

Microvascular failure is uncommon; however, given the small caliber of vessels in the pediatric population, there is always concern for clot or vascular spasm. Venous insufficiency is more common than arterial thrombosis and manifests with swelling and firmness of the gracilis long before a change in the arterial Doppler signal.

Unsatisfactory outcomes can arise from excess facial bulk, improper inset with abnormal oral commissure correction, and improper vector pull. In the absence of vascular compromise to the flap, flap failures, which are defined as less than 2 mm of smile excursion 4 to 12 months after the gracilis, are thought to result from lack of neural input. Infection after gracilis free muscle transfer is rare. All patients receive perioperative antibiotics and prophylactic oral antibiotics after discharge.

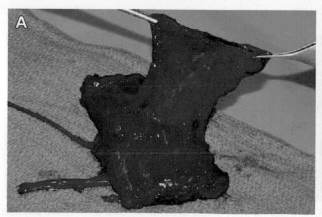
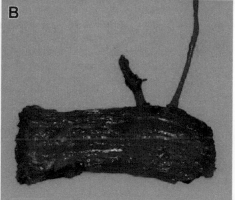

Fig. 13. (*A*) Thinning of the gracilis flap on the back table is performed to avoid excessive bulk in the face. (*B*) A 10-g gracilis muscle after aggressive thinning.

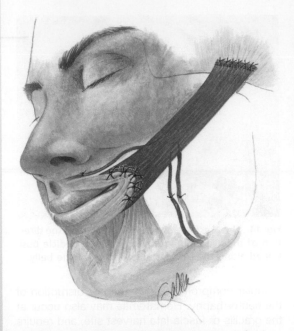

Fig. 15. Inset of the gracilis free muscle transfer.

Postprocedural care The patient is admitted, and the flap is monitored with Doppler every 4 hours. The patient is kept warm to prevent vasospasm. Foley catheter is removed at midnight, and the patient may ambulate the following morning. On postoperative day 1, duplex ultrasonography is performed to verify appropriate muscle perfusion. The face drain is removed on postoperative day 2. On postoperative day 3, the thigh drain is removed, and the patient is discharged home.

Rehabilitation, recovery, and follow-up Patients return in 1 week for suture removal. Facial swelling returns to baseline in several weeks, and patients can resume normal activity in 3 to 4 weeks. For a 1-stage gracilis, movement is expected in 2 to 6 months; for a 2-stage gracilis, movement typically begins in 5 to 12 months. A follow-up

appointment with the surgeon and with a physical therapist for muscle training is scheduled approximately 5 months after a 1-stage gracilis and 9 months after a 2-stage gracilis, or when movement is first appreciated.

Smile rehabilitation outcomes

Free muscle transfer for smile is a safe and successful procedure in children. Multiple studies have shown equivocal or superior results in children compared with adults. The senior author evaluated gracilis muscle transfer in patients 18 years of age or younger.[10] Mean smile excursion matched results seen in adults. There were fewer failures in the pediatric population. In addition, there were significant improvements in quality of life after dynamic smile reanimation. Terzis and Olivares[6] evaluated the long-term outcomes of free muscle transfer in children. All patients had improved function and symmetry at 2 years, despite their growing skeletons. They also found a trend toward superior results in children compared with adults. In a study of facial paralysis following tumor extirpation in pediatric patients, investigators found better EMG results in patients less than 10 years old and earlier reinnervation in the pediatric population.[7] Ueda and colleagues[2] found that children had earlier contraction of muscle and showed superior muscle function that was not affected by continued growth. Free muscle transfer is successful in special populations of pediatric facial paralysis. Zuker and colleagues[9] performed bilateral, 1-stage free gracilis transfers on children with Moebius syndrome. After surgery, all patients had active commissure movement bilaterally. **Table 1** provides a summary of clinical results for pediatric smile rehabilitation.

The cause of facial paralysis does not affect the outcome of smile reanimation.[6] Free muscle transfer has been shown to be successful in pediatric

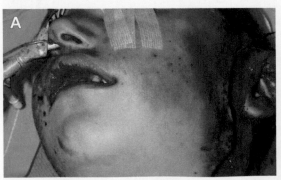
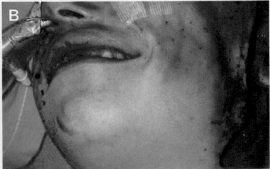

Fig. 16. Slight overcorrection of the oral commissure during inset of the gracilis. (*A*) Oral commissure position prior to gracilis inset onto the deep temporalis fascia. (*B*) Slight overcorrection of the oral commissure after inset of the gracilis onto the deep temporalis fascia.

Table 1
Summary of clinical results of free muscle transfer for smile reanimation in children

Study	Age Range (y)	Number of Cases	Type of Free Muscle Transfer (n)	Number of 1-Stage Procedures	Number of 2-Stage Procedures	Onset of Function (mo)	Measurement of Results	Results
Bianchi et al,[36] 2009	6–13	17	Gracilis (17)	13	4	3–6	Combination of patient response, clinical examination, and preoperative and postoperative videos	83% good symmetry while smiling; 83% patient satisfaction rate, 100% graft survival rate
Hadlock et al,[10] 2011	4–18	19	Gracilis (19)	6	13	NA	Change in oral commissure excursion >2 mm	89% success rate, 95% graft survival rate
Terzis et al,[6] 2009	2–15	34	Pectoralis minor (20) Gracilis (13) Latissimus dorsi (1)	0	34	3–9	Terzis functional and aesthetic grading system for smile; needle EMG	100% improvement in function and symmetry at 2-y follow-up; 100% graft survival rate
Zuker et al,[9] 2000	4–13	20	Gracilis (20)	20	0	NA	Third party interview of function, speech evaluation; measurement of commissure movement	100% active commissure movement bilaterally; 100% improvement in drooling
Ueda et al,[2] 1998	4–15	23	Gracilis (21) Latissimus dorsi (2)	0	23	6–11	5-category scale of muscle function based on clinical observation and needle EMG	83% grade 5 (symmetric at rest, sufficient voluntary contraction, EMG with full interference pattern); no complete failures

Abbreviation: NA, not available.
Data from Refs.[4,6,9,10,36]

patients with diverse causes of facial paralysis, including congenital, traumatic, infectious, tumor, Moebius syndrome, neurofibromatosis, and iatrogenic causes.[6–10,36,37]

Lip Rehabilitation

Paralysis of depressor labii inferioris (DLI) results in a superiorly malpositioned lower lip and asymmetry that is worse when speaking or smiling (**Fig. 17**A). Static and dynamic therapies are directed at correcting the asymmetry. Contralateral lower lip weakening to restore symmetry is accomplished by chemodenervation with botulinum toxin (see **Fig. 17**B). In patients who achieve good results with this technique, permanent weakening may be performed via transoral resection of DLI fibers under local anesthesia. The patient is placed in a supine position, and the mucosal surface of the lower lip is injected with 1% lidocaine with 1:100,000 epinephrine. A 1-cm incision in the lower lip mucosa is made with Bovie cautery. Dissection is carried down to the DLI, and a transverse segment of DLI muscle belly is removed. The incision is closed with absorbable monofilament suture.

Dynamic procedures address the ipsilateral lower lip. Direct depressor anguli oris muscle neurotization, coaptations of the cross-face nerve graft to selected branches of the depressor muscle, digastric muscle transfer, and platysma muscle transfer have been successful in pediatric patients.[5,7] Despite the beneficial results of dynamic procedures, most facial nerve surgeons prefer the simplicity and high success rates of static, contralateral lower lip weakening procedures.

Synkinesis Treatment

Synkinesis, defined as aberrant axonal regeneration resulting in involuntary muscle movements that accompany voluntary muscle contraction, is common after facial paralysis. Adjuvant therapy is directed at decreasing synkinesis, restoring symmetry, and improving facial function.

The treatment of synkinesis can be divided into surgical and nonsurgical therapies. Physical therapy and botulinum toxin injection are the primary nonsurgical treatments. Focused facial nerve physical therapy is given to pediatric patients who are old enough to cooperate with the treatment. The program consists of patient education, massage, neuromuscular retraining, and biofeedback. In children and teenagers who can tolerate injections, botulinum toxin is offered to treat ocular synkinesis, mentalis dimpling, platysmal banding.

Surgical procedures are available to treat synkinesis and are often used in conjunction with nonsurgical therapies. Terzis and Karypidis[3] investigated therapeutic strategies for pediatric patients who developed synkinesis after facial paralysis. Cross-face nerve grafting and secondary microcoaptations to selected distal branches of the affected facial nerve served to break the synkinesis cycle by providing appropriate neural signals from the cross-face nerve graft that seemed to override the aberrant signals causing synkinesis. The combination of cross-face nerve graft with secondary microcoaptations, biofeedback-assisted facial muscle reeducation, and botulinum toxin was extremely effective in the treatment of synkinesis and improved both facial function and symmetry.

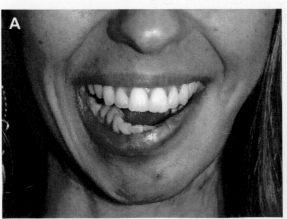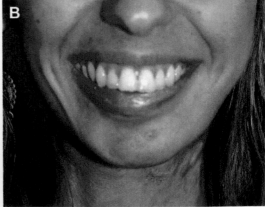

Fig. 17. Contralateral lower lip weakening with botulinum toxin. (*A*) Preprocedure left lower lip paralysis and lip asymmetry caused by hyperfunction of the contralateral DLI. (*B*) After injection of botulinum toxin to the right DLI. Note improved symmetry when smiling.

SUMMARY

Facial paralysis is a rare but severe condition in the pediatric population. Impaired facial movement has multiple causes and varied presentations, therefore individualized treatment plans are essential for optimal results. Special considerations in children make the treatment of facial paralysis especially challenging. Comprehensive management includes zone-based facial assessment and treatment in the setting of a specialized center equipped with a team dedicated to the treatment of facial nerve disorders.

REFERENCES

1. Harii K, Ohmori K, Torii S. Free gracilis muscle transplantation, with microneurovascular anastomoses for the treatment of facial paralysis. A preliminary report. Plast Reconstr Surg 1976;57(2):133–43.
2. Ueda K, Harii K, Asato H, et al. Neurovascular free muscle transfer combined with cross-face nerve grafting for the treatment of facial paralysis in children. Plast Reconstr Surg 1998;101(7):1765–73.
3. Terzis JK, Karypidis D. Therapeutic strategies in post-facial paralysis synkinesis in pediatric patients. J Plast Reconstr Aesthet Surg 2012;65(8):1009–18.
4. Terzis JK, Karypidis D. The outcomes of dynamic procedures for blink restoration in pediatric facial paralysis. Plast Reconstr Surg 2010; 125(2):629–44.
5. Terzis JK, Karypidis D. Outcomes of direct muscle neurotization in pediatric patients with facial paralysis. Plast Reconstr Surg 2009;124(5):1486–98.
6. Terzis JK, Olivares FS. Long-term outcomes of free muscle transfer for smile restoration in children. Plast Reconstr Surg 2009;123(2):543–55.
7. Terzis JK, Konofaos P. Reanimation of facial palsy following tumor extirpation in pediatric patients: our experience with 16 patients. J Plast Reconstr Aesthet Surg 2013;66(9):1219–29.
8. Zuker RM, Manktelow RT. A smile for the Möbius' syndrome patient. Ann Plast Surg 1989;22(3):188–94.
9. Zuker RM, Goldberg CS, Manktelow RT. Facial animation in children with Möbius syndrome after segmental gracilis muscle transplant. Plast Reconstr Surg 2000;106(1):1–8 [discussion: 9].
10. Hadlock TA, Malo JS, Cheney ML, et al. Free gracilis transfer for smile in children: the Massachusetts Eye and Ear Infirmary Experience in excursion and quality-of-life changes. Arch Facial Plast Surg 2011;13(3):190–4.
11. Jenke AC, Stoek LM, Zilbauer M, et al. Facial palsy: etiology, outcome and management in children. Eur J Paediatr Neurol 2011;15(3):209–13.
12. Leboulanger N, Maldent JB, Glynn F, et al. Rehabilitation of congenital facial palsy with temporalis
flap–case series and literature review. Int J Pediatr Otorhinolaryngol 2012;76(8):1205–10.
13. Barr JS, Katz KA, Hazen A. Surgical management of facial nerve paralysis in the pediatric population. J Pediatr Surg 2011;46(11):2168–76.
14. Manning JJ, Adour KK. Facial paralysis in children. Pediatrics 1972;49(1):102–9.
15. May M, Fria TJ, Blumenthal F, et al. Facial paralysis in children: differential diagnosis. Otolaryngol Head Neck Surg 1981;89(5):841–8.
16. Wang CH, Chang YC, Shih HM, et al. Facial palsy in children: emergency department management and outcome. Pediatr Emerg Care 2010;26(2):121–5.
17. Shih WH, Tseng FY, Yeh TH, et al. Outcomes of facial palsy in children. Acta Otolaryngol 2009;129(8): 915–20.
18. Grundfast KM, Guarisco JL, Thomsen JR, et al. Diverse etiologies of facial paralysis in children. Int J Pediatr Otorhinolaryngol 1990;19(3):223–39.
19. Evans AK, Licameli G, Brietzke S, et al. Pediatric facial nerve paralysis: patients, management and outcomes. Int J Pediatr Otorhinolaryngol 2005; 69(11):1521–8.
20. Harrison DH. The treatment of unilateral and bilateral facial palsy using free muscle transfers. Clin Plast Surg 2002;29(4):539–49, vi.
21. Ylä-Kotola TM, Kauhanen MS, Asko-Seljavaara SL. Facial reanimation by transplantation of a microneurovascular muscle: long-term follow-up. Scand J Plast Reconstr Surg Hand Surg 2004;38(5):272–6.
22. Terzis JK, Noah ME. Analysis of 100 cases of free-muscle transplantation for facial paralysis. Plast Reconstr Surg 1997;99(7):1905–21.
23. O'Brien BM, Pederson WC, Khazanchi RK, et al. Results of management of facial palsy with microvascular free-muscle transfer. Plast Reconstr Surg 1990;86(1):12–22 [discussion: 23–4].
24. Smith MF, Goode RL. Eye protection in the paralyzed face. Laryngoscope 1979;89(3):435–42.
25. Silver AL, Lindsay RW, Cheney ML, et al. Thin-profile platinum eyelid weighting: a superior option in the paralyzed eye. Plast Reconstr Surg 2009;123(6):1697–703.
26. Rose EH. Autogenous fascia lata grafts: clinical applications in reanimation of the totally or partially paralyzed face. Plast Reconstr Surg 2005;116(1): 20–32 [discussion: 33–5].
27. Terzis JK, Bruno W. Outcomes with eye reanimation microsurgery. Facial Plast Surg 2002;18(2):101–12.
28. Kinney SE, Seeley BM, Seeley MZ, et al. Oculoplastic surgical techniques for protection of the eye in facial nerve paralysis. Am J Otol 2000;21(2):275–83.
29. Alam D. Rehabilitation of long-standing facial nerve paralysis with percutaneous suture-based slings. Arch Facial Plast Surg 2007;9(3):205–9.
30. Hadlock TA, Greenfield LJ, Wernick-Robinson M, et al. Multimodality approach to management of the paralyzed face. Laryngoscope 2006;116(8):1385–9.

31. Harrison DH. Current trends in the treatment of established unilateral facial palsy. Ann R Coll Surg Engl 1990;72(2):94–8.

32. Bhama P, Weinberg J, Lindsay R, et al. Objective outcomes analysis following microvascular gracilis transfer for facial reanimation: a 10-year experience at the Massachusetts Eye and Ear Infirmary/Harvard Medical School. JAMA Facial Plast Surg 2014;16(2):85–92.

33. Collar RM, Byrne PJ, Boahene KD. The subzygomatic triangle: rapid, minimally invasive identification of the masseteric nerve for facial reanimation. Plast Reconstr Surg 2013;132(1):183–8.

34. Borschel GH, Kawamura DH, Kasukurthi R, et al. The motor nerve to the masseter muscle: an anatomic and histomorphometric study to facilitate its use in facial reanimation. J Plast Reconstr Aesthet Surg 2012; 65(3):363–6.

35. Urken ML. Atlas of regional and free flaps for head and neck reconstruction: flap harvest and insetting. 2nd edition. Philadelphia: Wolters Kluwer Health/Lippincott Williams & Wilkins; 2012.

36. Bianchi B, Copelli C, Ferrari S, et al. Facial animation in children with Moebius and Moebius-like syndromes. J Pediatr Surg 2009;44(11):2236–42.

37. Vakharia KT, Henstrom D, Plotkin SR, et al. Facial reanimation of patients with neurofibromatosis type 2. Neurosurgery 2012;70(2 Suppl Operative): 237–43.

Pediatric Septorhinoplasty

Jamie L. Funamura, MD, Jonathan M. Sykes, MD*

KEYWORDS

• Septorhinoplasty • Nasal surgery • Septoplasty • Children

KEY POINTS

• In the appropriately selected patient, septorhinoplasty can benefit a pediatric patient presenting with significant nasal trauma, abscess, or mass that would likely result in a progressive deformity in the growing nose or with negative functional or psychosocial effect.
• Clinical and experimental observations suggest that a conservative approach to pediatric septorhinoplasty is warranted.
• The long-term results of scoring and incisions in the cartilaginous nasal septum to realign the septum are not predictable, and intercartilaginous incisions should be avoided when possible.
• Intercartilaginous incisions should be avoided when possible.

INTRODUCTION

Performing nasal surgery on children has been the subject of controversy among facial plastic surgeons. Specifically, the indications for and timing of septorhinoplasty in children have been debated for the last several decades. Additionally, the extent of surgery and the appropriate approach and techniques to be used in children with congenital or acquired nasal deformities have been disputed. Central to the ongoing argument is that any surgical intervention in the growing nose can possibly cause severe growth inhibition that may not be evident until the child has achieved adult stature. Numerous observational and experimental studies on animal models and in clinical practice dating back to the early 1960s have attempted to elucidate normal nasal growth patterns. Implicit in these studies is that any surgical intervention should minimize disruption of these patterns of development of the bony-cartilaginous structures of the nose.

PATTERNS OF GROWTH IN PEOPLE

The external nose of the child has several characteristics that are distinct from that of the adult. Children typically display a larger nasolabial angle with a shorter, less projected dorsum. The nasal tip is also relatively flat and poorly projected with a short columella and round nares.[1,2] The present understanding of the nasal bony-cartilaginous framework that underlies these differences and the subsequent patterns of growth can largely be attributed to an interdisciplinary research group on craniofacial development in Amsterdam and Rotterdam. This group has demonstrated that infants, when compared to adults, have a greater cartilage-to-bone ratio. Newborn septal cartilage reaches from the nasal tip to the skull base. Similarly, early in life, the upper lateral cartilages extend under the complete length of the nasal bones. The pediatric bony structures are relatively underdeveloped when compared with those of adults, with an absent

Department of Otolaryngology–Head and Neck Surgery, University of California Davis Medical Center, University of California Davis Health System, 2521 Stockton Boulevard, Suite 7200, Sacramento, CA 95817, USA
* Corresponding author.
E-mail address: jonathan.sykes@ucdmc.ucdavis.edu

Facial Plast Surg Clin N Am 22 (2014) 503–508
http://dx.doi.org/10.1016/j.fsc.2014.07.005
1064-7406/14/$ – see front matter © 2014 Elsevier Inc. All rights reserved.

perpendicular plate and rudimentary vomer.[3,4] As the child grows, the upper lateral cartilages regress and the cartilaginous septum gradually ossifies. This ossification process results in the formation of the perpendicular plate, which then merges with the vomer between 6 and 8 years of age.[5]

The growth centers of the nose have been designated as the sphenodorsal zone and the sphenospinal zone. These zones are thought to increase the length and height of the nasal bones with the outgrowth of the maxilla, respectively. Trauma to these areas has been shown experimentally to interrupt growth in a predictable pattern and can lead to progressive nasal deformity.[1,2] Clinical evidence of traumatic growth inhibition of the nasal skeleton and maxilla was also demonstrated by Grymer and colleagues[6] in comparative observational studies of monozygotic twins.[7]

Nasal growth appears to continue until early adulthood with specific windows of accelerated growth. The 2 most significant nasal growth spurts occur in the first 2 years of life and during puberty.[1] The end of the nasofacial growth spurt was found to be at 12 to 16 years in girls and 15 to 18 years in boys.[8–10] For this reason, nasal surgeons often wait to perform elective nasal surgery until 15 to 16 years of age in girls and until 17 to 18 years of age in boys. Although the vast majority of growth appears to be complete by this age, a large-scale study in Switzerland of 2500 individuals showed some increase in nasal length and projection in women until 20 years and in men until 25 years of age, which may contribute to delayed postsurgical distortion.[1,11]

EARLY SURGICAL EXPERIENCE

Septorhinoplasty was described in children as early as 1902.[12] Resultant nasal deformities such as saddle nose deformities and growth inhibition with maxillary retrusion would later be noted as early as 1916.[13] Subsequent publications echoed the cautionary message. In 1958, Gilbert and Segal warned against resection of the quadrilateral keystone area of the immature nasal septum, and Farrior and Connolly in 1970 similarly recommended delaying septorhinoplasty in children until after growth was complete.[14,15] These clinical observations and practice recommendations inspired a plethora of experimental studies. The goal of these studies would be to examine the mechanisms of growth inhibition and the interventions that result in minimizing further growth distortions.

ANIMAL STUDIES

Although experimental animal studies involving nasal septal resection date back to as early as the 1850s, the most frequently cited early studies are from Sarnat and colleagues in the 1960s.[16,17] Sarnat and his group designed a series of experiments in growing rabbits in which the caudal aspect of the cartilaginous septum and overlying mucoperichondrium was resected with resultant underdevelopment of the snout and relative mandibular prognathism.[18] Significantly, Sarnat's experiments involved through-and-through resection of as much as the anterior half of the septum without preservation of overlying mucosa or mucoperiochondrial flaps.[16] His experiments, however, were the launching point for numerous investigations of nasoseptal interventions in various animal models. To date, conclusions have been drawn on the growth patterns and the role of trauma and surgical interventions on disrupting growth in rabbits, canine pups, baboons, and ferrets, to name a few. These studies highlighted the significance of submucosal and selective cartilage resection with careful preservation of mucoperichondrial flaps.[19–24] Unfortunately, animal studies have not been performed on animals simulating the conservative cartilage resection often required to straighten the nasal septum in children with nasal obstruction. These experiments may improve the predictive value of animal studies on nasal growth after pediatric nasal surgery.

CLINICAL STUDIES

Because of the aforementioned animal studies, the practice of pediatric septoplasty and septorhinoplasty has proceeded with caution. Evaluation of clinic results is largely limited by small sample size, variation in approach and technique, and lack of long-term follow-up. Keeping these limitations in mind, the literature does suggest that septorhinoplasty can be performed with minimal growth inhibition when performed selectively with specific indications. Using anthropometric measurements, external septoplasty has been shown to not affect most aspects of nasal and facial growth, when the mucoperichondrium is left intact and no large cartilaginous resections are made. One caveat, however, is that nasal dorsal length was noted to be decreased in multiple studies, although the difference was not statistically significant in these studies within the average follow-up period of 2 to 4 years.[25–27]

Although many surgeons have used results of animal studies to advocate delay in surgical treatment until full nasal growth, negative effects of delaying surgical intervention on a severely deviated nose have also been demonstrated. D'Ascanio and colleagues[28] reported facial and dental anomalies using cephalometric analysis in children who were obligate mouth breathers secondary to severe nasal septal deviations, compared with age- and sex-matched controls. The children who were obligate mouth breathers had larger gonial angles and a higher rate of class 2 skeletal malocclusion when compared with controls. Similarly, Penz and colleagues[29] demonstrated malocclusion in 13 of 14 neonates with uncorrected injuries to the bony and cartilaginous nose after long-term follow-up of 12 years.

CLINICAL INDICATIONS FOR PEDIATRIC SEPTORHINOPLASTY

Most authors continue to recommend postponement of septorhinoplasty until after the adolescent growth spurt in order to prevent nasal and midfacial growth inhibition and the scarring associated with surgery.[1,2,16,17,26,30,31] However, absolute and relative indications have been recognized based on potential for progressive deformity, functional deficits, and psychosocial effect. Christophel and Gross described septal abscess, septal hematoma, severe deformity secondary to acute nasal fracture, dermoid cyst, and cleft lip nasal malformation as absolute indications for pediatric septoplasty; a severely deviated septum causing significant nasal airway obstruction was identified as a relative indication.[30] Indications have also been divided into those requiring immediate intervention: acute nasal trauma, malignancy, septal abscess, and hematoma. Other indications that may be addressed in a delayed fashion—although

still before the adolescent growth spurt—would then include benign tumors such as dermoid cysts, progressive deformation, and children with nasal stigmata of orofacial clefting.[1]

Of particular note, primary rhinoplasty in the cleft lip population (rhinoplasty at the time of cleft lip repair) is now widely practiced (**Fig. 1**). Despite being contrary to early dogma, primary rhinoplasty in children with clefts was performed routinely by some cleft surgeons in the 1970s. Beginning in the 1990s, a new battery of techniques for addressing the nasal tip cartilages in a minimally invasive fashion generated a greater following of surgeons interested in early correction of cleft nasal deformity.[32] In most of these approaches, surgery on the nasal bones or nasal septum was not advocated. This conservative approach allows some correction of severe nasal tip and base asymmetries, while minimizing scarring and growth inhibition. The cleft patient population has now provided some of the best data regarding long-term follow-up and growth after childhood rhinoplasty. Longitudinal studies with length of follow-up of 10 years and beyond have shown that infants undergoing primary cleft rhinoplasty have demonstrated normal nasal growth after early repositioning of cartilaginous portions of the nose.[32–35]

GUIDELINES FOR PEDIATRIC SEPTORHINOPLASTY

In the appropriately selected patient, septorhinoplasty can therefore benefit a pediatric patient presenting with significant nasal trauma, abscess, or mass that will likely result in a progressive deformity in the growing nose or with negative functional or psychosocial effect. Clinical and

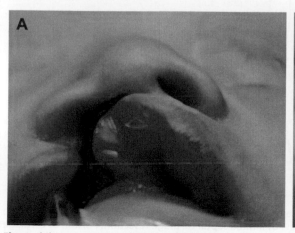
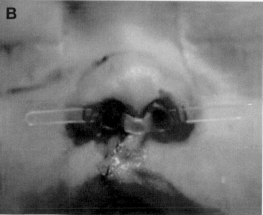

Fig. 1. (*A*) Preoperative photograph of a patient with unilateral complete cleft lip. (*B*) Immediate postoperative result after cleft lip repair with primary tip rhinoplasty and placement of nasal stents.

experimental observations do suggest that a conservative approach is warranted. A conservative septoplasty approach involving minimalist approach to septal cartilage resection is demonstrated in **Fig. 2**. A selection of other approaches and guidelines delineated by Nolst Trenité, Verwoerd, and Verhwoerd-Verhoef, has been reproduced below[1,14]:

- Elevation of the mucoperichondrium on one or both sides will not interfere with normal growth.[18]
- The long-term results of scoring and incisions in the cartilaginous nasal septum to realign the septum are not predictable.
- Incision of the posterior septum or separation from the perpendicular plate should be

avoided because of possible injury to the major growth center of the nasal septum.
- If resection of the cartilaginous septum is necessary, resection of the thinner central part has the least chance of causing growth inhibition.
- Residual crushed cartilage should be replaced in the resected septal bed to improve. regeneration of the cartilage and prevent septal perforations.[36]
- Dorsal hump reduction can lead to outgrowth of the septum anterior to the upper lateral cartilages and subsequent irregularities of the nasal dorsum.
- Osteotomies of the bony pyramid to realign the nasal dorsum do not create growth distrubances.[17]

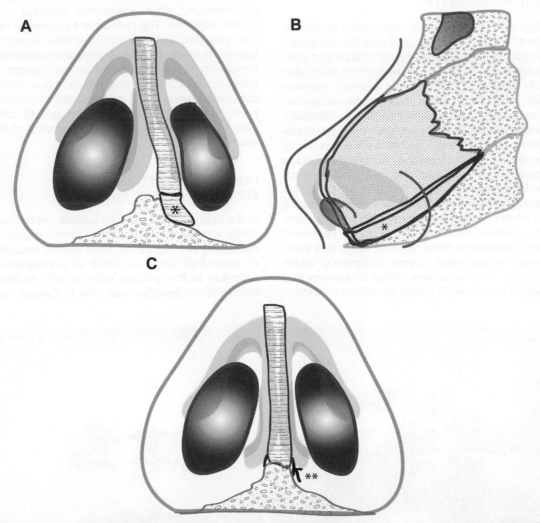

Fig. 2. (*A*) Base view of deviated cartilaginous nasal septum. Portion of cartilage to be resected, preserving the majority of the septal cartilage (*asterisk*). (*B*) Profile view of limited septal cartilage resection. Portion of cartilage to be resected to allow for midline repositioning of the septum (*asterisk*). (*C*) Base view of completed septoplasty. Absorbable suture shown securing the caudal septum to the anterior nasal spine (*double asterisk*).

- Transcolumellar incision (open approach), leaving the nasal skeleton intact, has not been shown to disturb nasal growth.[23–25]
- Intercartilaginous incisions should be avoided when possible.

REFERENCES

1. Nolst Trenité GJ. Rhinoplasty in children. In: Papel ID, Frodel JL, Larrabee WF, et al, editors. Facial plastic and reconstructive surgery. 3rd edition. New York: Thieme; 2009. p. 605–17.
2. Bae JS, Kim ES, Jang YJ. Treatment outcomes of pediatric rhinoplasty: the Asan Medical Center experience. Int J Pediatr Otorhinolaryngol 2013;77:1701–10.
3. Van Loosen J, Verwoerd-Verhoef HL, Verwoerd CD. The nasal septal cartilage in the newborn. Rhinology 1988;26:161–5.
4. Poublon RM, Verwoerd CD, Verwoerd-Verhoef HL. Anatomy of the upper lateral cartilages in the human newborn. Rhinology 1990;28:41–5.
5. Van Loosen J, Van Zanten GA, Howard CV, et al. Growth characteristics of the human nasal septum. Rhinology 1996;34:78–82.
6. Grymer LF, Pallisgaard C, Melsen B. The nasal septum in relation to the development of the nasomaxillary complex: a study a study in identical twins. Laryngoscope 1991;101:863–8.
7. Grymer LF, Bosch C. The nasal septum and the development of the midface. A longitudinal study of a pair of monozygotic twins. Rhinology 1997;35:6–10.
8. Van der Heijden P, Korsten-Meijer AG, Van der Laan BF, et al. Nasal growth and maturation age in adolescents. Arch Otolaryngol Head Neck Surg 2008;134:1288–93.
9. Meng HP, Goorhuis J, Kapila S, et al. Growth changes in the nasal profile from 7 to 18 years of age. Am J Orthod Dentofacial Orthop 1988;94:317–26.
10. Akguner M, Baratcu A, Karaca C. Adolescent growth patterns of the bony cartilaginous framework of the nose: a cephalometric study. Ann Plast Surg 1998;41:66–9.
11. Zankl A, Eberle L, Molinari L, et al. Growth charts for nose length, nasal protrusion and philtrum length from birth to 97 years. Am J Med Genet 2002;111:388–91.
12. Freer OT. The correction of deflections of the nasal septum with a minimum of traumatism. JAMA 1902;38:636–42.
13. Hayton CH. An investigation into the results of the submucous resection of the septum in children. J Laryng 1916;31:132–8.
14. Gilbert JG, Sogal S Jr. Growth of the nose and the septorhinoplastic problem in youth. AMA Arch Otolaryngol 1758;68:673–82.
15. Farrior RT, Connolly ME. Septorhinoplasty in children. Otolaryngol Clin North Am 1970;3:345–64.
16. Verwoerd CD, Verwoerd-Verhoef HL. Rhinosurgery in children: developmental and surgical aspects of the growing nose. GMS Curr Top Otorhinolaryngol Head Neck Surg 2010;9:1–29.
17. Lawrence R. Pediatric septoplasty: a review of literature. Int J Pediatr Otorhinolaryngol 2012;76:1078–81.
18. Sarnat BG, Wexler MR. Growth of the face and jaws after resection of the septal cartilage in the rabbit. Am J Anat 1966;118:755–67.
19. Verwoerd-Verhoef HL, Verwoerd CD. Surgery of the lateral nasal wall and ethmoid: effects on sinonasal growth. An experimental study in rabbits. Int J Pediatr Otorhinolaryngol 2003;67:263–9.
20. Verwoerd CD, Urbanus NA, Nijdam DC. The effects of septal surgery on the growth of the nose and maxilla. Rhinology 1979;17:53–64.
21. Meeuwis J, Verhoerd-Verhoef HL, Verwoerd CD. Normal and abnormal nasal growth after partial submucous resection of the cartilaginous septum. Acta Otolaryngol 1993;113:379–82.
22. Siegel MI. A longitudinal study of facial growth in Papio cynocephalus after resection of the cartilaginous nasal septum. J Med Primatol 1979;8:122–7.
23. Bernstein L. Early submucous resection of nasal septal cartilage. A pilot study in canine pups. Arch Otolaryngol 1973;97:273–8.
24. Cupero TM, Middleton CE, Silva AB. Effects of functional septoplasty on the facial growth of ferrets. Arch Otolaryngol Head Neck Surg 2001;127:1367–9.
25. Walker PJ, Crysdale WS, Farkas LG. External septorhinoplasty in children: outcome and effect on growth of septal excision and reimplantation. Arch Otolaryngol Head Neck Surg 1987;113:173–8.
26. Bejar I, Farkas LG, Messner AH, et al. Nasal growth after external septoplasty in children. Arch Otolaryngol Head Neck Surg 1996;122:816–21.
27. El-Hakim H, Crysdale WS, Abdollel M, et al. A study of anthropometric measures before and after external septoplasty in children. Arch Otolaryngol Head Neck Surg 2001;127:1362–6.
28. D'Ascanio L, Lancione C, Pompa G, et al. Craniofacial growth in children with nasal septum deviation: a cephalometric comparative study. Int J Pediatr Otorhinolaryngol 2010;74:1180–3.
29. Pentz S, Pirsig W, Lenders H. Long-term results of neonates with nasal deviation: a prospective study over 12 years. Int J Pediatr Otorhinolaryngol 1994;28:183–91.
30. Christophel JJ, Gross CW. Pediatric septoplasty. Otolaryngol Clin North Am 2009;42:287–94.
31. Healy GB, Tardy ME Jr. Septorhinoplasty in children. Operative Techniques in Otolaryngology-Head and Neck Surgery 1994;5:22–6.
32. Van Beek AL, Hatfield AS, Schnepf E. Cleft rhinoplasty. Plast Reconstr Surg 2004;114:57e–69e.
33. McComb H. Primary correction of unilateral cleft lip nasal deformity: a 10-year review. Plast Reconstr Surg 1985;75:791–9.

34. Millard DR Jr, Morovic CG. Primary unilateral cleft nose correction: a 10-year follow-up. Plast Reconstr Surg 1998;102:1331–8.

35. Salyer KE. Primary correction of the unilateral cleft lip nose: a 15-year experience. Plast Reconstr Surg 1986;77:558.

36. Nolst Trenité GJ, Verwoerd CD, Verwoerd-Verhoef HL. Reimplantation of autologous septal cartilage in growing nasal septum. II. The influence of reimplantation of rotated or crushed autologous septal cartilage on nasal growth: an experimental study in rabbits. Rhinology 1988;16:25–32.

Infantile Hemangiomas
Current Management

Marcelo Hochman, MD

KEYWORDS

• Infantile hemangioma • Surgery • Laser • Propranolol

KEY POINTS

- Management of infantile hemangioma (IH) includes a combination of observation, medical therapy, laser treatments, and surgery.
- The nomenclature to describe these lesions has been standardized and should be adhered to.
- The goal of treatment is to obtain the best possible result commensurate with known developmental milestones.
- Current knowledge of the biology of these tumors as well as experience allows obtaining this goal.
- "Leave it alone, it will go away" is no longer universally acceptable advice for treatment of IH.

Infantile hemangioma (IH) is a vascular anomaly and the most common benign tumor of infancy. In spite of it being so prevalent, there is still a widespread lack of understanding in the medical community leading to mismanagement of affected children. The purpose of this article is to review the current knowledge on pathogenesis, diagnosis, and management of IH.

Vascular anomalies are a group of disorders that are categorized as either tumors or malformations according to the accepted classification of the International Society for the Study of Vascular Anomalies (April 2014; http://www.issva.org). The tumors are further divided into benign, locally aggressive, or malignant entities. IH is one of the benign vascular tumors along with congenital hemangiomas, pyogenic granulomas, and a few other less common entities.

IH are true neoplasms of endothelial cell origin exhibiting up-regulated cell growth, increased mitosis, and cellular hyperplasia. Endothelial cells in IH have a clonal origin but the exact source of the progenitor cell is not clear. Striking commonality in the mRNA transcriptome have been found between IH and placental tissue, which suggests that progenitor cells from placenta may be associated with these tumors.[1] In addition to morphologic similarities between endothelial cells of IH and placenta, IH uniquely coexpresses glucose transporter protein 1 (GLUT-1) and other markers with placenta.[2] The only vascular anomaly that expresses GLUT-1 is IH, making this an important marker to histologically confirm a diagnosis of IH and distinguish from all other vascular lesions in the occasional case requiring a tissue biopsy. Endothelial and mesenchymal progenitor cells have been identified in both IH and placenta but the exact source of these progenitor cells is not clear. One theory suggests that fetal angioblasts differentiate into a placental vascular phenotype at locations that are prepared by circulating factors secreted by the placenta thus making the predisposed sites fertile ground for the growth of IH.[3] This metastatic niche theory has been shown to be true in some cancers. The other theory posits that embolic progenitor cells from the placenta deposit in the developing fetus and differentiate into IH.[4] These embolic cells may be more likely to deposit in the head and neck due to the increased vascularity in this region with the sites of predilection occurring at the end arteries of the developing facial placodes.[5] Neither theory

The author has no disclosures to make.

Hemangioma & Malformation Treatment Center, PO Box 80789, Charleston, SC 29416, USA

E-mail address: DrHochman@FacialSurgeryCenter.com

Facial Plast Surg Clin N Am 22 (2014) 509–521

http://dx.doi.org/10.1016/j.fsc.2014.07.003

facialplastic.theclinics.com

has yet to been proven or explains the peculiar natural history of IH, which consists of a period of rapid postnatal proliferation followed by a phase of involution.

Histologically, during proliferation, IH is characterized by a high mitotic activity in the endothelial cells and pericytes as the tumor enlarges. Involution is accompanied by an increase in apoptosis, endothelial cells flatten with enlargement of their lumina, and the lesions become dominated by fibrofatty stroma. Alterations in several cytokines important in angiogenesis have been demonstrated during the various phases. The proliferation phase is dominated by vascular endothelial growth factor (VEGF), which is a primary mitogen for benign and malignant vascular tumors and promotes cell survival while inhibiting apoptosis. Serum levels of VEGF are elevated in infants with proliferating IH compared with involuting IH and controls.[6] VEGF activates angiogenesis via the mammalian target of rapamycin (mTOR) signaling pathway. Also elevated during this time are basic fibroblast growth factor (bFGF), insulin-like growth factor (IGF)-2, matrix metalloproteinase (MMP)-9, and type IV collagenase, whereas levels of endogenous interferon are decreased. During involution, levels of VEGF, bFGF, and IGF-2 decline, whereas levels of regulatory cytokines such as interferon and tissue inhibitor of MMP-1 (TIMP-1) increase. These factors and pathways are potential targets for clinical intervention.

Clinically, these hallmark phases form the basis for diagnosis and management. IH are typically not visible at birth; however, up to 30% are evident as precursor lesions with variable findings including a telangiectatic macule, pale vasoconstrictor area, vascular stain, or bruised appearance. Within the first weeks of life, IH becomes visible as an erythematous macule or slightly raised papular lesion. The lesions then undergo a classic progression of rapid proliferative growth followed by involution that is variable in length and extent. The period of most rapid growth occurs in the early proliferative stage and is largely complete by about 4 to 6 months of age with tumors reaching roughly 80% of their final size at this point. Despite the increase in size during proliferation, IH tend not to expand beyond the defined anatomic site of the original lesion. The late proliferative phase is complete by 9 months in most children with very little growth occurring after this point as the lesion enters the plateau phase. Involution begins as early as 6 months and may last for several years. Clinically, lesions become lighter in color and softer to palpation with diminution in the volume of the mass. If one includes all IH (scalp to soles of feet) nearly 60% of IH will involute to aesthetically and functionally acceptable endpoints; however, 40% of lesions leave a remnant that may require further treatment.[7] They may appear as hypopigmented or telangiectatic macules, with loose, expanded soft tissue, and/or fibrofatty residual masses, depending on the nature of the original tumor. The threshold for what is considered acceptable varies with location and size. For example, a small focal lesion of the nasal tip will have a very different impact than a larger, segmental lesion of the lower back. For this reason, even though 100% of IH involute, a large number of patients will seek improvement as the threshold for acceptability is high because most occur in the face and head or neck areas (**Fig. 1**).

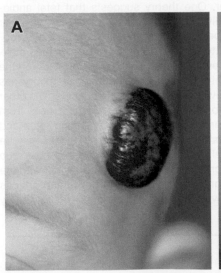 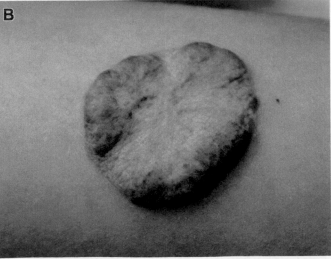

Fig. 1. Proliferating and involuting IHs. (*A*) Proliferating compound IH of the temple. (*B*) Involuting thick superficial IH of the arm.

Several risk factors for the development of IH have been identified. Fair-skinned individuals are at higher risk with rates up to 10% among white infants. Prematurity is associated with IH and the number of hemangiomas per infant increases with younger gestational age. Female children are more likely to develop IH than male children (3:1); however, this is less pronounced (1.8:1) among premature infants. Low birth weight, especially less than 1500 g, increases the likelihood of IH independent of gestational age. Every 500 g reduction in birth weight imparts a 40% increased risk of IH. A definite genetic link or pattern of inheritance has yet to be established with most IHs thought to be sporadic events.[8]

Adhering to standardized nomenclature is important to be able to communicate clinically relevant information. Terms such as cavernous hemangioma or strawberry should be abandoned as anachronisms. In addition to the phase of its natural history and anatomic site, IHs are described by the degree of cutaneous involvement. Superficial IHs are limited to the superficial dermis though they can be thick. Deep IHs involve the deep dermis and subcutaneous layers and present as masses without overlying skin involvement. Compound IHs involve both the superficial and deep layers (**Fig. 2**).

Additionally, IH are classified morphologically into (1) focal when a solitary lesion exists, (2) multifocal when multiple lesions are present, and (3) segmental when a lesion or cluster of lesions corresponds to a developmental subunit or dermatome. Focal lesions are the most common, occurring in 80% of affected patients. Although IHs can occur throughout the body, they most commonly affect the skin of the head and neck

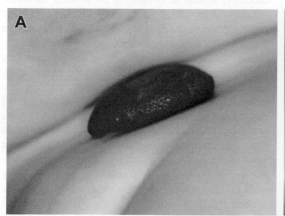
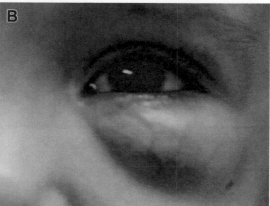
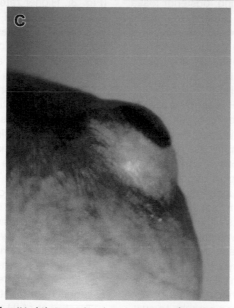

Fig. 2. Descriptive terminology for IH. (*A*) Superficial IH involving the upper layers of the dermis. (*B*) Deep IH involving the deeper layers of the dermis without involvement of the overlying skin. (*C*) Compound IH with both deep and superficial components.

(50%–60%), followed by the trunk (25%), and limbs (15%). Facial lesions are disproportionally distributed in the central face along lines of embryonic fusion with 60% of lesions occurring in the periorbital, nasal, and perioral zones.[5] The presence of more than five multifocal cutaneous lesions increases the chances of visceral organ involvement, particularly the liver, and further evaluation should be considered. Segmental IH are the least common subtype but are the most likely associated with other abnormalities, more difficult to treat, and have worse outcomes. These lesions loosely follow a dermatomal distribution. Segmental lesions have an even stronger predilection for involvement of the face than localized lesions and they are more common in nonwhite Hispanic infants at older gestational age and higher weight than localized lesions, suggesting there may be differences in pathogenesis. There is nearly twice the rate of female predominance among segmental IH (5.7–6.6:1) compared with the localized form (3:1). Segmental lesions of the so-called beard distribution or V3 dermatomal distribution have a unique association with IH in the airway. Most commonly this involves the subglottis. Conversely, more than 50% of patients with IH of the airway have a concomitant cutaneous IH. Segmental IH have a higher association with syndromes than focal IH. Lumbosacral segmental IH may be associated with underlying spinal dysraphia and urologic abnormalities. Beard distribution lesions also have an association with PHACE syndrome defined by the presence of a facial IH and one or more of the following: posterior fossa brain abnormalities, arterial anomalies, aortic coarctation or cardiac abnormalities, and eye anomalies. PHACE syndrome occurs in 20% to 33% of patients with segmental IH and nearly 50% of patients with airway IH but is much less common in infants with focal IHs.

The diagnostic workup for IH is simple because most cases can be diagnosed by history and physical examination. Imaging studies may be useful to evaluate for concomitant lesions in cases of greater than five visible cutaneous lesions, to assess the full extent of a lesion for surgical planning, and occasionally to lend support to an uncertain diagnosis. Ultrasonography can be helpful to examine for hepatic or abdominal IH in patients with multiple cutaneous lesions or to initially evaluate the spine in patients with overlying lumbosacral lesions. Children with concern for PHACE syndrome should undergo imaging of the brain with MRI to evaluate for posterior fossa lesions, echocardiogram, and possibly angiography or MR angiography to evaluate for aortic and cerebrovascular anomalies. When imaging is desired to determine the extent

of the tumor, contrast-enhanced MRI is the modality of choice and provides excellent evaluation of soft tissue without exposing the patient to ionizing radiation. On MRI, proliferating IH appear as a distinct, lobulated, enhancing soft tissue mass that is isointense to muscle on T1 and hyperintense on T2 images, often with a visible feeding artery and draining veins and intralesional flow voids. Involuting IH are heterogeneous masses with areas of increased T1 intensity corresponding to fibrofatty tissue and less robust enhancement than proliferating lesions.[9] Again, imaging studies are rarely needed for the diagnosis and treatment planning of most uncomplicated IH. Uncommonly, tissue biopsy may be necessary to confirm the suspected diagnosis or exclude other entities. IH can be positively identified based on characteristic histologic appearance and positive staining for GLUT-1, which is unique to IH among all other vascular anomalies. Laboratory blood tests play no role in the evaluation of patients with IH because there is no associated coagulopathy with this condition. As with imaging, biopsy and laboratory testing is not usually needed for uncomplicated IH.

Segmental lesions are more likely to develop complications than focal ones, with up to 50% of segmental lesions undergoing ulceration compared with 10% to 15% of localized lesions. Ulceration is the most common complication occurring in about 10% of cases overall almost all occur during proliferation. The cheeks, lip, and scalp are the most likely sites to ulcerate on the face, whereas the perineal area is the most common of the rest of the body (**Fig. 3**). Higher rates of complications (1.7 times) are seen among IH located on the face compared with other body sites and are more likely to require treatment.[10] Functional impairment most often interferes with visual axis, feeding ability, or respiration. Complications are more likely based on size, location, and morphology of the lesions but seem unrelated with patient characteristics or demographics. Larger lesions are more likely to develop complications, particularly ulceration, with a 5% increase in complications for every 10 cm^2 increase in size. Mixed IHs are more prone to ulceration than superficial lesions. The cause of ulceration is unknown but the speculation is that rapid expansion during proliferation exceeds the elastic capacity of the skin and the lesions outgrow their blood supply leading to ulceration. However, a small minority of lesions ulcerate during involution. Ulcerated lesions may become secondarily infected, are at higher risk for bleeding, and are more likely to result in scarring or require treatment.

Treatment of IH typically involves some combination of options including observation, medical therapy, laser treatments, and surgery. Treatments

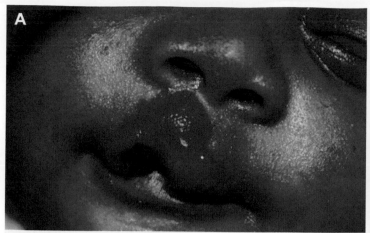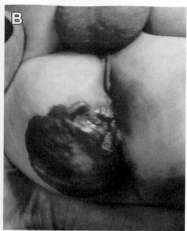

Fig. 3. IHs complicated by ulceration. (*A*) The most common site for ulceration on the face is the lip. (*B*) The most common site for ulceration elsewhere on the body is the perineal area.

may affect total resolution of the lesion, treat complications, and/or set the stage for further treatments. The management goal for IH is to achieve a functionally and aesthetically acceptable final result with the least amount of morbidity and lowest likelihood of complications. For some infants this involves serial observation and reassurance during the phases of growth, whereas others require active treatment at various stages. At least 40% of IHs do not involute to an acceptable result and require additional treatment. Roughly half of IHs take more than 6 years to involute and 80% of these have aesthetically unacceptable results. Because IHs are most common in the head and neck, the potential aesthetic consequences are quite high and nearly 50% of patients who require treatment cite disfigurement as the primary reason (**Fig. 4**). The goal is to achieve the best possible result before a child's development of self-image, which begins at age 2.5 to 3 years, or before the social pressures of school at 5 to 6 years, to minimize the psychological effects of these lesions.[7] Impending or active complications may mandate earlier treatment. Studies of children with IH suggest that those treated at young ages are not psychologically affected by the appearance of their tumors, despite significant distress felt by their family members about concerns for public scrutiny. This argues for a paradigm shift away from the adage that IH should be managed with benign neglect because they eventually go away. Because the eventual extent of involution is not predictable, intervention should be considered for any lesion whose treatment would result in an outcome as good or better than would be expected if the tumor was allowed to follow its natural history.

Observation is not an open-ended message to the parents to "leave it alone it will go away." It is an active process of watching the IH at arbitrary periods of time depending on the problem. For example, an infant seen very early for initial consultation may have a lesion that would be difficult to assess in terms of prognosis. Seeing the child within a few weeks would be reasonable to reevaluate and determine the next step of therapy.

A variety of medical treatments have been used through the years to treat IH with varying rates of success. Corticosteroids, the mainstay of medical treatment in the past have been supplanted by propranolol. Despite the overwhelming positive clinical response of propranolol treatment and its widespread use due to its wide safety margins, studies demonstrating efficacy have so far been limited to uncontrolled case studies. The only prospective, randomized double-blind study led to Food and Drug Administration approval of Hemangeol, a proprietary formula of propranolol hydrochloride specially formulated for pediatric dosing and approved for treatment of proliferating IH requiring systemic therapy (www.accessdata.fda.gov).

Propranolol is a nonselective β-antagonist that inhibits β_1 and β_2 receptors with equal affinity and has known effects of decreasing heart rate and blood pressure. The exact mechanism of action is unknown for propranolol's effect on IH but several mechanisms have been put forth. In addition, β receptors have been documented in tissue of proliferating and involuting IH.[11] The early effects of propranolol occur within 1 to 3 days of initiating therapy and are manifested as softening and flattening of the lesions with some diminution in redness if there is a superficial component. These effects most likely occur via vasoconstriction due to inhibition of vasodilation by blocking nitrous oxide production. Propranolol blocks the adrenergic stimulation of VEGF production and decreases

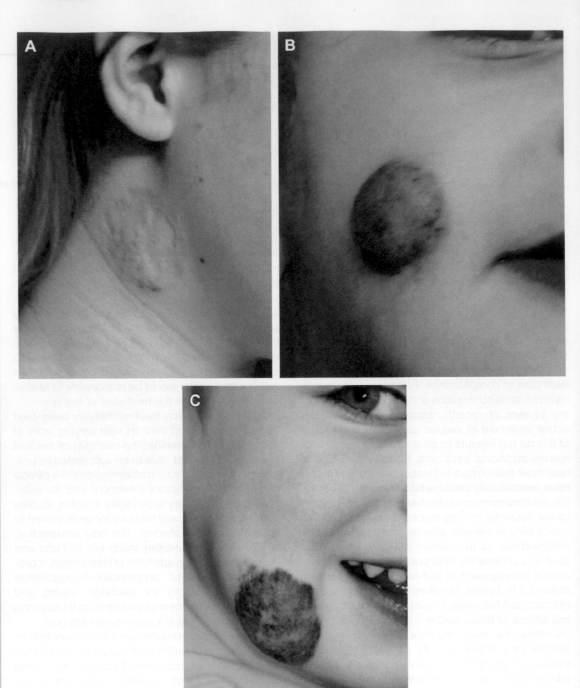

Fig. 4. (A–C) Examples of involuting IHs in patients who sought further treatment after being told to "leave it alone, it will go away." The threshold for acceptability is very high in the face, head, and/or neck area.

expression of MMP-9, which is thought to inhibit angiogenesis and slow proliferation. Finally, propranolol may speed involution through induction of apoptosis via the β₂ receptors. Propranolol is available as an oral suspension and is relatively well tolerated with no documented death or serious cardiovascular morbidity related directly to β-blocker

use in children in over 40 years of clinical experience. There are several well-known side-effects of propranolol that should be considered and discussed with parents, including bradycardia; hypotension; bronchial constriction with exacerbation of underlying reactive airways; hypoglycemia, especially among the premature or during times of limited oral intake or active infection; sleep disturbance; and gastrointestinal upset. Contraindications to propranolol therapy include preexisting bradycardia, hypotension, heart block or failure, asthma, or sensitivity to the drug. Protocols for pretreatment evaluation and drug initiation vary widely between clinicians with some pursuing a full cardiac work up and hospital admission to initiate therapy, whereas others start the drug in an outpatient setting. Recently, a multispecialty consensus panel released guidelines on propranolol use in IH, which are summarized herein.[12] Before initiating therapy a targeted history and physical examination should be performed of the cardiovascular and pulmonary systems to assess for underlying heart failure, arrhythmia, or asthma. No definitive consensus could be reached on the need for a pretreatment EKG for all children but it is recommended for children with baseline bradycardia, arrhythmia, or family history of congenital heart condition or connective tissue disease in the mother. Routine echocardiogram in the absence of abnormal clinical findings is not indicated. Children with PHACE syndrome should be evaluated by a pediatric cardiologist before starting propranolol because there is an increased risk of ischemic stroke in these children with associated cerebrovascular abnormalities. Random glucose measurements have not been shown to predict hypoglycemia with propranolol therapy and are not indicated. The maximum effect of propranolol is seen 1 to 3 hours after a dose so parents should be instructed to keep their child on a regular feeding regimen and avoid taking the medication during times of active infections to minimize the risk of hypoglycemia. The general dosing regimen used ranges from 1–3 mg/kg/d with most investigators advocating for 2 mg/kg/d divided in two or three daily doses. This may be slowly escalated from a lower starting dose to minimize adverse effects but these doses are significantly lower than typical doses used in children for cardiovascular indications. The dose should be adjusted periodically to keep up with the child's weight gain. Inpatient monitoring is suggested on initiation for infants who are 6 weeks old or younger or those with comorbid conditions affecting the cardiopulmonary system or increasing the risk of hypoglycemia. In older infants without these comorbidities and with good social support, initiation is done as an outpatient. These patients should have baseline vital signs, including pulse and blood pressure, and be observed in the office with repeat measurements within 2 hours after the first dose and every dose increase of greater than 0.5 mg/kg/d. The greatest response is seen within the first 8 weeks of therapy and patients who demonstrate a 20% drop in heart rate within the first 2 weeks seem to have a more

profound response than those whose heart rate is unchanged.[13] Treatment is generally continued through the proliferative phase and can be tapered off or discontinued after that point. Some lesions will demonstrate rebound growth and require resumption of the medication for a time. The goal is to treat with the drug beyond the time in the tumor's natural history in which it is proliferating. The deep component responds better than the superficial component. For superficial cutaneous involvement, the pulsed dye laser is used. This, in combination with propranolol, seems to give a better response than the drug alone (Fig. 5).[14]

Propranolol is most often started during the proliferative stage to limit IH growth and speed involution; however, some investigators have reported success with treatment initiated during the involution stage, likely related to the suspected effect on apoptosis. Treatment started at this phase does not produce as dramatic results but does accelerate the rate of involution compared with the untreated state and may allow for more conservative surgical resections of residual deformities. Topical β-blockers have also demonstrated efficacy versus placebo for early, proliferating superficial lesions.

Corticosteroids are an alternative medical therapy and represented the first-line option for treatment before the discovery of propranolol. Their use is now reserved for difficult IHs that do not respond to propranolol. Corticosteroids are effective only during the proliferative growth phase but have been shown to stabilize growth or promote involution and are thought to act by decreasing VEGF-A expression through the NF-κB pathway. No direct, randomized, head-to-head comparison between corticosteroids and β-blockers has been carried out thus far. However, there are two ongoing phase 2 trials (NCT01072045 and NCT00967226; ClinicalTrials.gov). A meta-analysis comparing individual studies, however, suggests superior efficacy with β-blocker treatment: 97% pooled response at 12 months compared with 69% for corticosteroid-treated lesions.[15] This clinical experience coupled with a more tolerable side-effect profile has led to wide-spread use of propranolol as the first-line medical therapy for problematic IH. Intralesional steroid injections have been used with some success for small isolated, deep, proliferating IH especially in children in whom systemic therapy does not seem appropriate. The author uses intralesional triamcinolone acetonide and betamethasone for focal, deep IH in which the injections may be the definitive treatment. Otherwise, other options are considered. Older therapies that demonstrated some efficacy in treating IH include interferon-α and vincristine. These are rarely, if

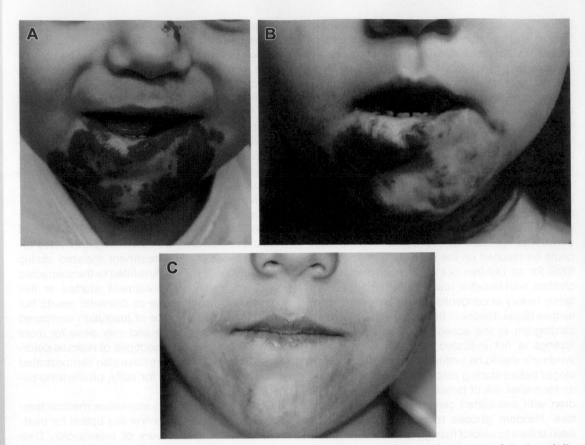

Fig. 5. Propranolol plus pulsed dye laser (PDL) treatment. (*A*) Segmental later proliferating IH of the beard distribution. There is no associated airway lesion in this patient. (*B*) Same patient during treatment with propranolol and PDL. (*C*) Two-year follow-up after termination of treatments.

ever, used anymore owing to unacceptably high rates of complications in infants with IH. Continued research, however, is identifying promising targets for newer therapies such as systemic or topical rapamycin, an mTOR inhibitor that has demonstrated efficacy for IH in culture and animal models.

Laser therapy has defined roles in the management of IH. The most commonly used laser for IH treatment is the pulsed-dye laser (PDL). This laser emits short pulses of yellow light (wavelength of 585–595 nm) that are absorbed preferentially by oxyhemoglobin. This allows for selective thermal destruction of vascular lesions without damage to surrounding tissue, a process known as selective photothermolysis. Treatment is often used for superficial, proliferating lesions to decrease redness, limit the full size of growth, and potentially prevent complications. Regimens for PDL treatment vary but often include a series of treatments at 2 to 6 week intervals until the desired response is achieved, with the appearance of purpura around the lesion serving as the endpoint for individual treatment sessions. Owing to the limited depth of penetration (1–2 mm), treatment is less

effective for thicker superficial lesions but can lighten the color of the lesion. PDL is ineffective for deep lesions without a surface component. Laser treatment with PDL is very effective for managing ulcerated lesions and has been shown to decrease bleeding, infection, and pain associated with ulceration while promoting more rapid epithelialization. More than 90% of ulcerated IHs are successfully treated with PDL, often with as few as one to two treatments. The goal of treatment is to heal the ulcer and set the stage for further treatment as needed. Residual telangiectasias after involution and erythematous scars following serial or near-total excision are also successfully managed with PDL. Clinically, the PDL effectively treats the superficial component's color and can effect resolution of the lesion if it is less than 2 mm in thickness during proliferation. The use of alternative lasers to treat complicated IH have been reported but have not gained as widespread use as the PDL owing to increased rates of scarring. The erbium or neodymium:yttrium-aluminum-garnet (Er:YAG and Nd:YAG, respectively) laser and the potassium-titanyl-phosphate

(KTP) laser have both been used interstitially to treat deeper IH, especially on mucosal surfaces. Although both lasers have demonstrated effectiveness, a comparison of multiple laser types revealed that the PDL laser demonstrated the best combination of effectiveness with the least amount of scarring for these lesions. The addition of a dynamic cooling device to the PDL has allowed for treatment of very young infants' skin, providing protection for the epidermis and allowing for the safe use of higher fluences. Again, laser therapy can effect total resolution of the superficial, proliferative lesion, treat complications such as ulcerations, and/or set the stage for further treatment such as surgery.

Surgical excision of IH was historically approached with reticence due to concern for significant intraoperative bleeding that was likely based on misdiagnosis of other vascular anomalies, such as venous malformations, as hemangiomas. In fact, IHs are solid masses rather than amorphous bags of blood that have identifiable feeding vessels that are readily controlled thus limiting blood loss from the tumor itself. Additionally, surgical planes are uniformly present between the tumor and normal tissues and can be created within the tumor itself or between the superficial and deep components. Successful surgery for proliferating lesions requires removal of the entire lesion because any residual tumor will continue to proliferate. This is most commonly done for smaller lesions that can easily be completely excised or occasionally as a debulking procedure to limit growth of large lesions that are functionally impairing, typically affecting the visual axis. The latter scenario often involves concomitant systemic therapy. Surgery on these lesions can be performed safely in a relatively bloodless fashion with meticulous dissection that includes needlepoint or bipolar cautery and close attention to surgical planes. For proliferating IHs that cannot be totally excised but do not threaten function, consideration could be made for treating medically while the lesion proliferates and addressing further deformities surgically once the final state of the lesion is known.

Surgical treatment[16] of involuting lesions is much more common than of those in proliferation. During involution it may be necessary to deal with persistent skin changes such as scarring or fibrofatty residuum, or to address persistent deformities in slowly involuting tumors. Excision should follow accepted facial plastic surgical techniques with preservation of as much normal skin as possible (**Fig. 6**). Conservative resection with primary closure is the goal and incisions should be camouflaged at natural boundaries of facial subunits or within relaxed skin tension lines. Rarely, large complicated lesions require management with tissue expanders or free tissue transfer to achieve adequate reconstruction of the resulting defect. However, advanced reconstructive techniques and complex local tissue rearrangement should be avoided in young patients with preference given to serial excision for removal of larger lesions.[17] The first excision should be performed along the axis of the planned final scar and entirely within the IH, sparing the surrounding skin. Closure should be performed under moderate tension to promote tissue creep and further excisions can follow after a 3 to 4 month interval. Most lesions can be managed in this way with an average of three excisions (**Fig. 7**). For deep lesions that do not involve the cutaneous surface, a plane of dissection can be created between the mass and the overlying normal skin. This allows for removal of all or a portion of the lesion without disrupting the uninvolved skin. Often, it is prudent to leave a portion of the deep residuum in situ to prevent a contour deformity that would result from removal of the entire lesion, especially in the lips. It is always better to err on the side of conservatism in these very young patients. IHs of the nasal tip and lips are two of the most cosmetically sensitive and potentially problematic locations on the face due to their prominent central position and low social tolerance for any residual lesion or scar. Lesions of the nasal tip often have significant redundancy of overlying skin that requires careful excision for proper redraping after removal of the residuum. Attempts should be made to respect nasal subunits when planning incisions but involvement of the nostril margin creates difficulty in redraping the skin if traditional external rhinoplasty incisions are made. Consideration should be given instead to leaving the nostril margin intact and placing incisions along the columellar edge and superior to the soft tissue triangles.[18] Deep lesions tend to laterally displace the lower lateral cartilages, which should be preserved and repositioned to their native location following tumor removal. Tumors involving the lip have a higher tendency to ulcerate and scar than other sites on the face. These lesions inherently expand the involved lip in either a vertical or horizontal direction, or both. Surgical excision during involution should follow a subunit-based principle, with incisions placed along natural boundaries, and a complete muscular sphincter should be restored. Careful attention should be paid to perfect alignment of the vermillion border and symmetric lip height.[19] As with other locations, serial excision is preferred for large lesions rather than advanced flap reconstruction whenever possible.

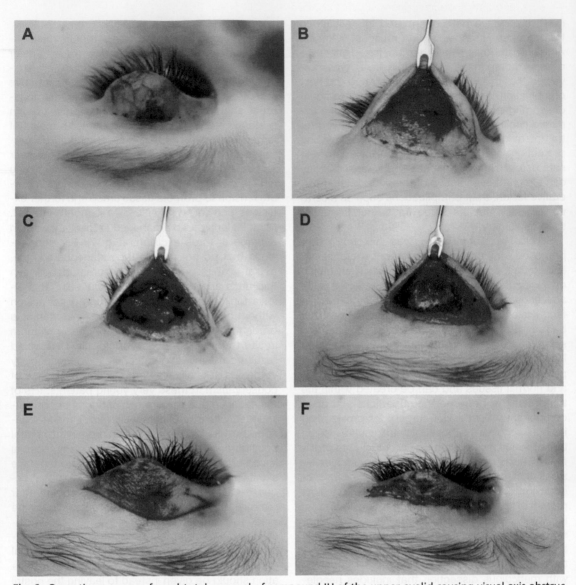

Fig. 6. Operative sequence for subtotal removal of compound IH of the upper eyelid causing visual axis obstruction. (*A*) Incision planned and marked in natural supratarsal crease. (*B*) Creation of dissection plane between the superficial component and the deep component of the IH. (*C*) Tumor completely exposed. (*D*) After subtotal removal of tumor by dissection between deep component and normal structures (tarsal plate or septum). The inferior-most portion of the tumor was left in place so as to not compromise the eyelash follicles. This portion of the IH will be allowed to continue involuting. (*E*) Redraping of the expanded soft tissue envelope. (*F*) Conservative resection and closure of the expanded skin so as to not create eye-closure problems. The involved skin may be treated with the PDL in the future if necessary.

IHs that require treatment are often managed with a combination of the treatments described above, including serial observation, systemic therapy, laser treatment, and surgical excision for various phases of IH growth. The treating clinician should be familiar with all treatment options and demonstrate flexibility in combining these options to achieve the best possible end result for the patient (**Fig. 8**). This is best facilitated through open communication with the family throughout the process and involvement of other specialties when needed. The prevailing dogma of "leave it alone it will go away" is no longer universally acceptable advice for IH at the time of this publication. Multiple treatment options exist that can achieve excellent results within the confines of developmental milestones for those lesions that merit intervention, thus sparing children and their families the stigma of living with a facial difference.

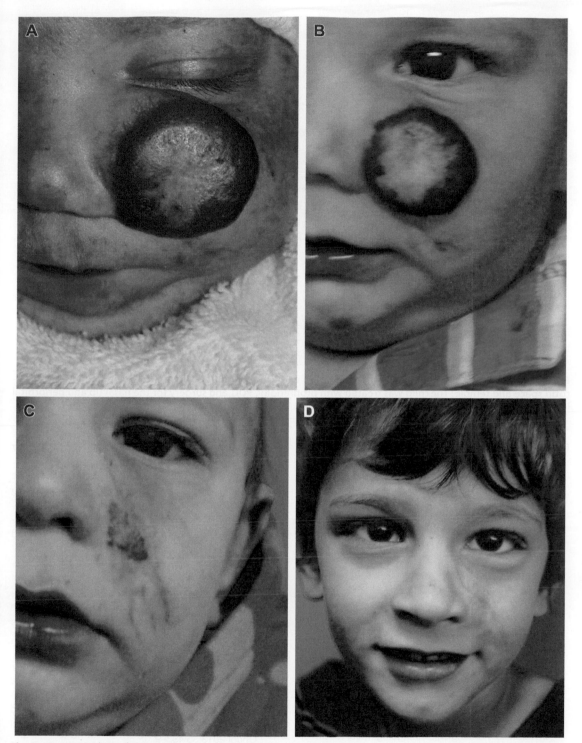

Fig. 7. Compound IH of the cheek treated with serial excision. (*A*) Large proliferating compound IH of the cheek in weeks-old infant. This child was seen before the advent of the use of propranolol and the parents opted not to use corticosteroids at the time. (*B*) Same infant several months later in early involution. The central pale area is a healed ulceration. (*C*) After two serial excisions and before PDL treatments. (*D*) A 4-year follow-up after serial excision and PDL treatments.

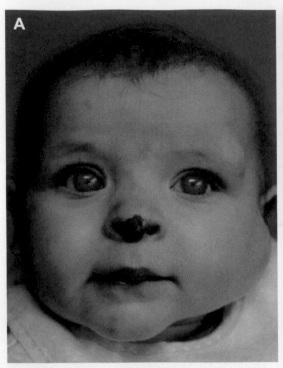
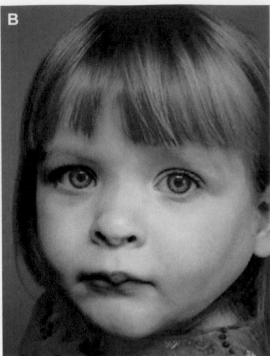

Fig. 8. IH of the nasal tip. (*A*) At time of presentation with compound IH of the nasal tip and deep IH of the parotid space and temple. The child was treated with propranolol, PDL, and surgery for the nasal tip and periorbital lesion. (*B*) Two-year follow-up after combined therapy.

REFERENCES

1. Phung TL, Hochman M, Mihm MC. Current knowledge of the pathogenesis of infantile hemangiomas. Arch Facial Plast Surg 2005;7:319–21.
2. North PE, Waner M, Mizeracki A, et al. A unique microvascular phenotype shared by juvenile hemangiomas and human placenta. Arch Dermatol 2001; 137:559–70.
3. Mihm M, Nelson JS. The metastatic niche theory can elucidate infantile hemangioma development. J Cutan Pathol 2010;37(1):83–7.
4. Barnés CM, Christison-Lagay EA, Folkman J. The placenta theory and the origin of infantile hemangioma. Lymphat Res Biol 2007;5:245–55.
5. Waner M, North PE, Scherer KA, et al. The nonrandom distribution of facial hemangiomas. Arch Dermatol 2003;139:869–75.
6. Przewratil P, Sitkiewicz A, Andrzejewska E. Local serum levels of vascular endothelial growth factor in infantile hemangioma: intriguing mechanism of endothelial growth. Cytokine 2010;49:141–7.
7. Hochman M, Adams DM, Reeves TD. Current knowledge and management of vascular anomalies: I. Hemangiomias. Arch Facial Plast Surg 2011;13: 145–51.
8. Haggstrom AN, Drolet BA, Baselga E, et al. Prospective study of infantile hemangiomas: demographic, prenatal, and perinatal characteristics. J Pediatr 2007;150:291–4.
9. Chaudry I, Manzoor M, Turner R, et al. Diagnostic imaging of vascular anomalies. Facial Plast Surg 2012;28(6):563–74.
10. Thomas RF, Hornung RL, Manning SC, et al. Hemangiomas of infancy: treatment of ulceration in the head and neck. Arch Facial Plast Surg 2005;7:312–5.
11. Storch CH, Hoeger PH. Propranolol for infantile haemangiomas: insights into molecular mechanisms of action. Br J Dermatol 2010;163:269–74.
12. Drolet BA, Frommelt PC, Chamlin SL, et al. Initiation and used of propranolol for infantile hemangioma: report of a consensus conference. Pediatrics 2013; 131:128–40.
13. Sondhi V, Patnaik SK. Propranolol for infantile hemangioma (PINCH): an open-label trial to assess the efficacy of propranolol for treating infantile hemangiomas and for determining the decline in heart rate to predict response to propranolol. J Pediatr Hematol Oncol 2013;35:493–9.
14. Reddy K, Blei F, Brauer JA, et al. Retrospective study of the treatment of infantile hemangioma using a combination of propranolol and pulsed dye laser. Dermatol Surg 2013;39(6):923–32.
15. Izadpanah A, Izadpanah A, Kanevsky J, et al. Propranolol versus corticosteroids in the treatment of

infantile hemangioma: a systematic review and meta-analysis. Plast Reconstr Surg 2013;131:601–13.

16. Hochman M. Management of vascular tumors. Facial Plast Surg 2012;28:584–9.

17. Kulbersh J, Hochman M. Serial excision of facial hemangiomas. Arch Facial Plast Surg 2011;13:199–202.

18. Hochman M, Mascareno A. Management of nasal hemangiomas. Arch Facial Plast Surg 2005;7:295–300.

19. O TM, Scheuermann-Poley C, Tan M, et al. Distribution, clinical characteristics, and surgical treatment of lip infantile hemangiomas. JAMA Facial Plast Surg 2013;15:292–304.

Craniofacial Anomalies

Laszlo Nagy, MD[a], Joshua C. Demke, MD[b],*

KEYWORDS

- Craniosynostosis • FGFR mutations • Scaphocephaly • Dolichocephaly • Trigonocephaly
- Brachycephaly • Plagiocephaly • Minimally invasive surgery

KEY POINTS

- Craniofacial anomalies are common (1:2000 for isolated suture synostosis) but syndromic craniosynostosis is relatively rare.
- FGFR mutations underlie most syndromic craniosynostosis, whereas nonsyndromic synostosis frequently involves a variety of genetic and environmental risk factors.
- Single-suture synostosis is often an isolated finding, and intracranial hypertension, developmental delays, and strabismus, though less likely in isolated synostosis, are more frequent in multisuture and syndromic forms of craniosynostosis.
- Minimally invasive approaches are most successful when done between ages 3 and 6 months, and often require many months of molding-helmet therapy postoperatively.
- Surgery after age 8 to 9 months usually requires open cranial vault reconstruction whereby the skull is surgically osteotomized; bone grafts are reshaped and repositioned, then fixated in anatomically improved and often overcorrected positions.

 Videos related to pediatric craniofacial surgical procedures (Video 1: Open approach for sagittal synostosis subtotal cranial vault recon without bone grafting and Video 2: Depicts endoscopic-assisted strip craniectomy with wedge craniectomy) accompany this article at http://www.facialplastic.theclinics.com/

OVERVIEW

Craniosynostosis, the premature closure of cranial sutures, may be isolated or nonsyndromic, affecting 1 in 2000 live births[1] (typically single-sutured), or syndromic, affecting 1:30,000 to 1:100,000 live births[2] (frequently multisutured), and primary or secondary. Multifactorial, genetic, and environmental influences may be involved. Regardless of etiology, the fused suture(s) typically cause(s) a restriction in skull growth and subsequent skull characteristics, skull base, and asymmetries and disturbances at the time of facial growth. Three theories have been proposed:

1. Virchow's theory that sutural fusion precedes other events

2. Moss's idea that primacy lies with primary skull-base growth restriction preceding synostosis
3. Others have suggested that brain growth restriction is the primary factor that subsequently leads to premature fusion[3]

It is now generally accepted that underlying mechanical force signaling pathways and cytokines mediate cranial suture patency, and premature fusion is thought to occur secondary to mutations in these genes.[4] Secondary synostosis is evidenced in both microcephalic and overshunted individuals, and in certain hematologic disorders.[5]

The majority or craniofacial growth and development occurs during the first year of life and growth potential, with the brain doubling in size

---

[a] Pediatric Neurosurgery, Department of Pediatrics, Texas Tech Health Sciences Center, 3601 4th Street, STOP 9406, Lubbock, TX 79430-9406, USA; [b] Facial Plastic and Reconstructive Surgery, Department of Surgery, Texas Tech Health Sciences Center, 3601 4th Street, STOP 8312, Lubbock, TX 79430-8312, USA
* Corresponding author.
E-mail address: joshua.demke@ttuhsc.edu

Facial Plast Surg Clin N Am 22 (2014) 523–548
http://dx.doi.org/10.1016/j.fsc.2014.08.002
1064-7406/14/$ – see front matter © 2014 Elsevier Inc. All rights reserved.

by 1 year of life and tripling by 2 years.[6] This rapid growth of the brain and resultant bone growth are determined by complex growth factor pathways regulated by genes that code for fibroblast growth factor receptor (FGFR) and transforming growth factor (TGF)-β, among others, and are at the core of the principles of craniofacial surgery, including the duration and timing of surgical intervention.[7] There are clearly both environmental and genetic factors at play for isolated, single-suture, nonsyndromic forms of synostosis (Fig. 1).

PATHOPHYSIOLOGY

Multiple environmental associations have been described, including paternal occupations such as agriculture and forestry, maternal age, exposure to tobacco smoke, and medications, including nitrofurantoin and warfarin use during pregnancy. Malpositioned fetal lie and intrauterine constraint or, at times, metabolic factors can also be associated, including mucopolysaccharidosis, mucolipidosis, rickets, and hyperthyroidosis.[5,8]

MOLECULAR GENETICS

A variety of mutations in transcription derived growth factors, FGFR1,2 and 3 are known to be involved in syndromic craniosynostosis (Table 1).[1,7,9,10]

Scaphocephaly

Scaphocephaly (boat-shaped head) (Fig. 2) can occur without synostosis; however, it is the most common manifestation of sagittal synostosis in up to 50%[1] of isolated synostosis. Calvarial bone growth is limited perpendicular to the affected sagittal suture, resulting in narrowing of the head transversely, and resultant brain growth anteroposteriorly leads to frontal bossing and/or occipital cupping. Shape may vary depending on the duration or timing of synostosis, whether partial or complete suture involvement, and whether other sutures are involved (Figs. 3 and 4).[2,3,11]

Trigonocephaly

Metopic synostosis may result in mild metopic ridging in the midline forehead or a combination of ridging, bitemporal narrowing, and hypotelorism, which together make the forehead appear triangular (Fig. 5C, D). The metopic suture fuses as early as age 3 to 6 months and, unlike other cranial sutures, normally disappears; hence, the diagnosis largely depends more on clinical shape and less on computed tomography (CT) findings.[12,13]

Deformational Plagiocephaly

Meaning twisted or slanted, deformational plagiocephaly (DP) refers to flattening of the head.

The most common type of plagiocephaly is positional, namely DP. DP results when the skull is

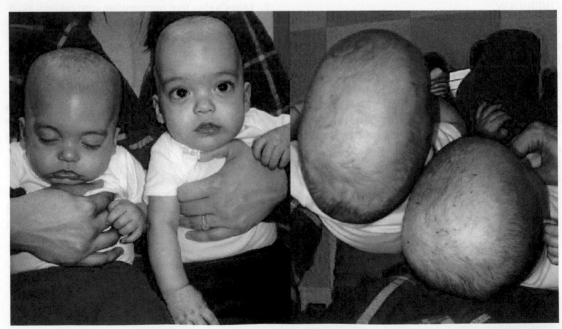

Fig. 1. Four-month-old identical twins, frontal and vertex views. Twin on left lap with sagittal synostosis and scaphocephaly.

subject to pressure either in utero or, more commonly, as a result of supine positioning. Favored fetal and postnatal lie are thought to underlie DP. Congenital torticollis is associated with and likely responsible for this condition one-third of the time,[14,15] leading to characteristic head tilt on the side of the affected sternocleidomastoid muscle and twisting of the neck such that babies tend to prefer sleeping on the contralateral occiput. Repositioning maneuvers and repositioning pillows work by keeping babies off the affected flat area(s), and are fairly effective in ameliorating DP when used in the first 4 to 6 months of life. Neck physiotherapy is important when congenital torticollis is present. When severe flattening persists beyond the first 5 to 6 months of life, orthotic molding bands or helmets (**Fig. 6**) have been shown to improve cranial symmetry, especially when used before age 12 months.[16,17] A recent randomized controlled study showed no differences in 5- to 6-month-old babies with moderate asymmetries treated for 6 months with or without helmets. Of note, these investigators excluded babies with the most severe cranial asymmetries.[18]

Although DP is more commonly unilateral, bilateral DP is not uncommon and presents with brachycephaly or bilateral occipital flattening. This condition leads to a head that is short anteroposteriorly and wide transversely, which makes both the head and face look round in appearance (see **Fig. 10**).

Anterior Plagiocephaly

Unilateral coronal synostosis results in anterior plagiocephaly. The affected frontal bone is underprojected, and the contralateral frontal bone bulges anteriorly (**Fig. 7**), which can push the orbit inferiorly, resulting in orbital asymmetry or vertical dystopia.

The superior orbital rim is elevated (Harlequin eye) (**Fig. 8**); in severe and late presenting coronal synostosis the nasal root deviates toward the fused suture and the mandible can be similarly shifted, with additional associated ipsilateral temporal narrowing.

Posterior Plagiocephaly

Like DP, lambdoid suture synostosis results in unilateral occipital flattening, but with concomitant ipsilateral mastoid bulging and posterior inferior displacement of the ipsilateral ear. There are no frontal bony changes, whereas in DP there is concomitant ipsilateral frontal bone shift anteriorly, and in DP the ipsilateral ear is often more anterior than the unaffected side. When viewed from above these differences are described as parallelogram

deformity in the case of DP and trapezoid deformity for unilateral lambdoid synostosis (see **Fig. 2**). It is worth remembering that whereas DP is common (20% to 50% of all babies are affected to some degree), lambdoid synostosis is extremely rare (1:100,000).[2,14,15,23]

Brachycephaly

Although the most common cause of brachycephaly (short head) is deformational and related to supine positioning, bilateral coronal synostosis needs to be ruled out (**Fig. 9**).

Usually a detailed history will reveal progressive flattening in positional brachycephaly, whereas syndromic brachycephaly will often present with characteristic syndromic facies and digital/pedal deformities (see **Table 1**). A noncontrasted head CT with 3-dimensional reconstruction (**Fig. 10**) will confirm the diagnosis.[16,23–25]

Cloverleaf skull

Cloverleaf skull is the result of fusion of all cranial sutures, except the metopic and squamosal. Because the brain is restricted in multiple planes, characteristic compensatory bulging occurs as brain and bone growth are forced across the 2 opened sutures, yielding the characteristic cloverleaf shape. Cloverleaf is perhaps the most challenging and dangerous craniosynostosis because of the severe bony growth restriction and limited intracranial volume, leading to problems with increased intracranial pressure (ICP), brain dysfunction, and hydrocephalus. Because of the severity of proptosis and orbital hypoplasia, impaired vision is common, especially in the case of extensive manipulation.[26]

History of craniofacial surgery

History of craniofacial surgery is beyond the scope of this article **Table 2** for brief overview.

EVALUATION AND DIAGNOSIS OF CRANIOSYNOSTOSIS

It is important to obtain detailed history of pregnancy, birth, family, and medications or drug exposure in utero. The duration and timing of head shape is important because progressive flattening would suggest DP, with deformities that are present since birth and relatively unaffected by positioning more likely to suggest synostosis. The head should be observed from all possible views and photographic documentation obtained, fontanelles and sutures should be palpated, fronto-occipital circumference measured, and calipers used to measure cephalic index (CI) (the ratio of width/length of the skull). Careful examination of

Table 1
Summary of the most common syndromic craniosynostoses

Syndrome	Skull Deformity	Craniofacial Abnormalities	Signs and Symptoms	Genetics	Hand and Feet Abnormalities	Incidence
Apert	Turribrachycephaly Acrocephaly Opened metopic suture Bitemporal bulging Bilateral coronal Bilateral lambdoid Sagittal synostosis	Orbital hypoplasia and orbital rim retrusion Hypertelorism Proptosis Downslanting palpebral fissures Cranial bony defects Short "beaked" nose Midface hypoplasia Mandibular prognatism Highly arched palate	Mental retardation Intracranial hypertension Cerebral atrophy Wide subarachnoid spaces	FGFR2 Autosomal dominant Mainly sporadic (paternal), some familial	Pansyndactylies of hands and feet	1:65,000–100,000 live births
Crouzon	Acrocephaly Coronal, lambdoid, and basilar synchondroses/synostosises	Shallow orbit, orbital proptosis Hypertelorism Strabismus Beaked nose Maxillary hypoplasia Mandibular prognatism Highly arched palate Enlarged sella turcica Jugular foramina stenosis	Hydrocephalus Symptomatic chronic tonsillar herniation Syringomyelia Intracranial hypertension Optic atrophy Mental retardation	FGFR2, FGFR3 if associated with acanthosis nigricans Autosomal dominant Sporadic and familial cases are almost equal	Usually unaffected	1.6 per 100,000
Pfeiffer	Type I: Turribrachycephaly Bilateral coronal Frontosphenoidal synostoses Type II: Cloverleaf deformation Type III: Severe turribrachicephaly Bilateral coronal Frontosphenoidal sagittal, metopic, and bilateral metopic synostoses	Orbital proptosis and stenosis Palpebral retraction Jugular foramen stenosis Midfacial hypoplasia Mandibular prognatism Highly arched palate Bifid uvula External ear duct atresia	Intracranial hypertension Hydrocephalus Symptomatic chronic tonsillar herniation Optic atrophy Severe mental retardation (Types II and III) Transmission hearing loss Respiratory insufficiency Sleep apnea	FGFR2 FGFR1 Autosomal dominant Sporadic and familial cases are close to equal	Brachdactyly, limited variable syndactyly	1:100,000

Syndrome	Skull	Facial features	Neurologic/other	Genetics	Limb anomalies	Incidence
Saethre-Chotzen	Acrocephaly Plagiocephaly Scaphocephaly Unilateral coronal, bilateral coronal, metopic, and bilateral lambdoid synostoses	Low-set frontal hairline Flat forehead Hypertelorism Eyelid ptosis Tear duct stenosis Highly arched palate Mandibular prognatism Angulated and small round ears	Mental retardation Conductive hearing loss	*TWIST* Gene mutation Chr 7 Autosomal dominant Mainly familial, one-third is sporadic	Partial cutaneous syndactyly, some brachydactyly	1:25,000–1:50,000
Carpenter syndrome	Sagittal and lambdoid synostosis	Downsloping palpebral fissures, low-set ears, short neck	Often short in height Obesity Mental retardation in many, normal intelligence in some	Autosomal recessive *RAB23* or *MEGF8* mutations	Variable polysyndactyly, clinodactyly, brachydactyly	1:1,000,000
Muenke syndrome	Unilateral or bilateral coronal synostosis	Variable hypertelorism Mild to moderate midface hypoplasia, low-set ears, associated hearing loss	Usually normal intelligence	Autosomal dominant *FGFR3* mutations	Variable carpal and tarsal fusions	1:30,000

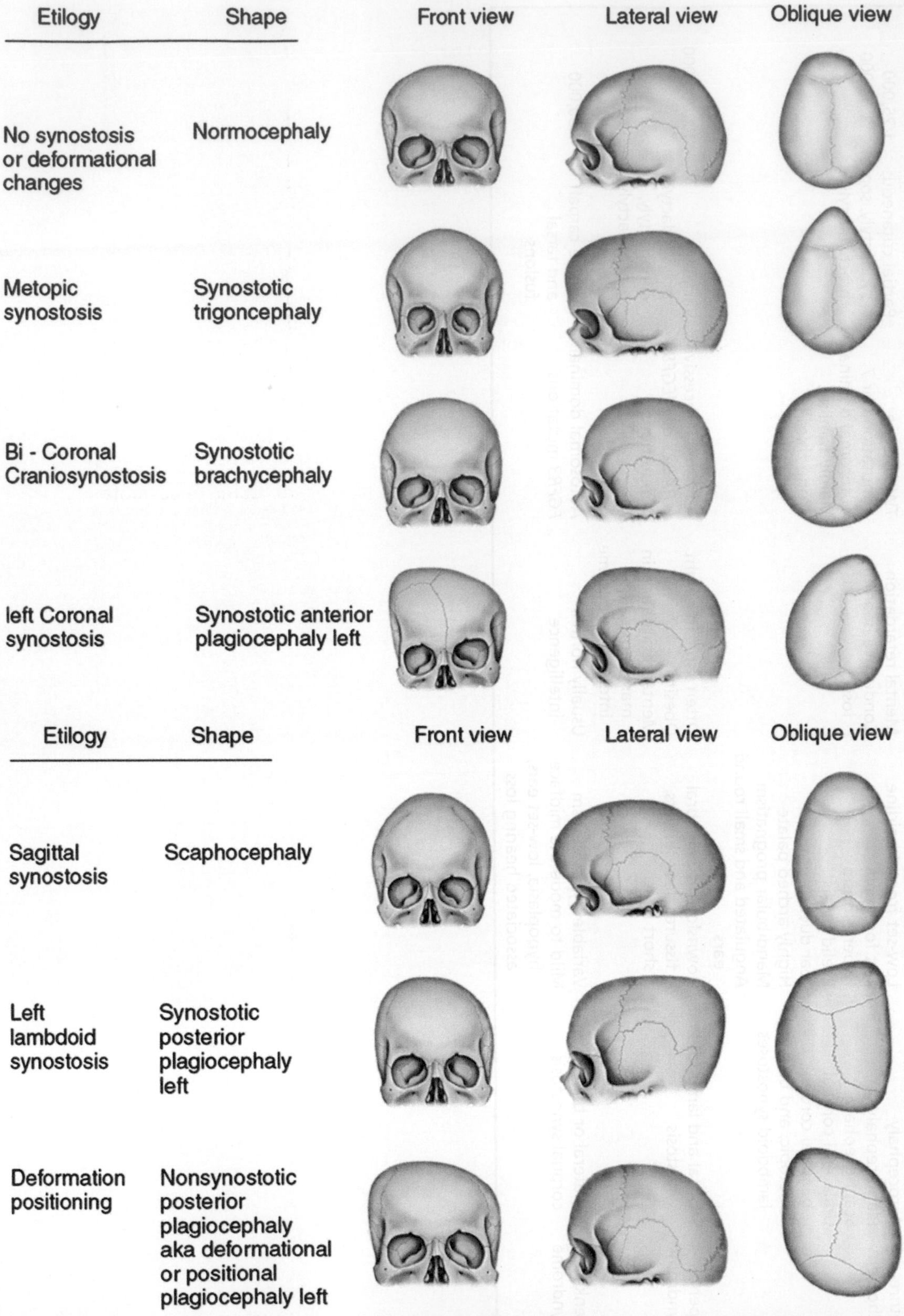

Etiology	Shape	Front view	Lateral view	Oblique view
No synostosis or deformational changes	Normocephaly			
Metopic synostosis	Synostotic trigoncephaly			
Bi - Coronal Craniosynostosis	Synostotic brachycephaly			
left Coronal synostosis	Synostotic anterior plagiocephaly left			

Etiology	Shape	Front view	Lateral view	Oblique view
Sagittal synostosis	Scaphocephaly			
Left lambdoid synostosis	Synostotic posterior plagiocephaly left			
Deformation positioning	Nonsynostotic posterior plagiocephaly aka deformational or positional plagiocephaly left			

Fig. 2. Normocephaly and common forms of craniosynostosis and deformational plagiocephaly, with representative shapes.

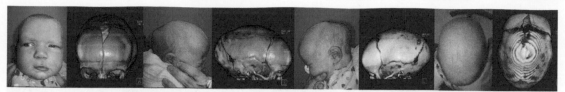

Fig. 3. Preoperative frontal, lateral, and vertex views, and 3-dimensional (3D) computed tomography (CT) demonstrating sagittal synostosis and, in this case, predominantly occipital deformity.

the face including orbital size, presence of asymmetry, ptosis, lagophthalmos, hypertelorism or hypotelorism, or pseudohypertelorism is warranted. Ear position, size, and any associated deformities, and facial paresis or paralysis should be noted. Full body examination is important to evaluate for findings involved in syndromic craniosynostosis, such as cardiac anomalies, respiratory difficulties as a result of mandibular or midface hypoplasia, and ocular exposure from exorbitism/proptosis. Hand/foot and finger/toe anomalies are common (see **Table 1**) with many of the syndromic craniosynostoses.[27]

Microcephaly, venous anomalies and pressure elevation, hydrocephalus, and cerebellar tonsillar herniation all can lead to increased ICP and can present acutely, subacutely, or chronically. It is important to look for nonspecific signs and symptoms such as irritability, feeding difficulties, inconsolable crying, or insomnia as red flags for ICP

elevation. A bulging fontanelle and engorged scalp veins are also often predictive. Pediatric ophthalmology evaluation to examine for strabismus and rule out papilledema is useful, and even in the absence of papilledema ICP monitoring should be considered if there is a strong suspicion for ICP elevation.[8,28–33]

Imaging in Craniosynostosis

Skull series are sometimes obtained when evaluating for abnormal head shapes. Thumbprinting or copper-beaten appearance on plain films, representing inner table scalloping (**Fig. 11**), is one warning of potential increased ICP.

CT scans are used to confirm a diagnosis of craniosynostosis and though not necessary for every craniofacial deformity, CT can be used with computer-aided design and modeling

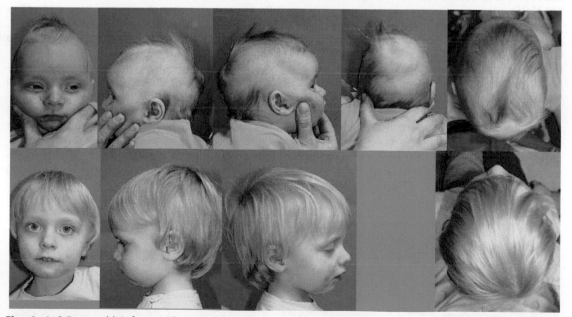

Fig. 4. A 3.5-year-old infant with predominantly frontal boxiness and bitemporal narrowing: Preoperative frontal, lateral, occiput, and vertex views, and 20 month postoperative view following extended sagittal strip craniectomy with biparietal wedge craniectomies and outfracture of parietal bones at 4.5 months of age and 4 months of postoperative molding helmet.

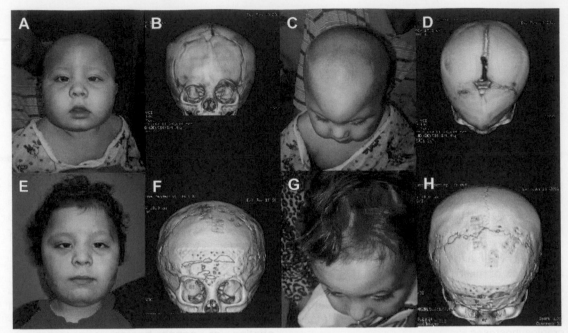

Fig. 5. Preoperative frontal and vertex views and 3D CT demonstrating severe trigonocephaly and hypotelorism at age 9 months (*A–D*), 21 months after bi–fronto-orbital advancements and frontal cranioplasties (*E, G*), and 3D CT 9 months postoperatively (*F, H*).

(CAD-CAM) for preoperative planning to create stereolithographic models, make miters, optimize osteotomies, and create custom CAD-CAM patient-specific implants designed to exactly match bony defects (**Figs. 12 and 13**).[34–37]

Some centers obtain immediate baseline postoperative CT scans following cranial vault reconstruction. Owing to the risks of ionizing radiation, the authors defer on ordering these unless the patient has neurologic deterioration; otherwise follow-up CT scans are obtained about 12 to 18 months postoperatively. For postoperative fluid collections, hematomas, or hydrocephalus, rapid magnetic resonance imaging (MRI) or lowered-radiation CT of the brain is the choice of diagnostic testing. MRI is useful for evaluating the brain for abnormalities such as Chiari malformations

(**Fig. 14**), venous anomalies, and hydrocephalus (see **Table 2**).[8,28,38–40]

THE CONCEPT OF THE CRANIOFACIAL TEAM

Because craniosynostosis is often part of a syndrome and many systems are often affected, an interdisciplinary team approach is now the standard of care for such complicated patients.

This team can include a plastic surgeon, pediatric otolaryngologist, or facial plastic surgeon trained in craniofacial surgery, a pediatric neurosurgeon, an oral-maxillofacial surgeon, a pediatric anesthesiologist and intensivist, a pedodontist orthodontist, a prosthodontist, a pediatric ophthalmologist, a psychologist, a geneticist, an audiologist, a speech pathologist, pediatrician, among others.[3]

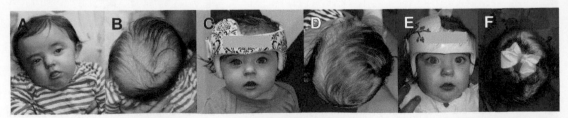

Fig. 6. Frontal and vertex views of a 4-month-old female with right torticollis and positional plagiocephaly (right > left) (*A, B*), after 6 weeks of orthotic molding band (*C, D*), and after 4 months of banding, pictured with the second band (*E, F*).

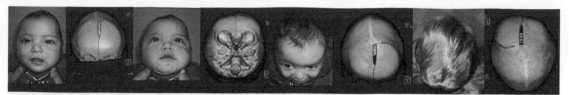

Fig. 7. Frontal, basal, fronto-vertex, and vertex photos, and 3D CT of a 9-month-old infant with right coronal and sagittal synostosis.

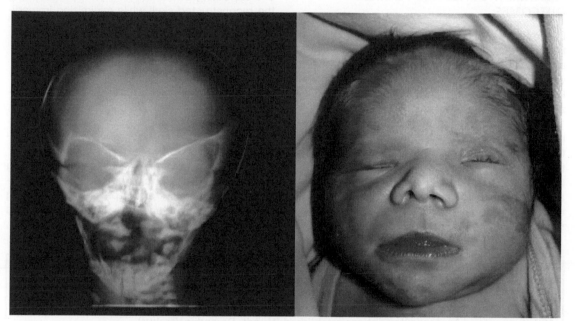

Fig. 8. Note the left frontal flattening and vertical dystopia on this 2-day-old baby with characteristic Harlequin sign on plain radiograph of the skull.[19–22]

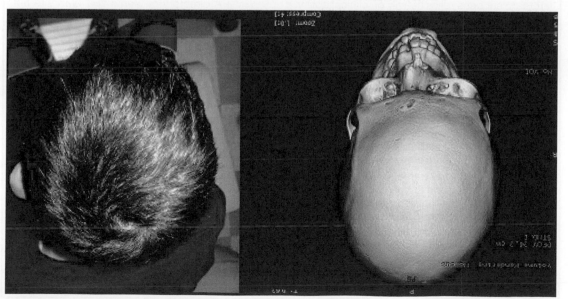

Fig. 9. A 13-year-old child with syndromic multisuture synostosis including bicoronal and brachycephalic head (vertex view).

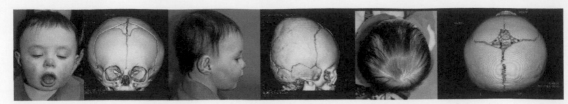

Fig. 10. A 16-month-old infant with positional brachycephaly.

TREATMENT GOALS AND PLANNED OUTCOMES

Determining which patients have or might develop functional problems as a result of increased ICP, and developmental delays, strabismus, or loss of vision as result of optic disc atrophy or exposure keratopathy is important in efforts to avoid the sequelae of these problems.

Improving outcomes from a functional standpoint is primary, but aesthetic improvements in form are not only important for cosmesis but also for improving psychosocial attitudes and perceptions, and minimizing teasing. Reconstruction aims to approximate normal size, shape, and symmetry by surgically removing synostotic bone, reconstructing the cranio-orbital asymmetries, overcorrecting when necessary, and stabilizing the reconstructed skull while minimizing immediate postoperative and/or late complications.[4,41,42]

PREOPERATIVE PLANNING AND PREPARATION

Physical examination is equally important in evaluating the head from all sides and from above, noting any head tilt and any associated maxillofacial, orbital, dental, or auricular asymmetries or abnormalities (Fig. 15).

Several investigators have described using normative CAD-CAM templates to design fronto-orbital bandeaus and presurgical cutting guides,[35,36] noting shorter intraoperative times and excellent immediate postoperative shape.

Table 2
Brief review of historical development of diagnosis and surgical treatment

762 BC	Homer in *Iliad*. Hippocrates and Galen delineate the shape
16th Century	Anatomic descriptions established (Hundt, Dryander Vesalius)
1851	Virchow describes basics of abnormal and compensatory skull growth. Names condition as craniostenosis, also known as Virchow's Law. Sear proposes title craniosynostosis in 1937
1912	Apert and Crouzon publish syndromic craniosynostosis
1890, 1892	First reported interventions for treatment; published in Paris and San Francisco
1921	Mechner publishes first modern surgical approach
1940s	Surgery available for those who present late in course of disease. Investigators propose polyethylene and tantalum to prevent suture reunion
1956	Anderson coagulates dura, based on assumption that it gives pathologic signal, but technique causes seizures. Matson applies pericraniectomy to help inhibition of bone reproduction at strip suture resection. Further development not possible without concurrent advent of modern anesthesiology and transfusion techniques. Leads to 2 deaths in 394 operations. From this point on, safety level and cosmetic outcome emerge as goals of surgery
1960–1990	Total cranial vault reconstruction with wedge craniectomies added to strip resections and Pi procedure for advanced sagittal and orbital rim. Extensive strip removal proposed and developed by Epstein, and extensive operations, new techniques, and classifications published by McComb
1971	Tessier further develops and makes safer existing surgical techniques by providing basis for safety and successful outcome
Today	Distraction craniotomies, endoscopic approach, and minimally invasive techniques make repertoire more colorful with obvious contribution to safety, less operative time, diminished blood loss, and shortened hospital stay

Data from Mehta VA, Bettegowda C, Jallo GI, et al. The evolution of surgical management for craniosynostosis. Neurosurg Focus 2010;29(6):E5. 1–7.

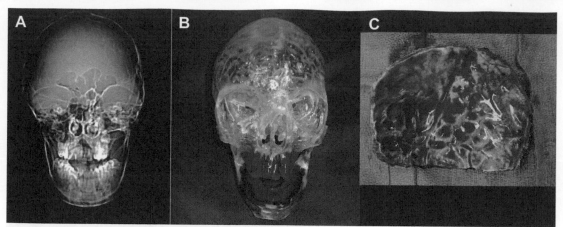

Fig. 11. Plain skull film (*A*) and stereolithographic model (*B*) demonstrating thumbprinting/copper-beaten appearance in child with syndromic multisuture craniosynostosis and brachycephaly. (*C*) intraoperative view of inner table of frontal calvarium depicting bony changes that are typical of chronic elevation of intracranial pressure.

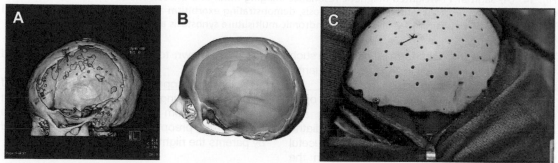

Fig. 12. (*A*) A 7-year-old child with large left fronto-temporo-parietal defect following decompressive craniectomy. (*B*) Proposed CAD-CAM model with allograft implant. (*C*) Intraoperative view with CAD-CAM PEEK implant reconstructing the defect.

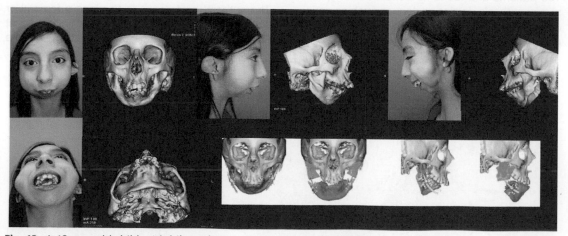

Fig. 13. A 13-year-old child with bilateral craniofacial microsomia, bilateral grade 2 microtia, and micrognathia with occlusal plane abnormalities. 3D model and preoperative planning session with proposed mandibular osteotomies and curvilinear distraction simulated.

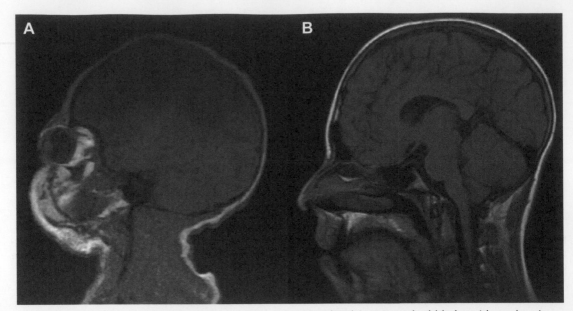

Fig. 14. (*A*) Sagittal T1-weighted magnetic resonance imaging (MRI) in a 2-week-old baby with syndromic cra-niosynostosis and bicoronal and metopic synostosis, demonstrating exorbitism and ocular proptosis. (*B*) Sagittal T1-weighted MRI depicting 13-year-old with syndromic multisuture synostosis and Chiari I malformation.

The authors question long-term outcomes on such templates, as overcorrecting (**Fig. 16**) is frequently needed for longer-lasting results.

Optimizing surgical outcomes includes open and frequent communication before, during, and after surgery with pediatric anesthesia, pediatric intensivists, and all surgeons involved. It is useful to have cross-matched blood available in the room at time of surgery, although some centers use minimally invasive approaches, or alterna-tively cell-saving/scavenging autologous blood transfusions.[43] Fearon and colleagues[44] recently published their prospective randomized study of 100 patients and found no benefit from hypoten-sive anesthesia. Lysine analogues such as amino-caproic acid and tranexamic acid bind to plasminogen and prevent binding to fibrin, which

has been shown to reduce intraoperative blood loss.[45–47]

Reviewing preoperative imaging on the day of surgery and having scans and photos visible in the operating room are also helpful. Chlorhexidine scalp scrubs preoperatively can be administered by parents the night before surgery.

PATIENT POSITIONING

Under mask anesthesia a single peripheral line is started and the child is orotracheally intubated, although nasal intubation may be necessary with certain craniofacial and orthognathic procedures. The authors' preference is to place a femoral or subclavian triple-lumen central line, although at times 2 large peripherals and an arterial line are

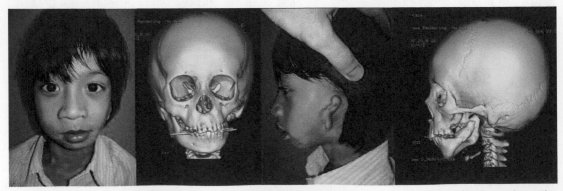

Fig. 15. A 6-year-old child with Pruzansky type III craniofacial microsomia, demonstrating occlusal cant, hypoplas-tic mandible, and grade III microtia with canal atresia.

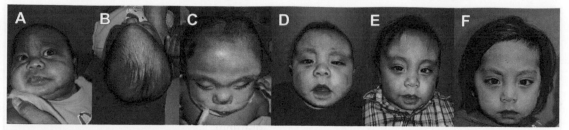

Fig. 16. (*A, B*) Frontal and vertex preoperative views at 3 months demonstrating severe trigonocephaly. (*C*) Intraoperative view at 9 months demonstrating overcorrection (overly boxy appearance). (*D*) 1 month postoperatively. (*E*) 3 months postoperatively. (*F*) 18 months postoperatively.

appropriate. For minimally invasive approaches these may be unnecessary.[20]

Depending on the deformity, the patient is positioned prone if working on the occiput, supine when working frontally, or at times a modified prone or "sphinx position" is used, whereby the head is extended while prone. When working on both the front and back, the authors prefer avoiding this position with extended neck because of the potential for air embolism. A 2-stage approach to surgery is preferred if severe occipital and frontal deformities are present.

- A Foley catheter and warming blanket are placed, in addition to a core temperature probe, and the child is rotated 180° (**Fig. 17**).
- The surgical suite is kept warm, especially early on when the child is exposed during venous and/or arterial access placement.
- Preoperative antibiotics and steroids are given; the authors' approach is to infuse aminocaproic acid (Amicar), 50 mg/kg loading dose then 25 mg/kg/h during the prodcedure.[45,46,48]
- The child's head is placed on a horseshoe head frame for optimal exposure.
- The eyes are protected with moisturizing eye ointment and sterile dermal plastic adhesives

placed over the eyes after skin preparation, although temporary tarsorrhaphies are at times helpful. The face and eyes should be carefully protected and padded, especially when the patient is prone.

- A wavy-line or zig-zag bicoronal incision (Video 1) is marked out, or a minimally invasive incision(s) marked out with marking pen, injected with 0.5% lidocaine with epinephrine 1:200,000 per pediatric weight guidelines, and tattooed with methylene blue.
- The whole head and at times upper face, including upper pole of ears and orbits, are prepped after limited hair clipping.
- The endotracheal tube is secured so that anesthesia has easy access if needed during surgery.
- Sterile drapes and collecting bags are placed to more accurately keep track of blood loss, and awareness of irrigation used during the case also helps to this end. A 180° turn from anesthesia provides access for surgeons and assistants, medical students, and residents, and allows anesthesia access to ventilation circuit and lines.

Anesthetists and surgeons should be in continuous communication regarding the patient's general status and be proactive in estimating blood loss,[46] discussing intraoperative hemoglobin/hematocrit, electrolytes, and pH assessment. Hemodynamic parameters such as low central venous pressure, tachycardia, and hypotension, though important, can be late indicators of hypovolemia; therefore, early transfusion or attempts to match cubic centimeter (cc) for cc of blood are useful.

Necessary assistance and access to implants, grafts, and plating systems should be coordinated before the day of surgery. An experienced nurse and surgical assistant or technician and product support representatives are welcomed and useful, especially in complex reconstructive surgeries. Blood and fluid supply should be in the room and kept appropriately warmed.

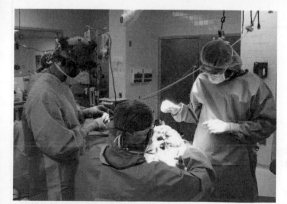

Fig. 17. Patient supine and rotated 180° from anesthesia for anterior cranial vault reconstruction for trigonocephaly.

Table 3
Open versus minimally invasive approaches to cranial reconstruction

Minimally Invasive	Open Approaches
Indication: first 3–6 mo of life and less severe deformities	*Indication:* >6 mo of life or severe deformities (extended strip craniectomies, subtotal cranial vault reconstruction, Pi procedure, or total cranial vault reconstructions with bone grafting)
1–3 small incisions placed so as to provide maximal exposure to suture involved	Bicoronal (wavy-line or zig-zag) incision
Strip craniectomy of synostotic suture; can be done under endoscopic visualization or using lighted retractors depending on preference and size of incision	Remove synostotic bone, osteotomize asymmetric bone, remove and reshape then replace and fixate in more natural/normalized or overcorrected position either with wires (less common in last 20 y), absorbable suture (often takes more time and less rigid fixation), or more commonly resorbable plates and screws (more expensive) which are hydrolyzed and disappear over about 18 mo
Placement of springs negates need for helmeting but requires second surgery 3–6 mo later to remove hardware	
Postoperative molding helmet for 6–12 mo to affect change after strip craniectomy	May still benefit from postoperative molding helmeting if only bone removed and final shape not locked in

DISTRACTION OSTEOGENESIS

Distraction osteogenesis is used for Monobloc, posterior cranial vault, or midface distraction, and is performed by external or internal distractors (**Table 4**). In these instances osteotomies are made as with any open approach, the distractors placed, then a bone segment is advanced slowly over days to weeks allowing soft tissues to gradually stretch, and thereby slowly achieve greater volume

enhancements. This approach is particularly useful in syndromic patients with brachycephaly in whom adequate advancement is difficult to achieve through conventional surgery.[21,49–51]

INDICATION AND TIMING OF OPERATION

Deciding when to operate depends on factors including age of the child at initial presentation, presence or absence of functional problems

Table 4
Neurosurgical complications of craniosynostosis

Pathology	Underlying Factors	Diagnosis	Therapy
Elevated intracranial pressure	Jugular vein obstruction Sleep apnea Chronic tonsillar herniation Hydrocephalus	CT scan MRI scan Ophthalmology Beaten-copper sign on radiograph Clinical signs and symptoms	Skull reconstruction Insertion of ventriculoperitoneal (VP) shunt
Ventriculomegaly/ hydrocephalus	Jugular vein obstruction/skull compliance (can be induced by early surgery)/chronic tonsillar herniation (obstructive)	MRI scan CT scan	VP shunt Endoscopic third ventriculostomy
Chronic tonsillar herniation	Small posterior fossa/primary or secondary lambdoid synostosis/ venous engorgement (jugular vein obstruction)	MRI scan	Chiari decompression during posterior vault reconstruction or as a separate surgery

including increased ICP, upper airway obstruction (UAO), severity of the deformities, and surgeon preferences. UAO requires intervention. Treatments may include:

- Continuous positive airway pressure
- Tracheostomy
- Reduction of airway soft tissue
- Distraction osteogenesis of the maxilla or mandible

Elevated ICP and related visual and neurodevelopmental impairments require close surveillance and intervention when necessary. Intelligence quotient has been shown to be negatively affected in babies older than 1 year with uncorrected synostosis,[52] whereas operating on babies earlier than 6 months potentially affects skull growth more adversely. Many surgeons try to balance these issues by operating when the patient is around age 9 to 12 months. Proponents of early surgery advocate that minimally invasive surgery leads to decreased costs, decreased blood loss and transfusion needs, smaller scars, shorter hospital stays, and comparable outcomes, although, at least for endoscopic approaches, without springs there is a need for up to 1 year of postoperative helmeting.[33,41,53,54]

SYNDROMIC CRANIOSYNOSTOSIS

More than 150 syndromes featuring craniosynostosis (**Fig. 18**) are currently described.[2,8,55,56]

Patients with syndromic craniosynostosis and multisuture synostosis are more likely to have increased ICP. Patients with syndromic craniosynostosis are more likely to have ventricular enlargement, hydrocephalus, enlarged subarachnoid space, and cerebellar tonsillar herniation than patients with sporadic single-suture synostoses. Each of these is associated with decreased cognitive functioning and lower intelligence quotients (**Table 3**).

Cognitive impairment is very common in Apert syndrome and cloverleaf deformities, and is present about 20% of the time in Crouzon, Pfeiffer, and Saethre-Chotzen type I.

Timing of surgery in syndromic patients depends on the presenting symptoms, the degree of exorbitism, and signs and symptoms of elevated ICP. There is a known higher incidence of hydrocephalus following early surgery, which is one consideration for delaying surgery, but it is known that surgery delayed beyond 1 year results in a higher likelihood of elevated ICP, cognitive deficits, and behavioral problems.[57–60] Therefore decompression, adding intracranial volume, and addressing ICP before age 1 year is a common goal.[28,30]

There is greater likelihood with syndromic patients to require several or even multiple surgeries, not only to improve cranial volume and shape early on but also to address in early childhood and adolescence the midface, orbital, and other facial deformities that often persist and/or recur as a result of poor bone growth. Diagnosing and treating UAO and early, timely decompression and reconstruction of the skull are all crucial in syndromic patients.[61]

PROCEDURAL APPROACH

Timing of synostosis surgery falls into 3 main periods (**Table 5**). In babies younger than 6 months, minimally invasive strip craniectomies or suturectomies can be done with endoscopic assistance or through small incision(s) using lighted retractors for visualization. Molding helmets are needed postoperatively for 4 to 7 months, and some investigators advocate up to 12 months of postoperative helmeting[53] unless implantable springs are used to affect change.[62–64] Springs allow such minimally invasive techniques to be done up to age 7 to 8 months, although they do require a second surgery for removal.[4] Windh and colleagues[62] demonstrated some relapse in their series, with postoperative CI changing from 72% at 1 year to 71% at 3 years postoperatively in 20 patients treated with springs, although some return to original deformity is a common trend regardless of

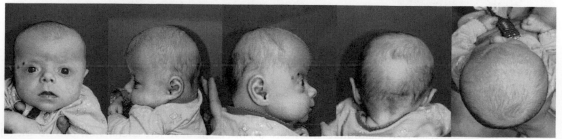

Fig. 18. Frontal, lateral, occipital, and vertex views of a 2-month-old female infant with syndromic bicoronal synostosis, brachycephaly, and midface hypoplasia.

Table 5
Craniofacial surgery parameters

Procedure	Age
Cranial vault decompression, suturectomy/strip craniectomy (with spring assistance or postoperative molding helmet)	Birth–6 mo
Fronto-orbital reshaping and advancement	6 mo–3 y
Correction of midface deformities, secondary cranial vault surgeries, adjunct procedures	4–8 y
Late correction of midface, secondary deformities, adjunct procedures	9–12 y
Adjunct procedures and orthodontic therapy	13–17 y
Orthognathic surgery	>17 y

Adapted from Warren SM, Proctor MR, Bartlett SP, et al. Parameters of care in craniosynostosis: craniofacial and neurologic perspectives. Plast Reconstr Surg 2012;129(3):731–7.

which technique is used, and is thought to be related to poor bony growth over time. Posterior vault expansion using springs across patent sutures has also been described.[65]

Fronto-orbital advancement and cranial vault reconstruction is optimally performed between age 9 and 12 months. Distraction osteogenesis (DO) has been used for fronto-orbital advancements coupled with midface advancement including monobloc distraction (**Fig. 19**), to improve eye exposure/exorbitism, increase intracranial volume, and advance the midface to improve UAO. Some centers perform this in the first 12 to 18 months of life, but other centers use posterior vault DO in syndromic patients younger than 12 months to increase intracranial volume and address intracranial hypertension, reserving midface advancements for after age 4 years.[48,66]

Surgical Treatment of Sagittal Synostosis

There are multiple surgical techniques addressing sagittal synostosis and scaphocephaly, which vary depending on the age of the patient at the time of surgery and surgeon preference.[67]

Simple strip craniectomy/suturectomy
Simple strip craniectomy/suturectomies alone have largely been abandoned unless coupled with spring assistance or postoperative molding helmets. The authors have previously highlighted several theoretic advantages to minimally invasive options including shorter hospital stays, decreased bleeding and transfusion requirements, and low numbers of reoperations.[20,53] Potential disadvantages include increased risks of anesthetic-related complications in babies younger than 1 year and the need for prolonged use of molding helmets, which can cause pressure sores, ulceration, and scalp alopecia.[4,16] The authors' experience has been that in cases with severe frontal bulging, temporal narrowing, and occipital coning, although the CI improves after a course of postoperative molding helmeting, the frontal, temporal, and occipital deformities often persist.

Endoscopic-assisted strip craniectomy with wedge craniectomy
The authors offer endoscopic-assisted strip craniectomy with wedge craniectomies (Video 2) if patients present at age between 3 and 6 months and for milder deformities, although some parents opt for an open approach in this age group (Video 1). Total cranial vault reconstruction (TCVR) at around age 9 to 12 months is appropriate for patients who present later than 6 months or who have severe

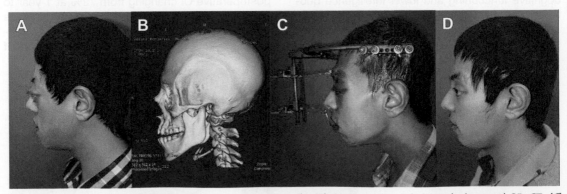

Fig. 19. A 13-year-old child with multisuture synostosis. (*A, B*) Preoperative left lateral view and 3D CT. (*C*) 1 month postoperatively with RED device for external distraction following Monobloc osteotomies. (*D*) 18 months postoperatively, left lateral view.

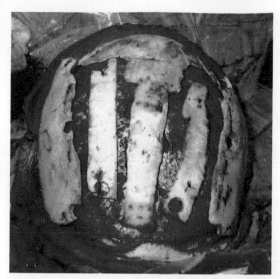

Fig. 20. Vertex view of prone baby after undergoing modified Pi procedure (note barrel staving of occiput). (*Photo courtesy of* Dr. John van Aalst, MD, University of North Carolina, Chapel Hill, BC.)

deformities. The authors counsel families that a 2-stage procedure is often needed to address both occipital and fronto-temporal deformities with the first surgery done early, in the first 3 to 6 months, followed by a second surgery at around 12 months to address any persistent deformities.[68,69]

Pi procedure or "squeeze" procedure

The Pi procedure (squeeze procedure) (**Fig. 20**) consists of 2 parasagittal craniectomies coupled with a transverse craniectomy. The procedure aims to shorten the skull in the anteroposterior (AP) plane, and squeezing the brain in AP direction plus bone grafting parasagittally adds to increased biparietal width. Together these changes result in immediate postoperative improvements in CI.

Minimally invasive procedures work best when used in babies younger than 6 months,[20,53,70] and prolonged postoperative molding helmeting is paramount unless springs are used in these

situations. Occasionally these patients are left with residual calvarial defects requiring further procedures. TCVR with suture or resorbable plate fixation is definitely helpful if severe deformities are present or when the patient is older than 6 months (**Fig. 21**).[69,71]

Fronto-orbital advancement

Fronto-orbital advancement (FOA) with reshaping is the keystone maneuver in trigonocephaly reconstruction and both unilateral (**Figs. 22 and 23**) and bicoronal synostosis. The principle is to advance, unilaterally or bilaterally, the flattened superior orbital rim anteriorly and secure it in place. This newly advanced construct becomes the foundation for the remainder of the cranial vault reconstruction, which is achieved by dissecting the pericranium around the supraorbital rims and superior orbital roofs. The neurovascular bundles of the supraorbital and supratrochlear neurovascular bundles are released from their bony foramina or notches.[1,13,72]

- The midline dissection is carried down to the nasofrontal suture.
- A frontal bone flap is designed, osteotomized, and removed.
- The dura is freed up from the inner table down to the anterior skull base.
- A fronto-orbital bar/bandeau is marked out at least 1 to 2 cm above the superior orbital rims and then cut while protecting the brain from above and the eyes from below using malleable retractors.

Surgical note: These cuts can be made with an unguarded craniotome, reciprocating saw, oscillating saw, or osteotome. The authors have moved to making these cuts with a piezosurgery bone-cutting device (**Fig. 24**C, D).

- The cuts are carried around the superior orbital roofs, the medial orbital walls, slightly superior to the nasofrontal suture, out

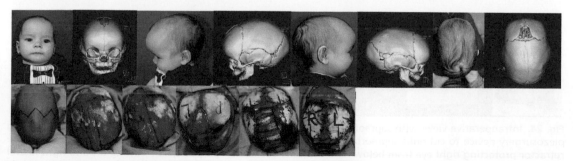

Fig. 21. Preoperative frontal, lateral, and vertex views, and 3D CT of a 6-month-old infant with sagittal synostosis and deformities involving both frontal and occipital bones. Intraoperative views show 2-cm sagittal strip craniectomy, biparietal anterior and posterior wedge craniectomies, and frontal bones flipped.

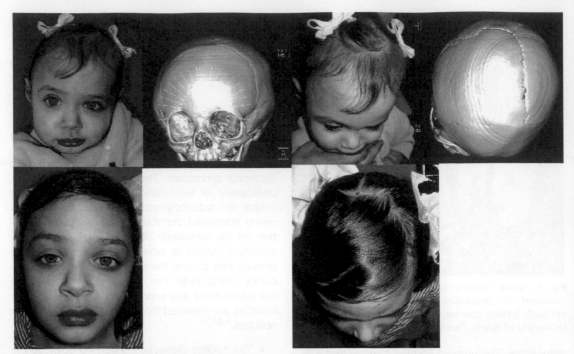

Fig. 22. An infant with unilateral right coronal synostosis. (*Top*) Preoperative frontal and vertex view at age 11 months. (*Bottom*) Three years postoperative frontal and vertex views.

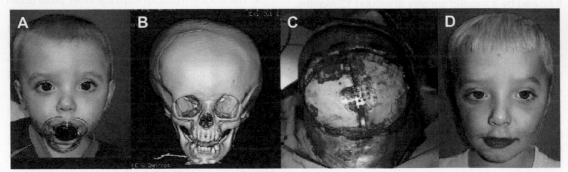

Fig. 23. (*A, B*) A 20-month-old infant with left unilateral coronal synostosis. (*C*) intraoperative fronto-vertex view at age 23 months. (*D*) Frontal view at 33 months postoperatively.

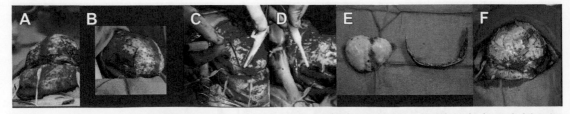

Fig. 24. Intraoperative views with supraorbital bar/bandeau marked out. (*A*) Frontal. (*B*) Right lateral. (*C*) Using piezosurgery device to cut right supraorbital roof (malleable retractor protecting brain from above, malleable retractor protecting right eye from below removed for visualization purposes). (*D*) Cutting around right lateral extent of supraorbital bar with tongue in groove and tab depicted. (*E*) frontal bone flap flipped 180° before barrel staves and reshaping, and supraorbital bar after reshaping. (*F*) Bone flaps and bandeau secured with resorbable plates and screws.

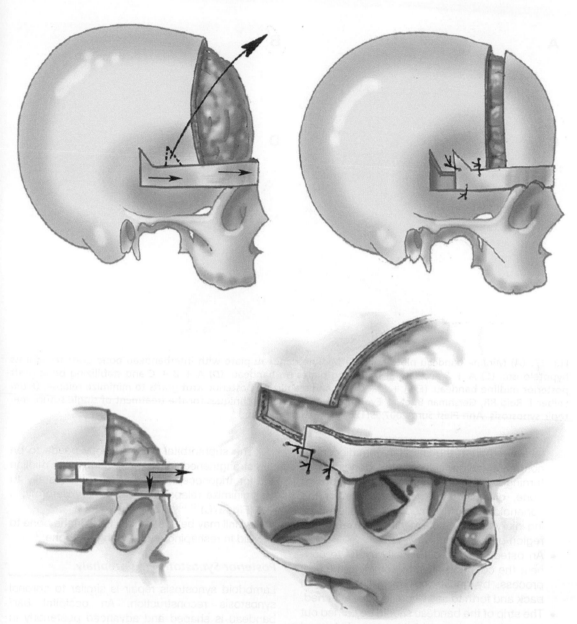

Fig. 25. Bandeau modifications. (*Adapted from* Fearon JA. Beyond the Bandeau: 4 variations on fronto-orbital advancements. J Craniofac Surg 2008;19(4):1180–2; with permission.)

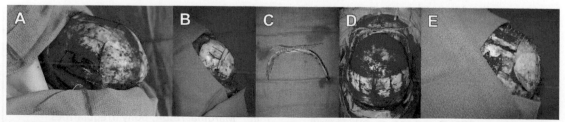

Fig. 26. Right lateral views of different patients with 2 differing bandeau designs: (*A*) rectangular and (*B*) triangular tenon-and-mortise concept to stabilize fronto-orbital bar after advancement. (*C*) Bandeau removed, bent to new shape with resorbable plate fixation. (*D*) Bandeau in situ, demonstrating advancement bilaterally in this trigonocephalic patient. (*E*) Right lateral view showing bandeau advanced into anterior triangle, providing additional stabilization to resorbable plates.

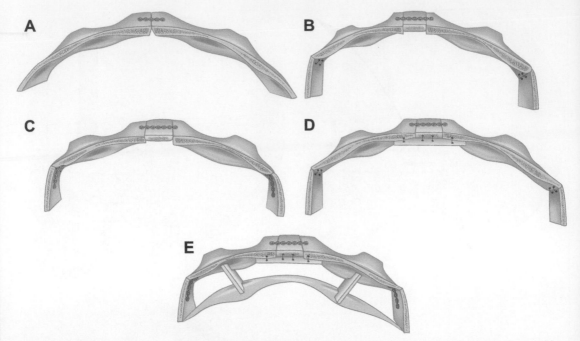

Fig. 27. (*A*) Midline bandeau plate only. (*B*) Midline bandeau plate with interbandeau bone graft to address hypotelorism. (*C*) *A* + *B* and lateral stabilizing plates on bandeau. (*D*) *A* + *B* + *C* and stabilizing bone graft posterior midline bandeau. (*E*) *A* + *B* + *C* + *D* and stabilizing posterior strut grafts to minimize relapse. (*From Selber J, Reid RR, Gershman B, et al. Evolutions of operative techniques for the treatment of single suture metopic synostosis. Ann Plast Surg 2007;59(1):6–13; with permission.*)

laterally though the lateral zygomaticosphenoid and zygomaticofrontal bones, then turning laterally into the temporal regions of bone, dissecting the lateral portion of the sphenoid wing off its medial part while avoiding injury to the middle meningeal artery in the region of the pterion.

- An osteotome is occasionally useful to connect the cuts and often to complete the final process, by gentle rocking of the bandeau back and forth to see where it is still attached.
- The strip of the bandeau should be carried out bilaterally in cases of trigonocephaly and brachycephaly, and unilaterally in single-sided coronal synostosis, into the squamous area of the temporal bone in a tongue-in-groove fashion or tenon-in-mortise manner.
- Adding a triangular or rectangular tab either inferiorly or superiorly that is advanced and locked into a defect of identical size of stable anterior bone after advancing the bandeau adds stability to the FOA and theoretically reduces relapse of the advanced bandeau over time (**Figs. 25**A, B and **26**A, B, D)[12,13,73–76]
- Once removed, the bandeau is reshaped. In trigonocephaly this may require dividing the bandeau in the midline and adding a small bone graft in attempt to address hypotelorism.

The supraorbital bar frequently needs to be strengthened with bone grafting in the midline for trigonocephaly and also out laterally to minimize relapse and secondary deformities (**Fig. 27**C)[12,13,73]

- A drill may be used to drill kerfs in the bone to aid in reshaping and bending the bone[73]

Posterior Synostotic Plagiocephaly

Lambdoid synostosis repair is similar to coronal synostosis reconstruction. An occipital bar/bandeau is shaped and advanced posteriorly in the region of flattening, and the occipito-parietal region is reshaped to reach symmetry in the

Table 6 Whitaker classification: need for surgical revision	
I	*Excellent result*, no need for revisions
II	*Satisfactory result*, soft-tissue revision needed
III	*Marginal result*, bony irregularities requiring contouring/camouflaging with bone grafts or alloplastic materials
IV	*Poor result*, craniotomies and cranioplasties required

Table 7
Review of recent craniosynostosis literature and level of evidence[87]

Authors,[Ref.] Year	Study Design	Findings	Level of Evidence
van Wijk et al,[18] 2014	Randomized controlled comparison of orthotic helmets vs no helmeting for positional plagiocephaly	42 babies age 5–6 mo with 6 mo helmet treatment vs 42 without; 10/39 (26%) helmet treatment achieved full recovery and 9/40 (23%) nonhelmeted group; excluded most severe deformities	Single-blind randomized controlled
Le et al,[37] 2014	Retrospective case-control series comparing aesthetic improvements in shape and CI in open vs endoscopic strip craniectomy and postoperative helmeting	No statistically significant differences were found in any of the measured parameters	Retrospective case-control series
Bonfield et al,[77] 2014	Retrospective case series of sagittal synostosis status post extended strip craniectomy (ESC)	238 patients underwent ESC at average 4.5 mo; mean CI increased from 0.68 to 0.75 (P<.001)	Retrospective series
Oppenheimer et al,[46] 2014	Retrospective case-control series comparing patients treated with and without aminocaproic acid (ACA) during cranial vault reconstruction (CVR)	30/148 CVRs received ACA Average intraoperative EBL for ACA (322 mL) and control groups (327 mL). Patients treated with ACA, however, received lower average perioperative transfusion volumes (25.5 mL/kg) compared with control patients (53.3 mL/kg). ACA subgroup less likely to require a second unit of blood (21% vs 43%)	Retrospective case-control
Fearon et al,[44] 2014	Randomized controlled trial evaluating effects of hypotensive anesthesia in craniosynostosis surgery	100 patients: No statistically significant differences were noted in transfusion rates between the hypotensive (9/53, 17.0%) and standard anesthesia (6/47, 13%) groups	Randomized controlled
Doumit et al,[78] 2014	Survey of craniofacial surgeons on sagittal synostosis management	59/102 responses; 35% operated at 6 mo, TCVR most common 37%, endoscopic approach 35% for <4 mo, 10% spring-assisted strip craniectomy	Survey
Jiménez and Barone,[20] 2013	Retrospective case series of endoscopic strip craniectomy and postoperative molding helmet	128 coronal synostoses: mean EBL 20 mL, mean surgical duration 55 min, transfusion rate 1.7%. 97% discharged POD 1. Supraorbital rim advancement of the ipsilateral eye was obtained in 98%	Retrospective series
Goldstein et al,[66] 2013	Retrospective Review of posterior distraction	13/22 patients first operation, and 11 <1 y; average EBL 400 mL, average distraction 27 mm, intracranial volume increased 21.5%	Retrospective review
Driessen et al,[57] 2013	Prospective cohort MRI and PSG on children with syndromic/complex craniosynostosis	71 children pre foramen magnum decompression. Hindbrain herniation (HH) in 35% (63% Crouzon). No difference in PSG of children with craniosynostosis ± HH. OSA not caused by HH	Prospective cohort
Greig et al,[79] 2013	Retrospective case series of Aperts patients undergoing bipartition with monobloc distraction	19 Apert patients; this approach enabled differential central face advancement	Case series

(continued on next page)

Table 7
(continued)

Authors,[Ref.] Year	Study Design	Findings	Level of Evidence
Basta et al,[47] 2012	Meta-analysis of antifibrinolytics in major pediatric surgery	34 studies included in this review of which 21 provided level 1b evidence, 11 were level 2b, and 2 were level 3b. Antifibrinolytics are effective in reducing blood loss and transfusion requirements in major pediatric surgery	Meta-analysis
Jimenez and Barone,[53] 2012	Retrospective case series of patients with sagittal synostosis treatment with endoscopic wide vertex craniectomy and barrel staved parietal bones followed by postoperative molding helmet	256 patients with sagittal synostosis treated at mean 3.9 mo. Mean EBL 27 mL. Mean transfusion rate 7%. Mean surgical time: 57 min. Mean LOS in hospital 1.1 d. Excellent (CI >80), good (CI 80–70), or poor (CI <70). A total of 87% classified as excellent, 9% as good, 4% as poor	Retrospective case series
Van Veelen and Mathijssen,[80] 2012	Retrospective series of spring-assisted cranioplasty for sagittal synostosis	41 patients treated with springs following strip craniectomies. Mean CI of 75 postop, Mean EBL 54	Retrospective series
Warren et al,[4] 2012	Multidisciplinary Consensus Panel	Parameters/guidelines on best practices in craniosynostosis	Expert opinion
Kluba et al,[17] 2011	Prospective longitudinal comparison of DP outcomes with helmeting in 2 different age groups	24 infants started helmet <6 mo of age and 38 >8 mo of age. More and quicker improvements in <6 mo age group	Prospective longitudinal
Berry-Candelario et al,[81] 2011	Retrospective series.	173 patients status post endoscopic strip craniectomies and postoperative molding helmeting. Mean operative time 46 min. 4.6% of patients received blood transfusions. Average hospital LOS 1.35 d	Retrospective series
Czerwinski et al,[83] 2011	Retrospective series of "complex" multisuture/nonsyndromic synostoses	31 patients, 1.7 procedures/patient. Average hospital stay 2.3 d. 21% required blood transfusions. 40% developed acquired Chiari deformations	Retrospective series
Goobie et al,[45] 2011	Double-blind placebo-controlled trial of tranexamic acid (TXA) use in craniosynostosis	43 patients: EBL (65 vs 119 mL) and lower perioperative mean blood transfusion (33 vs 56 mL). TXA administration reduces perioperative EBL and transfusion needs in children undergoing craniosynostosis surgery	Double-blind placebo-controlled
Windh et al[62] 2008	Retrospective case-control series comparing spring-assisted cranioplasty with Pi procedure for sagittal synostosis	20 patients undergoing spring approach and 20 Pi procedure; mean CI at 3 y 71 for springs and 73 for Pi procedure	Retrospective case-control
Fearon et al,[43] 2004	Prospective series evaluating need for allogeneic and autologous blood transfusions using intraoperative autologous blood recycling	Mean EBL 356 mL (110 mL of cell-saver); 59 of 60 patients received transfusions, only 18 (30%) received allogenic blood (average, approximately 140 mL)	Prospective case-control series

Abbreviations: CI, cephalic index; DP, deformational plagiocephaly; EBL, estimated blood loss; LOS, length of stay; MRI, magnetic resonance imaging; OSA, obstructive sleep apnea; PSG, polysomnography; TCVR, total cranial vault reconstruction.
Data from Refs.[4,17,18,20,37,43–47,53,57,62,66,77–81,83]

posterior skull. The bone flaps are secured with absorbable plates and screws. It is important in posterior vault reconstruction to use a protective helmet or keep the baby off the reconstructed repair when sleeping, as relapse may develop as a result of supine positioning.[2,14,15]

Secondary Deformities

These deformities include bony deficiencies (lacunae), and soft-tissue and bony asymmetries such as temporal hollowing. The most common classification of secondary deformities is the Whitaker Classification (**Table 6**). Temporal hollowing is thought to occur as result of both bony deficiencies/asymmetries and, to lesser extent, temporalis fat/muscle atrophy. Bony asymmetries that are inadequately overcorrected at the time of initial repair will recur or develop over time as result of relapse caused by poor bandeau construction, poor fixation, and/or deficient postoperative bony growth.[74–76]

The take-home from these pearls is that stable bandeau construction coupled with overcorrection is necessary to maintain long-term results.[13,72–76]

EVIDENCE-BASED MEDICINE IN CRANIOFACIAL SURGERY
Controversies in Craniofacial Care

It is clear to the authors that there is a lack of level I and II studies in craniofacial surgery to draw conclusions about best-practice algorithms, as most of the literature in this field is retrospective analysis, which supplies evidence not much stronger than expert opinion (**Table 7**). Randomized controlled studies are difficult to perform given the complexities of multiple surgeons, differing locations, and limited patient populations. Based on several large case series, it is difficult to deny potential benefits from minimally invasive approaches in terms of decreased operative times, decreased blood loss, shorter hospital stays, smaller scars, and comparable outcomes. Controversies exist in terms of optimum timing and the role for minimally invasive approaches versus TCVR. There is also controversy regarding what constitutes mild, moderate, and severe DP, in addition to both when and which patients with DP should be helmeted. There is also debate among craniofacial surgeons regarding internal versus external distractors. A survey of 48 of 102 responding institutions found no consensus on perioperative management of children undergoing craniofacial reconstruction.[82]

A more recent report similarly revealed a lack of surgical consensus in terms of timing or approach, and this lack of consensus is viewed as a great obstacle in managing children with craniosynostosis.[76] A multidisciplinary consensus panel, however, was able to meet in the last few years and develop parameters of care and best practices for craniosynostosis, and these parameters and guidelines are useful for review.[4]

Trends and Future Horizons

Resorbable plate technology represents a real technical advancement in the last 20 years, as it allows for rigid fixation without the risks of transcranial hardware migration over time that is inherent in wires and metal plates in children. Advances in both neuroimaging modalities and surgical telescopes will continue to allow surgeons to see greater detail via narrower approaches. Robotic approaches to bony surgery are presently limited. Perhaps the day will come when cutting saws and tools will be wireless, allowing for robotic cutting instruments that could be preprogrammed to perform craniectomies based on neuroradiographic computerized data points, and allow for image-guided and minimally invasive craniectomies to be performed remotely.

The future holds promise for new advances in bone substitutes, biomaterials, and growth factors that mediate new bone growth. Using a 3-dimensional printer to print customized calvarial constructs with bioabsorbable scaffolds and osseoinductive properties is no longer science fiction, and will surely improve with time.[30]

There is hope that one day in utero delivery of gene-targeted therapy might obviate some, if not all, craniofacial deformities by replacing defective genes or downstream products such as growth factors needed for normal bone growth. Until that day, craniofacial surgeons are guided by the past and look to the future with optimism and hope.[84–86]

SUPPLEMENTARY DATA

Supplementary data related to this article can be found online at http://dx.doi.org/10.1016/j.fsc.2014.08.002.

REFERENCES

1. Albright AL, Pollack IF, Adelson PF. Principles and practice of pediatric neurosurgery. 2nd edition. New York, Stuttgart (Germany): Thieme; 2007. Chapter 17. p. 265.
2. McLone DG. Pediatric neurosurgery. Surgery of the developing nervous system. 4th edition. Philadelphia: Saunders; 2001. Chapters 27 and 31.
3. Mehta VA, Bettegowda C, Jallo GI, et al. The evolution of surgical management for craniosynostosis. Neurosurg Focus 2010;29(6):E5, 1–7.

4. Warren SM, Proctor MR, Bartlett SP, et al. Parameters of care in craniosynostosis: craniofacial and neurologic perspectives. Plast Reconstr Surg 2012;129(3):731–7.

5. Carmichael SL, Rasmussen SA, Lammer EJ, et al. Craniosynostosis and nutrient intake in pregnancy. Birth Defects Res A Clin Mol Teratol 2010;88:1032–9.

6. Sgouros S, Hockley AD, Goldin JH, et al. Intracranial volume change in craniosynostosis. J Neurosurg 1999;91(4):617–25.

7. Britto JA, Moore RL, Evans RD, et al. Negative autoregulation of fibroblast growth factor receptor 2 expression characterizing cranial development in cases of Apert (P253R mutation) and Pfeiffer (C278F mutation) syndromes and suggesting a basis for differences in their cranial phenotypes. J Neurosurg 2001;95:660–73.

8. Cinalli G, Renier D, Sebag G, et al. Chronic tonsillar herniation in Crouzon's and Apert's syndromes: the role of premature synostosis of the lambdoid suture. J Neurosurg 1995;83:575–82.

9. Chumas PD, Cinalli G, Arnaud E, et al. Classification of previously unclassified cases of craniosynostosis. J Neurosurg 1997;86:177–81.

10. Lajeunie E, Le Merrer M, Arnaud E, et al. Trigonocephaly: isolated, associated and syndromic forms. Genetic study in a series of 278 patients. Arch Pediatr 1998;5(8):873–9.

11. Agrawal D, Steinbok P, Cochrane DD. Reformation of the sagittal suture following surgery for isolated sagittal craniosynostosis. J Neurosurg 2006;105(2 Suppl):115–7.

12. Eppley BL, Sadove AM. Surgical correction of metopic suture synostosis. Clin Plast Surg 1994;21(4):555–62.

13. Fearon JA. Beyond the Bandeau: 4 variations on fronto-orbital advancements. J Craniofac Surg 2008;19(4):1180–2.

14. Robinson S, Proctor M. Diagnosis and management of deformational plagiocephaly. J Neurosurg Pediatr 2009;3:284–95.

15. David DJ, Menard RM. Occipital plagiocephaly. Br J Neurosurg 2000;53:367–77.

16. Gump W, Mutchnick I, Moriarty T. Complications associated with molding helmet therapy for positional plagiocephaly: a review. Neurosurg Focus 2013;35(4):E3.

17. Kluba S, Kraut W, Reinert S, et al. What is the optimal time to start helmet therapy in positional plagiocephaly? Plast Reconstr Surg 2011;128(2):492–8.

18. van Wijk RM, van Vlimmeren LA, Groothuis-Oudshoorn CG, et al. Helmet therapy in infants with positional skull deformation: randomised controlled trial. BMJ 2014;348:g2741. http://dx.doi.org/10.1136/bmj.g2741.

19. David L, Fisher D, Aregenta L. New technique for reconstructing the affected cranium and orbital rim in unicoronal craniosynostosis. J Craniofac Surg 2009;20(1):194.

20. Jiménez DF, Barone CM. Early treatment of coronal synostosis with endoscopy-assisted craniectomy and postoperative cranial orthosis therapy: 16-year experience. J Neurosurg Pediatr 2013;12(3):207–19.

21. Kobayashi S, Honda T, Saitoh A, et al. Unilateral coronal synostosis treated by internal forehead distraction. J Craniofac Surg 1999;10(6):467–71.

22. Stelnicki E, Heger I, Brooks CJ, et al. Endoscopic release of unicoronal craniosynostosis. J Craniofac Surg 2009;20(1):93–7.

23. Lin KY, Polin R, Gampper T, et al. Occipital flattening in the infant skull. Neurosurg Focus 1997;2(2):E8.

24. Losee JE, Mason AC, Dudas J, et al. Nonsynostotic occipital plagiocephaly: factors impacting onset, treatment, and outcomes. Plast Reconstr Surg 2007;119(6):1866–73.

25. Hutchison BL, Hutchison LA, Thompson JM, et al. Plagiocephaly and brachycephaly in the first two years of life: a prospective cohort study. Pediatrics 2004;114(4):970–80.

26. Manjila S, Chim H, Eisele S, et al. History of the Kleeblattschadel deformity: orgin of concepts and evolution of management in the past 50 years. Neurosurg Focus 2010;29(6):E7.

27. Anantheswar YN, Venkataramana NK. Pediatric craniofacial surgery for craniosynostosis: our experience and current concepts: part-1. J Pediatr Neurosci 2009;4(2):86–99.

28. Thompson DN, Harkness W, Jones BM, et al. Aetiology of hindbrain herniation in Craniosynostosis. An Investigation Incorporating Intracranial Pressure Monitoring and Magnetic Resonance Imaging. Pediatr Neurosurg 1997;26:288–95.

29. Hayward R, Gonsalez S. How low can you go? Intracranial pressure, cerebral perfusion pressure, and respiratory obstruction in children with complex craniosynostosis. J Neurosurg 2005;102:16–22.

30. Inagaki T, Kyutoku S, Seno T, et al. The intracranial pressure of the patients with mild form of craniosynostosis. Childs Nerv Syst 2007;23(12):1455–9.

31. Terner JS, Travieso R, Lee S, et al. Combined metopic and sagittal craniosynostosis: is it worse than sagittal synostosis alone? Neurosurg Focus 2011;31(2):E2.

32. Rollins N, Booth T, Shapiro K. MR venography in children with complex craniosynostosis. Pediatr Neurosurg 2000;32(6):308–15.

33. Seruya M, Boyajian MJ, Posnick JC, et al. Treatment for delayed presentation of sagittal synostosis: challenges pertaining to occult intracranial hypertension. J Neurosurg Pediatr 2011;8(1):40–8.

34. Probst FA, Hutmacher DW, Muller DF, et al. Calvarial reconstruction by customized bioactive

implant. Handchir Mikrochir Plast Chir 2010;42(6): 369–73.

35. Khechoyan DY, Saber NR, Burge J, et al. Surgical outcomes in craniosynostosis reconstruction: the use of prefabricated templates in cranial vault re-modelling. J Plast Reconstr Aesthet Surg 2014; 67(1):9–16.

36. Mardini S, Alsubaie S, Cayci C, et al. Three-dimensional preoperative virtual planning and template use for surgical correction of craniosy-nostosis. J Plast Reconstr Aesthet Surg 2013; 67(3):336–43.

37. Le MB, Patel K, Skolnick G, et al. Assessing long-term outcomes of open and endoscopic sagittal synostosis reconstruction using three-dimensional photography. J Craniofac Surg 2014;25(2):573–6.

38. Koral K, Blackburn T, Bailey AA, et al. Strength-ening the Argument for Rapide MRI imaging: esti-mation of reduction in lifetime attributable risk of developing fatal cancer in children with shunted hydrocephalus by instituting a rapid brain MR im-aging protocol in lieu with head CT. AJNR Am J Neuroradiol 2012;33:1851–4.

39. Morton R, Reynolds R, Ramakrishna R, et al. Low-dose head computer tomography in children: a sin-gle institutional experience in pediatric radiation risk reduction. J Neurosurg Pediatr 2013;12:406–10.

40. Cinalli G, Sainte-Rose C, Kollar EM. Hydrocephalus and craniosynostosis. J Neurosurg 1998;88:209–14.

41. Fearon JA, Ruotolo RA, Kolar JC. Single sutural cra-niosynostoses: surgical outcomes and long-term growth. Plast Reconstr Surg 2009;123:635–42.

42. Szpalski C, Weichman K, Sagebin F, et al. Need for standard outcome reporting systems in craniosy-nostosis. Neurosurg Focus 2011;31(2):E1.

43. Fearon JA. Reducing allogenic blood transfusions during pediatric cranial vault surgical procedures: a prospective analysis of blood recycling. Plast Re-constr Surg 2004;113(4):1126–30.

44. Fearon JA, Cook TK, Herbert M. Effects of hypoten-sive anesthesia on blood transfusion rates in cra-niosynostosis corrections. Plast Reconstr Surg 2014;133:1133–6.

45. Goobie SM, Meier PM, Pereira LM, et al. Efficacy of tranexamic acid in pediatric craniosynostosis sur-gery: a double-blind, placebo-controlled trial. Anesthesiology 2011;114(4):862–71.

46. Oppenheimer AJ, Ranganathan K, Levi B, et al. Minimizing transfusions in primary cranial vault re-modeling: the role of aminocaproic acid. J Craniofac Surg 2014;25(1):82–6.

47. Seruya M, Oh AK, Boyajian MJ, et al. Unreliability of intraoperative estimated blood loss in extended sagittal synectomies. J Neurosurg Pediatr 2011;8: 443–9.

48. Basta MN, Stricker PA, Taylor JA. Systematic re-view of the fibrinolytic agents in pediatric surgery

and implications of craniofacial use. Pediatr Surg Int 2012;28(11):1059–69.

49. Alonso N, Goldenberg D, Fonseca AS, et al. Blind-ness as a complication of monobloc frontofacial advancement with distraction. J Craniofac Surg 2008;19(4):1170–3.

50. Akizuku T, Komuro Y, Ohmori K. Distraction osteo-genesis for craniosynostosis. Neurosurg Focus 2000;9(3):E1, 1–7.

51. Kazuaki Y, Keisuke I, Takuya F, et al. Cranial distrac-tion osteogenesis for syndromic craniosynostosis: Long-term follow-up and effect on postoperative cranial growth. J Plast Reconstr Aesthet Surg 2014;67:35–41.

52. Starr JR, Kapp-Simon KA, Cloonan YK, et al. Presurgical and postsurgical assessment of the neurodevelopment of infants with single-suture cra-niosynostosis: comparison with controls. J Neuro-surg 2007;107(2 Suppl):103–10.

53. Jimenez DF, Barone CM. Endoscopic technique for sagittal synostosis. Childs Nerv Syst 2012;28:1333–9.

54. Vogel T, Woo A, Kane A, et al. Comparison of costs associated with endoscope assited craniectomy versus open cranial vault repair for infants with sagittal synostosis. J Neurosurg Pediatr 2014; 13(3):324–31.

55. Agrawal D, Steinbok P, Cochrane D. Long term anthropometric outcomes following surgery for iso-lated cranial synostosis. J Neurosurg 2006;105(5 Suppl):357–60.

56. Addo NK, Javadpour S, Kandasamy J, et al. Cen-tral sleep apnea and associated Chiari malforma-tion in children with syndromic craniosynostosis: treatment and outcome data from a supraregional national craniofacial center. J Neurosurg Pediatr 2013;11:296–301.

57. Driessen C, Joosten KF, Florisson JM, et al. Sleep apnea in syndromic craniosynostoses occurs inde-pendent of hindbrain herniation. Childs Nerv Syst 2013;29(2):289–96.

58. Renier D, Arnaud E, Cinalli G, et al. Prognosis for mental function in Apert's syndrome. J Neurosurg 1996;85:66–72.

59. Van Der Meulen J, Van der Vlugt J, Okkerse J, et al. Early beaten-copper pattern: its long-term effect on intelligence quotients in 958 children with craniosy-nostosis. J Neurosurg Pediatr 2008;1:25–30.

60. Pollack IF, Losken HW, Biglan AW. Incidence of increased intracranial pressure after early surgical treatment of syndromic craniosynostosis. Pediatr Neurosurg 1996;24:202–9.

61. diRocco F, Juca CE, Arnaud E, et al. The role of endoscopic third ventriculostomy in the treatment of hydrocephalus associated with faciocraniosy-nostosis. J Neurosurg Pediatr 2010;6:17–22.

62. Windh P, Davis C, Sanger C, et al. Spring-assisted cranioplasty vs pi-plasty for sagittal synostosis- a

long term follow-up study. J Craniofac Surg 2008; 19(1):59–64.

63. Davis C, Lauritzen CG. The biomechanical characteristics of cranial sutures are altered by spring cranioplasty forces. Plast Reconstr Surg 2010;125(4): 1111–8.

64. Tovetjärn R, Maltese G, Kölby L, et al. Spring-assisted cranioplasty for bicoronal synostosis. J Craniofac Surg 2012;23(4):977–81.

65. Arnaud E, Marchac A, Jeblaoui Y, et al. Spring-assisted posterior skull expansion without osteotomies. Childs Nerv Syst 2012;28(9):1545–9.

66. Goldstein JA, Paliga JT, Wink JD, et al. A craniometric analysis of posterior cranial vault distraction osteogenesis. Plast Reconstr Surg 2013;131(6):1367–75.

67. Tatum SA, Jones LR, Cho M, et al. Differential management of scaphocephaly. Laryngoscope 2012; 122(2):246–53.

68. Jiménez DF, Barone CM. Endoscopy-assisted wide-vertex craniectomy, "Barrel-stave" osteotomies, and postoperative helmet molding therapy in the early management of sagittal suture craniosynostosis. Neurosurg Focus 2000;9(3):1–6.

69. Fearon JA, McLaughlin EB, Kolar JC. Sagittal craniosynostosis: surgical outcomes and long-term growth. Plast Reconstr Surg 2006;117(2):532–41.

70. Murad GJ, Clayman M, Seagle MB, et al. Endoscopic-assisted repair of craniosynostosis. Neurosurg Focus 2005;19(6):E6, 1–10.

71. Jiménez DF, Barone CM. Multiple-suture nonsyndromic craniosynostosis: early and effective management using endoscopic techniques. J Neurosurg Pediatr 2010;5:223–31.

72. Mesa J, Fang F, Muraszko K, et al. Reconstruction of unicoronal plagiocephaly with hypercorrection surgical technique. Neurosurg Focus 2011;31(2):E11.

73. Selber J, Reid RR, Gershman B, et al. Evolutions of operative techniques for the treatment of single suture metopic synostosis. Ann Plast Surg 2007; 59(1):6–13.

74. Steinbacher DM, Wink J, Bartlett SP. Temporal hollowing following surgical correction of unicoronal synostosis. Plast Reconstr Surg 2011;128(1):231–40.

75. Fearon J. Discussion: temporal hollowing following surgical correction of unicoronal synostosis. Plast Reconstr Surg 2011;128(1):241–2.

76. Whitaker LA, Bartlett SP, Schut L, et al. Craniosynostosis. An analysis of the timing, treatment, and complications in 164 consecutive patients. Plast Reconstr Surg 1987;80:195–206.

77. Bonfield CM, Lee PS, Adamo MA, et al. Surgical treatment of sagittal synostosis by extended strip craniectomy: cranial index, nasofrontal angle, reoperation rate, and a review of the literature. J Craniomaxillofac Surg 2014. [Epub ahead of print].

78. Doumit GD, Papay FA, Moores N, et al. Management of sagittal synostosis: a solution to equipoise. J Craniofac Surg 2014;25:1260–5.

79. Greig AV, Britto JA, Abela C, et al. Correcting the typical Apert face: combining bipartition with monobloc distraction. Plast Reconstr Surg 2013; 131(2):219–30.

80. Van Veelen ML, Mathijssen IM. Spring-assisted correction of sagittal suture synostosis. Childs Nerv Syst 2012;28(9):1347–51.

81. Berry-Candelario J, Ridgway EB, Grondin RT, et al. Endoscopic-assisted strip craniectomy and postoperative helmet therapy for treatment of craniosynostosis. Neurosurg Focus 2011; 31(2):E5.

82. Czerwinski M, Kolar JC, Fearon JA. Complex craniosynostosis. Plast Reconstr Surg 2011;128(4): 955–61.

83. Stricker PA, Cladis FP, Fiadjoe JE, et al. Perioperative management of children undergoing craniofacial reconstruction surgery: a practice survey. Paediatr Anaesth 2011;21(10):1026–35.

84. Hankinson TC, Fontana EJ, Anderson RC, et al. Surgical treatment of single-suture craniosynostosis: an argument for quantitative methods to evaluate cosmetic outcomes, a review. J Neurosurg Pediatr 2010;6(2):193–7.

85. Piatt JH, Starly B, Sun W, et al. Application of computer-assisted design in craniofacial reconstructive surgery using a commercial image guidance system. J Neurosurg 2006;105 (1 Suppl):64–7.

86. Hochfeld M, Lamecker H, Thomale UW, et al. Frame-based cranial reconstruction. J Neurosurg Pediatr 2014. http://dx.doi.org/10.3171/2013.11. PEDS1369.

87. Wood JS, Kittinger BJ, Perry VL, et al. Craniosynostosis incision: scalpel or cautery? J Craniofac Surg 2014;25(4):1256–9.

Utilization of Free Tissue Transfer for Pediatric Oromandibular Reconstruction

Nicole M. Fowler, MD, Neal D. Futran, MD, DMD*

KEYWORDS

- Head and neck malignancy (pediatric) • Free tissue transfer (pediatric) • Mandibular reconstruction
- Craniofacial surgery • Microsurgical reconstruction • Maxillofacial surgery

KEY POINTS

- Pediatric free tissue transfer is safe and reliable.
- Primary consideration must be for long-term restoration of mastication, deglutition, and cosmesis.
- Long-term functional and cosmetic results require reestablishment of the normal maxillomandibular occlusion and condylar-cranial articulation for normal craniofacial development to occur.
- Fixed dental prosthodontic rehabilitation is favored in the pediatric population because it results in maintenance of the normal occlusal relationships and promotes normal craniofacial development.

Head and neck tumors, craniofacial trauma, or infections are the most common indications for large composite oromandibular resections. When encountered, the surgeon's primary focus should be on optimal restoration of function and cosmesis. In contrast to the adult population in which most oromandibular resections are due to malignancies, most pediatric conditions are benign, allowing for narrow margins and minimizing the need for complex reconstruction.[1]

Common neoplasms within this population include osteosarcoma, rhabdomyosarcoma, ameloblastoma, neuroblastoma, lymphoma, germ cell tumor, and teratoma. The two most common head and neck cancers involving the maxilla and mandible are osteosarcomas and rhabdomyosarcomas (through direct bone invasion).[1] Treatment algorithms have been difficult to create due to the low incidence combined with the wide variety of rare conditions. However, sarcoma studies have shown the importance of obtaining negative surgical margins as evidenced by local failure

and poor survival if positive margins remain.[2-7] Five-year survival dropped from 80% to 55% in pediatric sarcoma patients who had a positive surgical margin.[2,3] In addition, surgical resection is usually recommended after the patient has been treated with radiation therapy, chemotherapy, or both, resulting in compromise of the recipient bed and limiting the use of adjacent tissue transfer or bone grafts.

Free tissue transfer has been shown to be safe and effective in the pediatric patient population.[8-10] Unique to the pediatric population compared with adults is their continued craniofacial growth and development. It is essential that the pediatric reconstructive surgeon know the anatomic location of the growth centers and the normal oromandibular relationships. Disruption of the normal maxillary, mandibular, and cranial relationships results in abnormal midface, mandible, or skull base development, resulting in profound functional and cosmetic consequences. The use of free tissue transfer can restore normal

Disclosure Statement: The authors have no financial or nonfinancial relationships to disclose.

Department of Otolaryngology-Head and Neck Surgery, University of Washington, 1959 NE Pacific Street, Seattle, WA 98195, USA

* Corresponding author. Department of Otolaryngology-Head and Neck Surgery, University of Washington, 1959 Northeast Pacific Street, Box 356515, Seattle, WA 98195.

E-mail address: nfutran@uw.edu

Facial Plast Surg Clin N Am 22 (2014) 549–557

http://dx.doi.org/10.1016/j.fsc.2014.07.001

maxillomandibular occlusion and condylar-cranial articulation resulting in normal craniofacial development. In addition, free tissue transfer options, including the fibula, iliac crest, and scapula, provide sufficient bone volume to allow for osseointegrated implants.

CRANIOFACIAL DEVELOPMENT

Normal craniofacial development, including facial symmetry, requires the reestablishment of the normal maxillary and mandibular relationships. Growth of the mandible occurs through two mechanisms: epiphyseal proliferation and remodeling (**Fig. 1**). Epiphyseal proliferation is the dominant method of growth in both bone length and projection during the first 18 years of life. The mandibular epiphysis is located just beneath the condyle in the proximal subcondylar ridge. This growth center is what allows the intercondylar distance to widen as the skull base expands with growth. Therefore, if surgically feasible, it is preferred to preserve the condyle and this subcondylar growth center. Girls reach mature mandibular height and depth at a mean age of 13, whereas boys' maturation lags behind approximately 2 to 5 years.[10]

Even after the fusion of this growth center, bony remodeling continues to shape the mandible. Bone deposited at the posterior margin of the ramus (combined with anterior margin resorption) results in forward projection and buccal bone deposition (along with lingual bone resorption) increases mandibular width. The muscles of mastication create mechanical forces that promote bony remodeling throughout adult life. Therefore, limiting the amount of dissection on the native mandible (ie, restricting detachment of the masseter muscle) may promote normal growth and contouring.

The maxilla grows in both vertical height and width. The vertical height increases as the maxilla is displaced inferiorly and bony remodeling occurs along the suture lines. The maxilla does not contain any endochondral growth centers. Mature vertical height of the maxilla is achieved by girls at approximately 14-years-old and boys at approximately 16-years-old.[10] Fusion of the palate occurs at age 18.

Finally, normal maxillomandibular occlusion is essential for normal craniofacial development. Without normal occlusion, such as in cases were defects are left unreconstructed, midface and mandibular growth halts, resulting in facial asymmetry. This is unfavorable cosmetically and produces inferior functional outcomes. Therefore, to preserve facial growth, symmetry, and oromandibular function it is essential to restore the patient's baseline occlusion.

RECIPIENT CONSIDERATIONS AND OUTCOMES

In these complex composite surgical resections it is essential that the surgical teams work together to facilitate complete surgical excision while maintaining the best possible functional and cosmetic reconstruction. As described above, if the condyle and subcondylar epiphyseal growth center can be preserved without compromising the surgical margins, they should be. Consideration of the patient's current dentition and permanent dentition are also important with the goal of complete surgical resection while maintaining as much of the normal maxilla or mandible as possible. Based on the age of the patient and the current state of their dentition, it may not be possible to place the patient in mandibulomaxillary fixation. Furthermore, the disease burden or bony involvement may prevent preplating of the mandible. In these cases, craniomaxillomandibular relationships can be maintained by a temporizing external fixator, which can then be removed once the permanent plating is applied. An emerging option in these difficult cases involves the use of computer-aided prefabricated bone plates and surgical cutting guides. Regardless of the plate size or type, it is essential that the head and neck surgeon place the plates on the native mandible as low as possible to limit any injury to permanent dentition. The reconstructive surgeon may prefer to place the osteocutaneous bone flap flush with the superior edge of the mandible to assist with future osseointegrated implants; however, this may be impossible based on the location of the dental roots or permanent dentition buds. The head and neck surgeon should also consider if distal mental

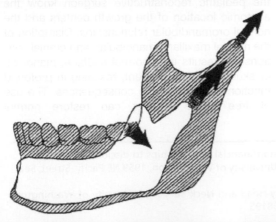

Fig. 1. Mandibular growth and expansion during development.

nerve and proximal inferior alveolar nerve can be preserved, allowing for possible nerve grafting. **Fig. 2** details an 8-year-old girl with a right mandibular alveolar osteosarcoma who underwent fibula osteocutaneous free flap reconstruction with greater auricular nerve graft to connect the proximal inferior alveolar nerve to the remaining distal mental nerve stump. Every effort should be made to maintain the marginal mandibular nerve while performing the primary resection and/or neck

dissection. In addition it is paramount that these structures be maintained on the contralateral side to avoid oral incompetence. When dissecting around the condyle and temporomandibular joint, care must be taken to ensure safety of the facial nerve, which may require complete identification and dissection.

Neck vessels should be chosen based on the length and direction of the free flap pedicle, vessel caliber, and location. Vessels can be obtained in

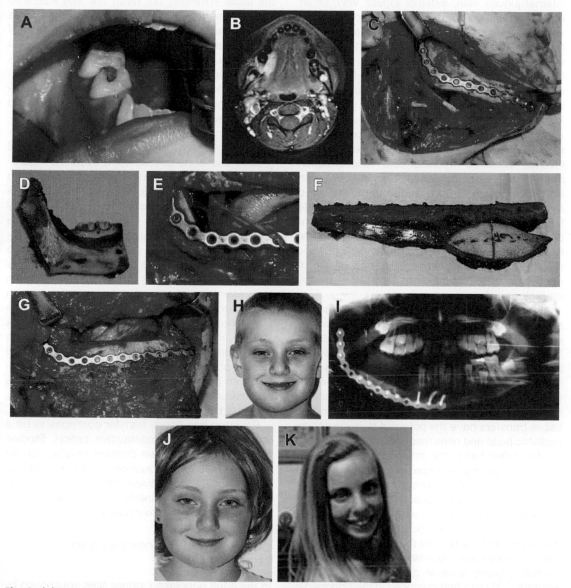

Fig. 2. (*A*) Intraoral view of an 8-year-old girl with a right mandibular alveolar osteosarcoma. (*B*) T2 axial MRI image showing the tumor after three cycles of chemotherapy. (*C*) Transcervical approach to the tumor. Reconstruction plate applied to the mandible before resection to maintain shape of the mandible. (*D*) Resected tumor specimen. (*E*) Plate reapplied. Greater auricular nerve graft used to connect proximal inferior alveolar nerve sump to mental nerve stump. (*F*) Fibula osteocutaneous free flap. (*G*) Flap inset. (*H*) 6-month follow-up. (*I*) 1-year panoramic radiograph follow-up. (*J*) 1-year follow-up. (*K*) 5-year follow-up.

the ipsilateral or contralateral neck based on the pedicle orientation and direction. Although the reconstructive surgeon may chose to avoid a previously radiated neck in adults, previously radiated tissue in pediatrics has been found to be of better quality and is less of a concern. The most commonly used arteries include the facial artery and superior thyroid artery but any branch off the external carotid or, in some cases, the external carotid artery itself can be used.[8] The same tenets are true when choosing a vein, any branch of the internal jugular vein, external jugular vein, or an end-to-side anastomosis to the internal jugular vein are options. Based on the age and size of the child, there may be significant differences in vessel size compared with the adult population that can result in technical difficulties. Successful osteocutaneous free flap reconstruction has been described in children as young as 10 months.[8] As previously noted, dissection for an appropriately sized vessel may require use of the external carotid artery or internal jugular vein. Overall, pediatric microsurgical reconstruction has fewer complications compared with adults,[8–10] which may be related to the improved nutritional status and overall better health despite the smaller vessel size. In the past, theoretic concerns regarding the rate of endothelial growth at the anastomosis site were concerning but have not shown to have any clinical significance, which may be because for weeks the flaps depend solely on their pedicle.

An algorithm has been proposed that recommends pediatric bony free tissue transfer be considered in cases involving a previous radiated bed in which greater than 6 cm of bone is resected, in composite soft tissue and bone resections, and in cases of failed bone grafts or when the periosteum is resected with the underlying bone.[8] Although less commonly indicated, pediatric free tissue transfers have the potential to revolutionize pediatric head and neck reconstruction by producing far better functional and cosmetic outcomes and, therefore, warrant consideration in any large composite resection, especially when prior radiation or postoperative radiation is planned.

There has not been adequate data on the long-term follow-up of the osteocutaneous free flap pediatric patient to determine the true growth rates of the neomaxilla and neomandible compared with the native bone; however, growth has been documented.[11–14] Data first compiled in the orthopedic literature involving limb reconstruction using the fibula epiphysis documented growth with near normal limb symmetry.[15] Animal studies then showed more reliable craniofacial development with the use of vascularized grafts compared with nonvascularized grafts. There have been concerns for disproportionate growth compared with the native mandible, resulting in facial asymmetry.[8] However, the current literature continues to show promising results. At this time, neomaxillary and neomandibular growth may be variable; however, as discussed above, if the craniofacial and occlusal relationships are maintained then gross symmetric growth can be achieved. Distraction osteogenesis or sagittal splitting osteotomies of the neomandible are theoretic options to improve the facial symmetry but rarely are they indicated or performed.[16] Some surgeons advocate for a second free flap reconstruction after maturity if the patients are doing well but need additional soft tissue or bony advancement.[8]

Controversy remains regarding long-term management of the bone fixation plates. Initial recommendations were for the removal of the plates and screws because it was believed they could interfere with mandibular growth and contouring. However, that was not found to be the case. Normal growth and bone development occurred regardless of whether the plates remained. Long-term follow-up has been published in studies with small numbers, and have consistently shown that bony growth and remodeling will continue around the plates. Some investigators continue to recommend removal of the plating system because they believe it may interfere with future surgery when it would be harder to remove. The decision to preserve or remove the plates remains with the reconstructive surgeon; however, the risks and benefits of additional surgery and anesthesia should always be considered in the pediatric patient population. There have been no published reports of the use of absorbable plates in conjunction with pediatric microvascular osteocutaneous reconstruction; however, with future development, this may become an option.

Pediatric free tissue transfer continues to be a safe and reliable reconstructive option. Studies have repeatedly shown positive results with no flap failures and no nonunions.[8,9] It is hoped that future studies will provide answers to questions regarding normal craniofacial and neomaxillary and neomandibular growth and development.

DONOR SITE DEVELOPMENT AND MORBIDITY

In the adult population, donor sites are chosen by considering the anticipated defect and the patient's comorbidities. In contrast, children are generally healthy. Therefore, the main considerations are the anticipated defect and donor site development and morbidity.

The fibula free flap has been widely accepted as one of the best options in mandibular reconstruction since the 1990s.[17,18] The fibula free flap has distinct advantages for use in the pediatric population as well. This is the most commonly used osteocutaneous free tissue option.[8,9,19] Understanding the normal fibula development will enhance placement and potential growth of the neomandible or maxilla. The fibula has three centers of endochondral growth: one at each of the distal and proximal epiphyses and one in the center of the fibula shaft.[20] The distal and proximal epiphyses are preserved, allowing for proportional growth and continued ankle stability after fibula harvest. The central ossification center is harvested and should be used to recreate the maxilla or mandible (see **Fig. 2**F, G), When designing the osteocutaneous reconstruction, the surgeon can design the neomaxilla or neomandible, maintaining the central ossification zone, providing at least a theoretic increased potential for growth. The fibula allows for the greatest length of harvested bone and is an excellent match for maxillary reconstruction. When reconstructing the mandible, however, the height will be deficient. This is especially true if the defect is located anteriorly. Options to improve the vertical height both for the

future use of osseointegrated implants and to decrease an intraoral step-off include using a double-barrel technique (by creating a midpoint osteotomy and folding the bone on itself), adding nonvascularized bony onlay grafts to the superior fibula edge, or even performing secondary vertical distraction osteogenesis.[8,9,21–23] As research continues into the creation and use of scaffolds, engineered growth factors, and bone morphogenetic proteins, new options for increasing neomandibular height and/or eliminating the need for a donor site may develop in the future. Currently, however, the need for a donor site remains and the fibula donor site has been found to have the lowest donor site morbidity. Although concern for asymmetric leg growth was theoretic, this has not been noted clinically. Postoperatively, patients should be expected to make a complete recovery with a normal gait and ankle stability (provided adequate fibula has been preserved both distally and proximally). The most common delayed complication is a valgus deformity of the donor ankle (particularly common in children <9 years of age at the time of harvest) but this does not result in any gait change or instability. There is the potential need for a skin graft, especially at the distal aspect of the incision, depending on

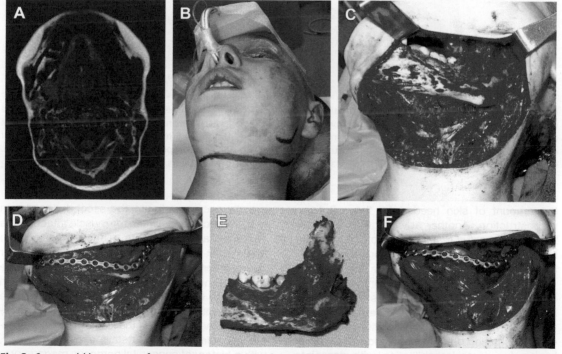

Fig. 3. 9-year-old boy status after preoperative chemotherapy for a left body, angle, and ramus osteosarcoma. (A) T1 axial MRI scan showing persistent tumor. (B) Outline of transcervical approach to the tumor. (C) Tumor fully exposed. (D) Reconstruction plate applied before tumor resection. (E) Resected tumor. (F) Plate reapplied before flap inset.

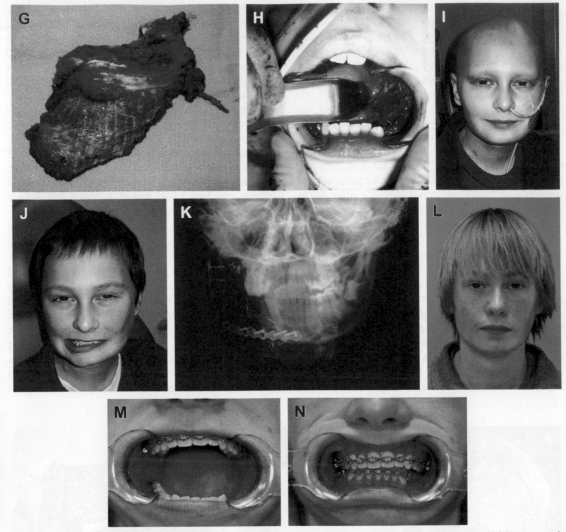

Fig. 3. (*continued*). 9-year old boy with ramus osteosarcoma. (*G*) Iliac crest free flap with internal oblique muscle used for reconstruction. Both fibulas not available due to congenital peroneus magnus presence bilaterally. (*H*) Internal oblique muscle used to restore intraoral mucosa and lining. (*I*) 6-month follow-up at completion of additional chemotherapy. (*J*) 1-year follow-up. (*K*) A-P mandibular radiograph at 1 year. (*L*) 5-year follow-up. (*M*) Maximum oral opening at 5 years. (*N*) Maintenance of occlusion at 5 years.

the amount of skin needed for the soft tissue reconstruction. Another advantage of the fibula free flap harvest is that it is able to occur simultaneously with the resection, allowing for decreased length of anesthesia and operative time.

In adults the second-most commonly used osteocutaneous free tissue option is the iliac crest. A large amount of both soft tissue and bone volume are available and a large variety of methods exist for shaping both the bone and soft tissue, allowing for dental rehabilitation with osseointegrated implants. Although an option in pediatric osteocutaneous reconstruction, the entire length of the iliac crest is cartilaginous at birth and pelvic growth occurs well into the second decade. In fact, interactions between the muscle attachments and the iliac crest create a traction ossification center that contributes to pelvic and acetabular development and gait stability. Gait disturbance is one of the major comorbidities associated with iliac crest harvest in adults and, therefore, the considerable concern for lifelong disability has resulted in the rare use of the iliac crest in the pediatric population. **Fig. 3** details a 9-year-old boy, with a history of congenital peroneus magnus preventing use of a fibula free flap, who was treated with an iliac crest osteocutaneous free flap for left ramus to body osteosarcoma.

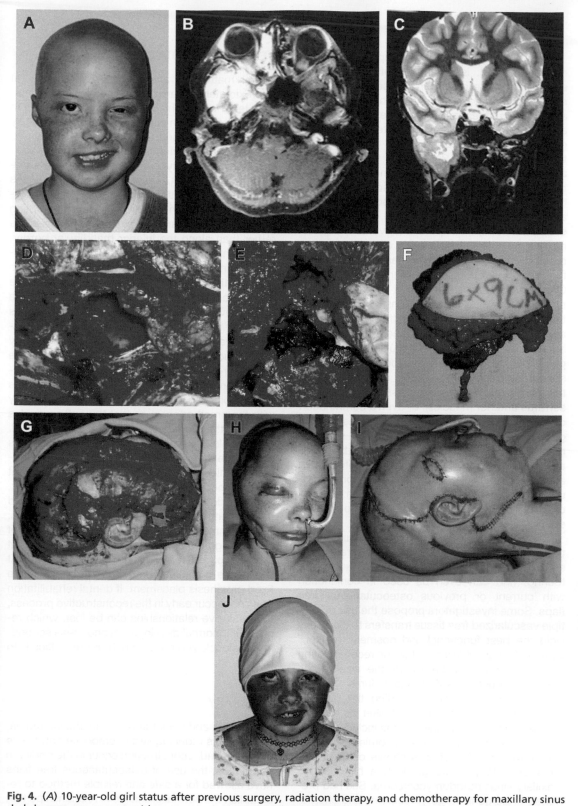

Fig. 4. (*A*) 10-year-old girl status after previous surgery, radiation therapy, and chemotherapy for maxillary sinus rhabdomyosarcoma now with recurrence in the right infratemporal fossa. (*B*) T2 axial MRI scan showing recurrent tumor filling the infratemporal fossa. (*C*) T2 coronal MRI scan showing tumor extending intracranially. (*D*) Surgical defect after craniofacial resection via lateral and intraoral approach. (*E*) Surgical defect after completion of dural repair. (*F*) Rectus abdominis free flap harvested for reconstruction. (*G*) Flap inset to obliterate the infratemporal defect, and seal the skull base and oral cavity. (*H*) Immediate postoperative frontal view. (*I*) Immediate postoperative lateral view. A small portion of the rectus flap is incorporated in the incision closure for monitoring. (*J*) 1-year follow-up.

A third osteocutaneous flap option, which is rarely indicated, is a variation off the scapular system. The lateral border and scapular tip are most commonly used. At birth these areas are composed entirely of hyaline cartilage and are encompassed in a large osteocartilaginous growth plate. Ossification begins in the superior to inferior direction. By age 10, the scapula is approximately 12 cm in length and the ossification center has decreased considerably in size but growth plate fusion will not occur until approximately 20 years of age. If the lateral scapula or scapular tips are harvested, this removes the inferior ossification center and does result in scapular size discrepancy but was not found to have an associated functional deficit.[24] One considerable advantage of the scapular osteocutaneous flap is that extensive variability in the harvest allows for many different soft tissue and bony options. Scapula bone options include harvesting of the lateral scapular border (supplied by the circumflex scapular artery), the scapular tip (supplied by the angular branch), the ribs (supplied by the latissimus dorsi and serratus anterior muscles), or even a combination of these. Dental rehabilitation using osseointegrated implants is an option when scapular bone is harvested in adults; however, in the pediatric population, the scapula may be quite thin. In a similar manner as described above for the fibula, the scapula can be augmented with nonvascularized bony onlay grafts to promote implant stability.

When bony reconstruction is not required, soft tissue free flaps can be used to obliterate large soft tissue resections, restore normal facial contouring, and can even be used in conjunction with current or previous osteocutaneous free flaps. Some investigators propose the use of multiple vascularized free tissue transfers to ultimately yield the best functional and cosmetic results.[8] Options for vascularized soft tissue reconstruction are decided mainly based on the size of the defect, amount of soft tissue volume needed, and type of soft tissue, including the differing needs for fascia, muscle, and skin as well as pedicle length. Soft tissue options include the anterolateral thigh flap, rectus abdominis flap, and latissimus dorsi flap. **Fig. 4** shows detailed pictures of a 10-year-old girl with a history of a maxillary sinus rhabdomyosarcoma. She had previously undergone surgery, radiation, and chemotherapy, and presented with a infratemporal fossa recurrence, which required soft tissue reconstruction of the surgical defect following combined neurosurgical head and neck craniofacial resection.

DENTAL REHABILITATION

Dental maturation and development begins at approximately 6 years of age when the first permanent teeth erupt. This progression from mixed to permanent dentition continues until approximately age 13. As discussed above, both the fibula and scapula osteocutaneous flaps provide for excellent bony continuity but do not have the same mandibular height, especially anteriorly. As mentioned, options include using the double-barrel technique (in fibular harvests), attempting to inset the neomandible along the lingual ridge rather than along the inferior mandibular border, placement of nonvascularized bony onlay techniques, and vertical distraction osteogenesis. The thick cortical bone of the fibula is very favorable for the placement of dental implants. It is favorable to achieve dental rehabilitation as early as possible, including primary placement of the osseointegrated implants at the time of the primary reconstruction. Another advantage of the computer-aided prosthetically guided reconstruction techniques is that osseointegrated implants can be planned and mapped out preoperatively with the prosthodontist so that the cutting guides will have the predetermined drilling sites marked. If possible, fixed osseointegrated prostheses should be heavily favored over removable implants, which can be difficult for the child or parent to insert or remove, pose a possible airway risk, require additional maintenance or cleaning, and have potentially higher psychological implications. It is recommended that, following the placement of osseointegrated implants, the prosthodontist wait 4 to 6 months before placing the prosthesis. At least three implants are required to achieve stable fixed prosthesis placement. If dental rehabilitation does not occur early in the reconstructive process, the occlusive relationships can be lost, which results in abnormal development and these secondary malocclusions are much more difficult to repair.

SUMMARY

When head and neck tumors, craniofacial trauma, or infections requiring large composite soft tissue resection and reconstruction occur in the pediatric population, the use of osteocutaneous free flaps have allowed for a safe and reliable method to reestablish the normal craniofacial relationships that allow for long-term functional and cosmetically pleasing results. It is essential to consider dental or prosthetic rehabilitation as early as possible to maintain normal occlusion and promote normal craniomaxillofacial development.

REFERENCES

1. Benoit MM, Vargas SO, Bhattacharyya N, et al. The presentation and management of mandibular tumors in the pediatric population. Laryngoscope 2013;123(8):2035–42.
2. Wanebo HJ, Koness J, MacFarlane JK, et al. Head and neck sarcoma: report of the head and neck sarcoma registry. Head Neck 1992;14:1–7.
3. Wanebo HJ. Head and neck sarcoma. Med Health R I 1997;80:26–30.
4. Daw NC, Mahmoud HH, Meyer WH, et al. Bone sarcomas of the head and neck in children. Cancer 2000;88:2172–9.
5. Zhang WL, Zhang Y, Huang DS, et al. Clinical character of pediatric head and neck rhabdomyosarcomas: a 7-year retrospective study. Asian Pac J Cancer Prev 2013;14(7):4089–93.
6. Tanaka N, Murata A, Yamaguchi A, et al. Clinical features and management of oral and maxillofacial tumors in children. Oral Surg Oral Med Oral Pathol Oral Radiol Endod 1999;88:11–5.
7. Gadwal SR, Gannon FH, Fanburg-Smith JC, et al. Primary osteosarcoma of the head and neck in pediatric patients. Cancer 2001;91:598–605.
8. Guo L, Ferraro NF, Padwa BL, et al. Vascularized fibular graft for pediatric mandibular reconstruction. Plast Reconstr Surg 2008;121:2095–105.
9. Genden EM, Buchbinder D, Chaplin JM, et al. Reconstruction of the pediatric maxilla and mandible. Arch Otolaryngol Head Neck Surg 2000;126:293–300.
10. Urken ML, editor. Multidisciplinary head & neck reconstruction: a defect-oriented approach. Philadelphia: Wolters Klower; 2010.
11. Weiland AJ, Phillips TW, Randolph MA. Bone grafts: a radiographic, histologic, and biomechanical model comparing autografts, allografts, and free vascularized bone grafts. Plast Reconstr Surg 1984;74:368–79.
12. Donski PK, Carwell GR, Sharzer LA. Growth in revascularized bone grafts in young puppies. Plast Reconstr Surg 1979;64:239–43.
13. Mizumoto S, Tamai S, Goshima J, et al. Experimental study of vascularized tibiofibula graft in inbred rats: a preliminary report. J Reconstr Microsurg 1986;3:1–11.
14. Tamai S. Experimental vascularized bone transplantation. Microsurgery 1995;16:179–85.
15. Yang YF, Zhang GM, Huo ZQ, et al. Reconstruction of the distal ulnar epiphysis with vascularized proximal fibula including epiphysis in children after osteochondroma resection: report of two cases. Plast Reconstr Surg 2013;132(5):784e–9e.
16. Visavadia BG, Heliotis M, Sneddon KJ, et al. Sagittal split osteotomy of a vascularized iliac crest free flap to correct residual asymmetry and malocclusion in the reconstructed mandible. Br J Oral Maxillofac Surg 2005;23(1):65–7.
17. Hidalgo DA. Fibular free flap mandibular reconstruction. Clin Plast Surg 1994;21:25.
18. Wei FC, Seah CS, Tsai YC, et al. Fibula osteoseptocutaneous flap for reconstruction of composite mandibular defects. Plast Reconstr Surg 1994;93:294.
19. Arnold DJ, Wax M. The Microvascular Committee of the American Academy of Otolaryngology-Head and Neck Surgery. State of the art in pediatric microvascular reconstruction—a report from the Microvascular Committee of the American Academy of Otolaryngology. Otolaryngol Head Neck Surg 2005;133:171.
20. Prichett JW. Growth and growth prediction of the fibula. Clin Orthop 1997;334:251–6.
21. Horiuchi K, Hattori A, Inada I, et al. Mandibular reconstruction using the double barrel fibular graft. Microsurgery 1995;16:450–4.
22. He Y, Zhang ZY, Zhu HG, et al. Double-barrel fibula vascularized free flap with dental rehabilitation for mandibular reconstruction. J Oral Maxillofac Surg 2011;69(10):2663–9.
23. Chang YM, Wallace CG, Tsai CY, et al. Dental implant outcome after primary implantation into double-barreled fibula osteoseptocutaneous free flap-reconstructed mandible. Plast Reconstr Surg 2011;128(6):1220–8.
24. Teot L, Bossé JP, Gilbert A, et al. Pedicle graft epiphysis transplantation. Clin Orthop Relat Res 1983;180:206–18.

Pediatric Craniomaxillofacial Trauma

Robert M. Kellman, MD[a], Sherard A. Tatum, MD[b],*

KEYWORDS

- Pediatric • Surgery • Maxillofacial • Craniofacial • Craniomaxillofacial • Trauma • Management
- Injury

KEY POINTS

- As children grow and develop, their craniomaxillofacial (CMF) structure changes dramatically.
- This change informs the location, pattern, and nature of CMF injury.
- Dental development stage significantly impacts management of fractures involving occlusion.
- Many pediatric fractures are amenable to conservative, nonoperative, or minimally invasive management.
- Growth effects from the injury as well as the management must be considered and monitored long term.

INTRODUCTION

Etiologies

Although trauma is a leading cause of death in pediatric age groups, pediatric craniomaxillofacial (CMF) trauma accounts for only about 15% of all CMF trauma, and that number includes teenagers. Younger children probably only account for about 5% of CMF trauma, and maxillofacial injuries in this age group are frequently associated with skull fractures and concomitant neurologic injuries.[1] Unique to the infant are facial fractures caused by traumatic delivery. In the newborn, this facial trauma can be owing to forceps being used to bring the baby down through the birth canal. This can result in neonatal injury, including fractures of the skull and facial skeleton, as well as soft tissue trauma, such as injury to the facial nerve. These injuries are less common today than previously owing to the increased use of Cesarean section when a difficult delivery is anticipated.

In the edentulous and deciduous dentition stage, skull fractures are much more common than maxillofacial fractures because the cranium is more prominent than the face. Falls are the most common cause, but abuse/neglect must remain a cause for which providers are vigilant, particularly with repeated injuries or sketchy histories.[2,3] In the nonambulatory child, being dropped or rolling off a bed or sofa are likely mechanisms of injury often leading to lateral as well as frontal skull and skull base injuries.[4] Small children also suffer injuries owing to motor vehicle accidents. The early ambulating child is more likely to fall forward, striking the chin and forehead on the ground. The most common soft tissue injuries are owing to dog bites that can be associated with fractures. However, primarily soft tissue injuries are beyond the scope of this article.

As the child grows, sports, motor vehicle, and bicycle accidents and fighting become more common causes. As children approach their teens,

No disclosures or conflicts.

[a] Department of Otolaryngology, Upstate Medical University, State University of New York, 750 E Adams Street, Syracuse, NY 13210, USA; [b] Departments of Otolaryngology and Pediatrics, Upstate Medical University, State University of New York; 750 E Adams Street, Syracuse, NY 13210, USA

* Corresponding author.

E-mail address: tatums@upstate.edu

they are more likely to be involved in trauma associated with more adult behavior. Teenagers are more likely to engage in risk-taking adventures and substance abuse that might lead to an increased risk of traumatic injury.[5] Falls from heights and vehicular trauma become more frequent during the teen years.[6] Like adults, common causes include recreational accidents, particularly with off-road vehicles like all-terrain vehicles and bicycles. Other sports-related injuries are more common, and interpersonal and industrial traumatic events increase in frequency.[5,7] Because the management of post puberty teenage trauma is similar to adult trauma, the rest of this article focuses primarily on prepubescent and pubescent patients.

Comparative and Developmental Anatomy

The pediatric age group includes everyone from birth to maturity, which is typically considered to occur around the age of 16 years, although some consider it to continue to age 18. During this time, the pediatric facial skeleton goes through progressive development and major changes. Some of these include[8]:

- Change in the size ratio of the cranium to the face;
- Change in the ratio of facial soft tissue to bone, dental eruption → shedding → eruption; and
- Pneumatization of the sinuses.

The softness of the infant bone results in more incomplete (greenstick) fractures in infancy, which changes as the child grows and the solidity of the bone increases. The growth centers are more cellular and therefore even softer and more susceptible to injury.[9]

Skull–Face Ratio

At birth, the cranium is much larger relative to the facial skeleton than it is at maturity. In the small child, the relative proportion of the craniofacial skeleton represented by the face, particularly the lower face, is still much less. As the child grows, the lower face lengthens and widens, developing to represent a greater proportion of the overall craniofacial skeleton. Similarly, the mid face, although larger than the mandible in early childhood, still represents a much smaller area relative to the skull.[9] As the child develops into adulthood, the relative growth of the face exceeds that of the skull, and the relative size of the facial skeleton increases (**Fig. 1**). Thus, in infancy, cranial injuries are far more common in proportion to those of the facial skeleton, and as children grow and mature, nasal, mid facial, and mandibular fractures become more common.[10] As the facial skeleton comes to represent a larger proportion of the craniofacial skeleton, it becomes more exposed to potential injuries. Therefore, mandible fractures are less frequent, owing to the small area of the mandible relative to the face and skull in the infant. However, the small ambulating child is likely to trip and fall forward, striking the chin and fracturing the mandible even if it is still relatively small. The nose also becomes more prominent with maturation, and the small, diminutive noses of infancy are typically displaced by the larger, adult nasal anatomy. In adulthood, the nose is the most frequently fractured facial bone, followed by the mandible.

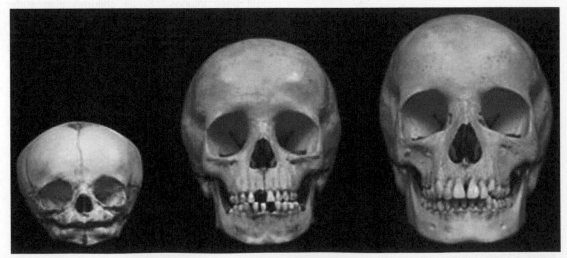

Fig. 1. Cranial to facial ratio comparison in a neonate, toddler, and adult. (*Courtesy of* Columbia University Medical Center, New York, NY; with permission.)

Small Sinuses

The paranasal sinuses are small in infancy, and the frontal sinuses in fact do not even begin to develop until the preteen years. The paranasal sinuses develop throughout childhood.[11] The newborn has small ethmoid sinuses and poorly aerated sphenoid sinuses, as well as typically small maxillary sinuses. The frontal sinuses generally do not even begin to form until 9 to 12 years of age. By the teenage years, the maxillary, ethmoid, and sphenoid sinuses tend to be well developed, with the frontals reaching full growth around age 16 to 18 years (**Fig. 2**). Sinus development corresponds with the enlarging size of the maxillofacial skeleton. As the face develops, it occupies a greater percentage of the head relative to the cranial vault. This is believed to contribute to the greater relative incidence of facial fractures compared with skull fractures as maturity is reached.

Brain and Ocular Injuries

The facial skeleton is smaller, making the cranial vault more exposed to injury. The sinuses are theorized to provide protection to the cranium, brain and eyes, among other structures, functioning as a "crumple zone" that can lead to facial fractures that might absorb energy upon impact and thereby minimize the damage to more vital structures. The less collapsible facial skeleton may lead to an increased number of cranial and neurologic injuries in infancy and early childhood.

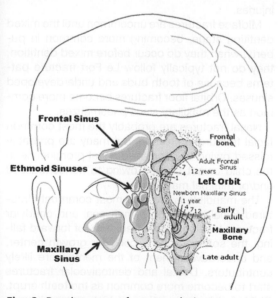

Fig. 2. Development of paranasal sinuses, birth to adult. (*Courtesy of* Dr Russell Faust, Franklin, MI.)

Tooth Buds

As children grow and develop, their facial structures grow and develop. This includes the teeth, which start out as germinal centers within the bones of the maxilla and mandible and occupy most of the bone in the lower maxilla and anterior mandible in early childhood (**Fig. 3**). As we develop, these form teeth that gradually erupt through the alveolar bone and through the gingiva. There are ultimately 20 deciduous teeth that generally erupt between ages 1 and 6 years, and these are then pushed out by the developing permanent dentition between the ages of 6 and 14 years. The final 4 posterior molars develop later and become the so-called wisdom teeth. There are ultimately 32 teeth in the full adult dentition. These are numbered 1 to 32, counting from the maxillary right posterior molar to the left, 1 to 16, then continuing around from the mandibular left posterior as number 17 to the right posterior molar, which is number 32. The deciduous teeth are designated in the same order with letters, A–J in the maxilla and K–T in the mandible.

The presence of deciduous and mixed dentition creates unique difficulties for the CMF surgeon, because the conical deciduous teeth do not hold wires and arch bars well. Also, as their roots resorb they are easily extracted with wires. The presence of the unerupted permanent dentition in the bone makes it difficult to properly position plates for repair of fractures. Once the permanent teeth have fully erupted, they provide excellent fixation points for wires that can be used to attach arch bars for stabilization of the occlusal relationships.

As noted, tooth buds are present in the bone of the maxillae and the mandible, making them prone to injury when facial fractures occur. If a tooth bud is injured, it is less likely to develop into a fully formed normal tooth, and eruption may be less likely. Tooth buds can be injured by trauma, particularly fractures, and they can be injured by the surgeon during the repair.

Softer Bone

The developing bone is less calcified and therefore less hard than fully mature calcified bone. The interosseous sutures are also softer and more flexible. This flexibility makes complete through and through fractures less likely, also contributing to the lower frequency of fractures needing repair in the pediatric age group. These incomplete fractures, known as 'greenstick' fractures are more often seen in children. This term 'greenstick' refers to the greater resilience seen in living (green) branches of a tree, compared with the easy-to-break, dried out dead branches.

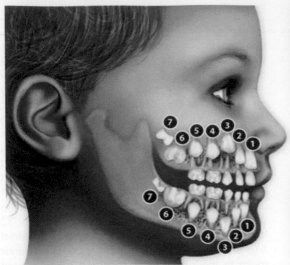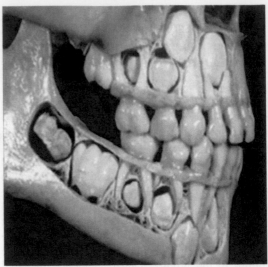

Fig. 3. Skulls with outer cortex removed showing deciduous and permanent dentition in early childhood. (*Courtesy of* McLoughlin Dental Care, Milwaukie, OR; with permission.)

Greenstick fractures are generally incomplete like bending of the bone, so that little or no reduction of the fracture might be needed. One cortex is fractured, and the fragments are held together by the second cortex of the bone. However, growth centers like the condylar region are relatively hypercellular and therefore softer, leading to greater susceptibility to burst-type fractures. Such fractures are rarely seen in adults.

More Soft Tissue

Children have more soft tissue both subcutaneously and in localized fat pads (baby fat) covering the maxillofacial skeleton than normal adults, which results in a greater likelihood of soft tissue injury.[12] As might be expected, owing to greater padding of the skeleton, this leads to fewer fractures. (Of course, the softer bone is less likely to break, adding to this effect.) However, severe soft tissue injuries are still common, and the facial nerve is in a more superficial anatomic position in the infant and young child.

Fracture Patterns

As in adults, any part of the pediatric CMF skeleton can be fractured, but certain fractures are more common. The difference in fracture patterns seen in children relative to adults is owing to a combination of the noted factors, namely, the mechanisms of injury, the softness and compliance of the bone, the presence of tooth buds, the smaller size of the paranasal sinuses, the relatively small size of the face compared with the skull, and the greater amount of facial soft tissue. Because of these differences between adult and pediatric anatomy and the differences in likely mechanisms of injury (low-energy short falls vs high-energy sports and motor vehicle injuries), the fracture mechanisms and patterns are different as well. All of these factors affect the exposure of the facial skeletal bones to trauma as well as their response to impact.

Skull fractures are more common than facial fractures, but orbital roof and other skull base fractures without calvarial fractures are also more likely. Upper facial fractures are typically associated with cranial vault fractures and are, therefore, often associated with more serious intracranial injuries.

Midface fractures are uncommon until the mixed dentition stage, becoming more common in puberty; when they do occur before mixed dentition, they do not typically follow Le Fort fracture patterns because of tooth buds and underdeveloped sinuses. Orbital floor fractures become more common as the maxillary sinus pneumatizes.

Nasal fractures are probably the most common facial fracture in children, but many are probably missed owing to decreased nasal prominence in the child or not studied owing to noncentralized and/or minimal management.

The mandible is the next most commonly fractured facial bone with symphyseal and condylar fractures leading.[4,5] The frequency of forward falling, the softness of the condylar growth center, and underdevelopment of the menton are likely contributors. Dental and dentoalveolar fractures start to become more common as the teeth erupt. Children who are victims of high-energy injuries can suffer pan facial fractures, as can adults.

FACIAL ANATOMY
Cranium

Cranial vault (skull) fractures are more common than maxillofacial bone fractures in infants and young children. The cranium is initially almost twice the area of the facial skeleton and the facial skeletal size does not usually begin to catch up in growth until about age 5 or 6 years, after which facial growth progresses significantly relative to the cranium to ultimately occupy about two thirds of the craniofacial skeletal area. Thus, cranial bone fractures are far more likely in infants and young children, as are intracranial injuries. The frontal bones occupy the region of the forehead, superior to the orbits. The temporal bones house the ears and their associated structures, as well as the facial nerves. The sphenoid bones contribute significantly to the anterior skull base and internal orbits, in particular housing the optic canals through which the important optic nerves pass.

Orbits

Like in adults, the orbits are complex structures, housing the globe, along with its surrounding musculature, vasculature, and nerves. Nine bones contribute to the orbital structure. Cranial nerves III, IV, V1, and VI pass through the superior orbital fissure, and the optic nerve passes through the neighboring optic canal, along with its vessels. The anterior and posterior ethmoid arteries come off the ophthalmic artery in the orbit and pass medially into the ethmoid sinuses just below the skull base. The medial and inferior orbital walls are very thin, allowing for globe trauma to be transmitted through them into the sinuses, which seems to be protective of the globe when it is directly traumatized.

Maxilla

The paired maxillae occupy the areas below the orbits, thereby encompassing the middle vertical one third of the face lateral to the nose. Essentially, the nose and maxillae occupy the area between the frontoorbital area and the mandible. As the maxillae lengthen and the maxillary sinuses enlarge, the face elongates and develops its adult length. The young maxilla contains a small maxillary sinus, and the bone inferiorly is filled with the germinal centers that will eventually form the maxillary dentition. As the infant matures, the deciduous dentition descends into the oral cavity, and as the adult teeth form and descend, they push the deciduous teeth out and ultimately replace them. The roof of the sinus

forms the floor of the orbit. The medial wall forms the lateral wall of the nose, and the floor contributes to the roof of the oral cavity. The infraorbital nerve (V2) exits the orbit through the floor (the roof of the sinus) and exits the maxilla anteriorly through the infraorbital foramen, after which it innervates the skin of the cheek, upper lip, and lateral nose.

Mandible

The mandible is an arch-shaped bone hinged bilaterally from the skull base by the temporomandibular joints, which sit in the glenoid fossae just inferomedial to the zygomatic roots of the temporal bones. It is the only moving bone of the maxillofacial skeleton, and it is critically important for mastication. The process of mastication involves both up-and-down and side-to-side movements that allow the teeth to grind food. The masticatory muscle slings stabilize the mandible and help to splint fragments after a fracture. Posteriorly, the vertical rami contribute to the vertical height of the face and serve to create the hinge that connects the mandibular bodies that house the dentition to the condylar heads, which articulate with the glenoid fossae. The inferior alveolar nerves enter the medial (lingual) sides of the mandibular rami at the lingula and then travel anteriorly within the mid portion of the mandibular bodies to exit through the mental foramina to innervate the skin of the lower lips and chin. Along the way, the nerves supply the mandibular dentition, including the anterior dentition via a continuing branch. The curved central anterior portion of the mandible is called the *symphysis*. The presence of the nerves and tooth roots as well as the germinal centers for developing teeth (tooth buds) add to the difficulty of repairing mandibular fractures. Obviously, any appliances placed into bone (ie, screws) have to be judiciously positioned to avoid these important structures.

Occlusion

The main goal of repair of maxillofacial fractures that involve either the maxilla or mandible or both is to reestablish normal or preinjury occlusion. Note that what is normal or preinjury occlusion might be abnormal occlusion in an individual patient, rather than the textbook normal occlusion. There is a normal relationship between the upper and lower teeth that is defined as normal occlusion. The maxillary dentition is supposed to override the mandibular dentition, so that the maxillary incisors extend forward of the mandibular dentition, called *overjet*, and the maxillary bicuspids and molars have buccal cusps that extend buccally (laterally) over the mandibular buccal (lateral) cusps. The maxillary canines also extend buccally (laterally) over the mandibular canines. The maxillary incisors also extend vertically over the mandibular incisors, and the distance of the vertical overlap is called *overbite*.

If the maxillary and mandibular incisors meet end to end it is *underjet* (usually called *negative overjet*), which is even worse if the maxillary incisors come down behind the mandibular incisors as an anterior cross-bite. The correct anterior–posterior relationship of the molars is defined by the relationship between the mesiobuccal cusp (anterior–lateral cusp) of the maxillary and mandibular first molars. If the mandibular first molar mesiobuccal cusp sits within the same groove of the maxillary first molar, it is defined as Angle's class I occlusion. If the maxilla sits anterior (mandible is posterior or distal), then it is class II, and if the maxilla sits posterior (mandible is anterior creating a prognathic appearance), then it is Angle's class III. If the maxillary teeth are more lingual (medial), then it is a cross-bite, which can be either unilateral or bilateral.

This discussion refers to occlusion for adult permanent dentition. The deciduous teeth have similar relationships, but a class II–like occlusion referred to as a flush terminal plane is more normal because of the relatively small mandibular arch in this age child (**Fig. 4**). In transitional or mixed dentition, assessment of the occlusion is difficult. The general alignment of the dental arches is a start. There should be appropriate relationships among the teeth present. Sometimes the anatomic alignment of the fracture lines is the best guide, with the understanding that minor occlusal abnormalities in this phase are common anyway and will often self-correct with natural dentofacial development.

FRACTURES
Frontoorbital Maxillary Fractures

Nasal/nasoorbital ethmoid/medial blowout
Central facial fractures are uncommon in small children, but they do occur. They are usually the result of major traumas, such as those seen in sporting vehicle accidents (all-terrain and other off-road vehicles) and when a child is unrestrained and in a motor vehicle accident. They may also occur in pedestrian or bike interactions with motor vehicles. The likelihood of these fractures increases as the face grows and the central face becomes anatomically larger and more exposed. The nasal fracture occurs with milder trauma and involves only the nasal bones. Most childhood nasal fractures are minimally displaced and often

do not require any treatment. However, if the nose is deformed, an attempt at closed reduction is reasonable. Open reduction, that is, rhinoplasty, is usually reserved for bony maturity, unless the airway is so severely compromised that it affects airway function significantly (**Fig. 5**).

Nasoorbital ethmoid (also called nasoethmoid complex) fractures occur when the nasal root is hit hard enough to force it posteriorly. It telescopes between the orbits, collapsing the ethmoids. The bones holding the medial canthal ligaments are released, allowing the lids to move laterally and creating the appearance of hypertelorism, called telecanthus or pseudohypertelorism. Damage to the ethmoids includes the medial orbital walls.[13]

Note that when the anterior skull base is involved in fractures, the subcranial approach can be used, just as it is in adults. This approach includes removal of the nasal root for access to the ethmoids and removal of the inferior frontal bones for access to the anterior skull base for direct repair of dural defects.

Inferior blowout/zygomaticomaxillary fracture
The inferior wall of the orbit "blows out" when there is direct trauma to the globe (and sometimes to the inferior orbital rim as well). The orbital floor gives way and "blows out" into the maxillary sinus, allowing the globe to decompress into the sinus rather than rupture. If the inferior rectus is entrapped, there is inability to look up, typically creating diplopia. In the so-called white-eye blowout fracture, the inferior rectus entrapment leads to a marked vagal response, including nausea and vomiting, and often marked discomfort. This is considered an urgent case, and urgent release of the entrapment is indicated.[13]

The zygomaticomaxillary complex fracture refers to the dislocation or separation of the malar eminence from the temporal bone, frontal bone, and the maxilla on a given side of the face. The attachment of the zygoma (which includes the malar eminence) to the temporal bone is via the zygomatic arch, the anterior portion of which is the zygoma and the posterior portion of which is the temporal bone, the frontal bone along the lateral orbital rim and the maxilla inferomedially up to and including the inferior orbital rim. In addition, there is an attachment to the sphenoid wing in the lateral wall of the orbit. Because of the broad attachment to the maxilla, which is usually the most shattered portion of this fracture, it is generally called a zygomaticomaxillary fracture.

LeFort I, II, and III fractures
Le Fort fractures are named after Rene LeFort, who first described these patterns in cadavers.

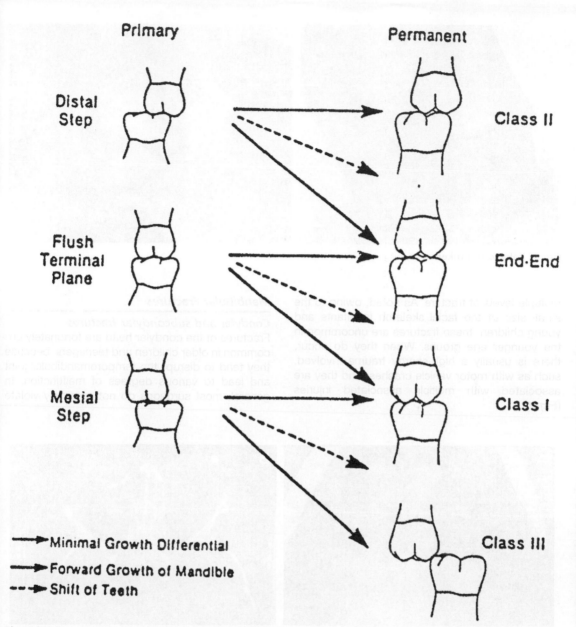

Fig. 4. Various deciduous occlusal relationships and their respective adult occlusal relationships. (*From* Proffit WR, Fields HW, Sarver DM. Contemporary orthodontics. New York: Elsevier; 1993. p. 81–4; with permission.)

All 3 types refer to a separation of the bones bearing the maxillary dentition from the bones superior to them. Designations I, II, and III refer to the level at which this separation takes place. A horizontal fracture across both maxillae that completely separates the entire maxillary alveoli from the remaining maxillae above, mobilizes the alveolar arches and dentition along with the palate, and is called a Le Fort I fracture. Of course, it has to transect the maxillary sinuses and the nasal septum, as well as fracture the pterygoid plates, something common to all Le Fort–level fractures.

The Le Fort II or pyramidal fracture typically breaks through the maxillae laterally, but then traverses the infraorbital rims and floors as well as the medial orbits, completing the separation at or near the nasal root, and also including the nasal septum and pterygoid plates. The Le Fort III fracture, or classical "craniofacial separation" crosses the zygomatic arches and lateral orbital walls and floors, as well as the medial orbits and nasal roots, again including the nasal septum and pterygoid plates. Typically, few fractures precisely mimic these patterns, and most are a combination of

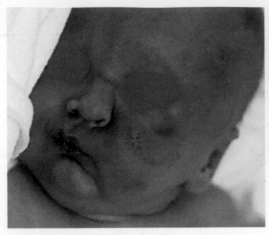
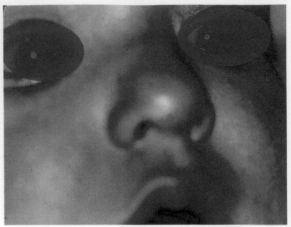

Fig. 5. Baby with broken nose.

multiple levels of fracture. As noted, owing to the small size of the facial skeleton in infants and young children, these fractures are uncommon in the younger age groups. When they do occur, there is usually a high-energy trauma involved, such as with motor vehicle crashes, and they are associated with multiple associated injuries (**Fig. 6**).

Manbibular Fractures

Condylar and subcondylar fractures

Fractures of the condylar head are fortunately uncommon in older children and teenagers, because they tend to disrupt the temporomandibular joint and lead to various degrees of malfunction. In general, most surgeons do not surgically violate

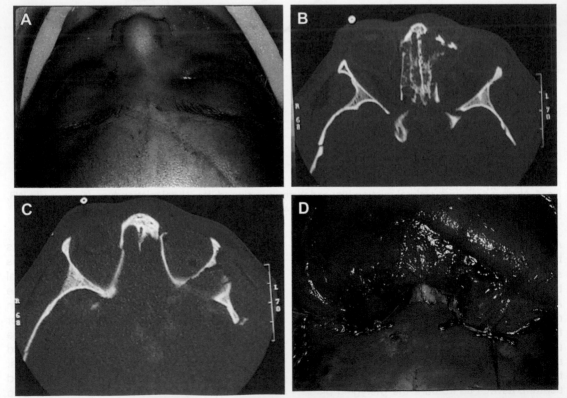

Fig. 6. Le Fort fracture. (*A*) Preoperative, (*B*) and (*C*) Preoperative imaging, (*D*) Intraoperative.

the joint for repair of these fractures, although there is controversy regarding this management, particularly in Europe. Fractures below the joint are generally referred to as subcondylar fractures, so long as the anterior extent of the fracture falls within the sigmoid notch and the posterior extent is behind the angle of the mandible. If the fracture crosses below the coronoid, it is considered a ramus fracture, and if it extends anterior to the angle, it is considered a vertical ramus fracture.

Most surgeons advocate conservative (non-open) repair of subcondylar fractures in children, although again, this course of action is controversial as well.[14] In younger children, probably younger than 14 years, and certainly younger than 12 years, there is a greater propensity for remodeling of the joint and subcondylar area, so that even unreduced fractures, so long as the occlusion is reduced, typically heal with what seems to be normal or near-normal anatomy after 1 to 2 years.

Coronoid fractures

The coronoid fracture occurs when the coronoid process is separated from the remainder of the ramus of the mandible. It is a horizontal fracture of the ramus above and anterior to the sigmoid notch. It may sometimes be associated with a subcondylar fracture, making it a complete fracture across the ramus area but above the sigmoid notch. Coronoid fractures are uncommon, and most often they do not require repair. If the patient is having extreme discomfort or significant dysfunction, some people advocate repair.

Ramus fractures

Fractures of the ramus of the mandible may be horizontal, vertical, or a combination thereof, including various patterns of diagonal fractures. As noted, if the fracture occurs between the posterior ramus and the sigmoid notch, it is a subcondylar fracture. Depending on the degree of discomfort and dysfunction caused, many of these can be managed conservatively, particularly in children.

Angle fractures

Angle fractures of the mandible occur behind the mandibular dentition and typically extend posteriorly toward the actual angle of the mandible. Because they are behind the dentition, they are not well stabilized by conservative measures, that is, fixing the occlusion. Fortunately, as noted, fractures in children are often incomplete (greenstick fractures), in which case the lack of instability may allow for conservative treatment to be effective. However, when there is instability, more definitive (open) treatment is usually indicated.

Mandibular body fractures

Fractures of the mandibular body and symphysis occur along areas of dental occlusion. This makes the precise realignment critically important owing to the importance of dental occlusion for the patient. However, the presence of the tooth roots and tooth buds can make rigid fixation very difficult and risky, so that all options must be considered. Sometimes, when possible, dental splints can be crafted and used to stabilize the occlusion and thereby the bone fragments, which leads to healing with proper occlusion.

Symphysis and parasymphysis fractures

The symphysis is an extension of both mandibular bodies, and like the bodies, it contains dentition. However, it is less stable owing to its curvature, so that the forces that occur across fractures in this area are directed in multiple directions, and therefore more fixation is generally required to stabilize this area adequately. Again, dental splints often can stabilize the occlusion effectively and lead to satisfactory healing.

Dentoalveolar fractures

Dentoalveolar fractures occur when a trauma directly involves the dentition and the alveolar bone holding the teeth. These are typically treated by gentle closed reduction and stabilization with adjacent teeth, and this is often done by dentally trained professionals. All efforts are made to maintain teeth, even deciduous teeth, because they serve an important role as "spacers," preventing migration of remaining teeth. Alveolar fractures can often be stabilized by cementing solid wires to the teeth, which stabilizes both the teeth to each other and the bones that hold them.[15,16]

PHYSICAL EXAMINATION

The injured child is likely to be anxious and resistant to vigorous palpation of their injured head and face. Much can be gleaned from pupillary and extraocular movement, patterns of ecchymosis and edema, scalp, face, and oral lacerations and occlusion. Findings such as altered consciousness, globe injury, hyphema, septal hematoma, and dental avulsion should be ruled out because of the urgent nature of their management. Gentle palpation for deformities and stop-offs can be attempted, but should be done patiently and with awareness of the impact on the child. More complete physical examination can be done if the child is sedated for a procedure or imaging. This is also a good time for an ophthalmologic evaluation, if warranted.

IMAGING AND DIAGNOSIS

There is a greater concern for the long-term effects of radiation on the growing child than the adult. This has led to more attention being paid to the amount of radiation being delivered to pediatric patients being imaged particularly in those cases where repeat imaging is required. That being said, the standard of care for imaging of most significant pediatric CMF trauma is computed tomography. Children's and other hospitals' radiology departments have begun to minimize radiation dosage in their imaging protocols, using rapid sequence spiral and other techniques. The brain is generally imaged as well as the CMF skeleton because of the chance of associated neurologic injury. Depending on the age and anxiety of the child sedation is frequently required for quality scans. Multiplanar and 3-dimensional image reformatting is often helpful in complicated cases.[17]

SURGICAL APPROACHES TO THE CMF SKELETON
Timing

Although certain injuries such as uncontrolled hemorrhage, large dural tears, globe injuries, and extraocular muscle entrapment require emergent management, most facial skeletal fractures can be repaired nonemergently. However, the robust inflammatory response and relatively rapid bone healing of the pediatric patient must be considered. A fracture that can easily be reduced at 1 week might be quite difficult to reduce at 2 weeks. This also applies to immobilization. A maxillomandibular fixation period as brief as 3 days might be adequate to stabilize a (sub) condylar fracture and prevent temporomandibular joint ankylosis with early function.

Airway Management

Depending on the severity of the injury, an airway might have already been established in the field or emergency department. Also depending on injury severity, consideration should be given to conversion to tracheostomy when prolonged intubation is anticipated. When the airway is to be established in the operating room, there are several options. Standard orotracheal intubation is adequate if the patient does not have to be put into occlusion as part of the trauma management. If there is adequate space, a retromolar positioning of the orotracheal tube allows the jaws to be brought into occlusion. A temporary surgical airway alternative to tracheostomy that has been suggested by some is the submental airway. Nasotracheal intubation has been feared in maxillary, ethmoid, and skull base fractures owing to the possibility of the tube passing through fractured bone into the brain, so-called intracranial intubation. Although this possibility should be respected, it is very unlikely in all but the most severe trauma, if appropriate technique is employed. The first point is to direct the tube parallel to the palate, not the nasal dorsum. Lifting the nasal tip helps with this. Second, a finger in the nasopharynx can intercept the tube tip and guide it through the turn in the nasopharynx. Orienting the angle of the tube tip open superiorly facilitates this passage of the tube through the nasopharynx and inferiorly toward the larynx. The tube should be well secured with tissue adhesive and tape to reduce the chance of intraoperative extubation.

Coronal Approach

The coronal approach is the workhorse for access to the upper facial skeleton, including the frontal region, the superior and upper lateral orbits, and the zygomatic arches (see **Fig. 6**). It is also the best access for reaching the nasal root region, particularly for repair of nasoorbital ethmoid fractures and fractures that extend into the anterior skull base.

The incision is generally carried from over 1 ear across the scalp to the other. It can be extended either into the preauricular crease if needed, or some surgeons prefer to extend it inferiorly just behind the auricle, although some find this location more difficult when inferior exposure is needed. The incision may be straight or curvilinear ("sine wave" or "W-plasty"), to make the scar less visible when the hair grows.

The incision can be carried down to the periosteum, which can be elevated secondarily in case a pericranial flap is needed, or it can be taken down to bone, and the pericranium is thus preserved in the flap itself for later separation if needed. The incision then reaches the bone from temporalis to temporalis, and over the muscle the incision is taken down to the level of the deep temporal fascia, but not through it. In the temple area, when the fat is seen between the layers of the temporalis fascia, the surgeon has the option of hugging the fascia or opening the outer layer and elevating over or under the temporal fat pad to minimize risk of injury to the temporal branches of the facial nerve. Elevation can then be carried forward at these levels to the orbital rims, where great care is used to preserve the supraorbital nerves. Access to the nasal root and medial orbits as well as the upper lateral orbits and zygomatic arches is then possible.

Note that the coronal approach provides broad access to the inferior frontal bones and nasal root and if needed the ethmoid areas for performance of the above-noted subcranial approach, when repair of the anterior skull base is indicated.

Periorbital Approach

Access to the frontozygomatic suture and lateral orbit can be achieved via an upper lid lateral blepharoplasty incision or via the coronal incision, as described. The inferior orbit is generally accessed via a lower lid incision of some type. Today, most surgeons utilize transconjunctival approaches, either preseptal or postseptal. Subciliary and infraorbital incision are sometimes used, but are less popular today. The medial orbit can be accessed via a transcaruncular incision.

Intraoral Approach

Intraoral exposure of maxillary and mandibular fractures is performed through the mucosa just above and just below the gingiva, usually about 5 mm from the gingival margin. The oral vestibular incisions are then taken down to the bone, and the bone is exposed by elevating deep to the periosteum. Care is taken not to injure the infraorbital nerve when exposing the maxillary bone. Similarly, care is taken to avoid injury to the mental nerves when exposing the mandible.

Transcervical Approach

As in adults, the mandible can be exposed using external incisions. The submandibular, Risdon, retromandibular, and submental incisions provided good exposure when needed. Such incisions are carefully placed in the relaxed skin tension lines to minimize visibility of future scars. Care should also be taken to preserve the mandibular branches of the facial nerves.

REDUCTION OF THE OCCLUSION/ MAXILLOMANDIBULAR FIXATION

As in adult maxillofacial fractures, the most important aspect of reduction of maxillary and mandibular fractures is to assure that the occlusion is reestablished. This can be more difficult in young children, particularly those with mixed dentition. When available, dental splints may prove helpful in stabilizing the occlusion.[15] Splints are fixed to the maxilla by placing wires from the splint to the maxillary and/or zygomatic bones. Fixing a splint to the mandible generally requires the placement of 2 or 3 circummandibular wires. When 2 separate splints are used, arch bars or hooks in the splints will allow fixation of the occlusion (ie, maxillomandibular fixation) by wiring the splints together after they are fixed to the bones (Fig. 7).

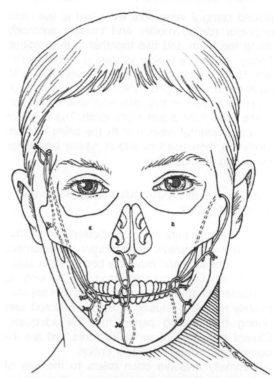

Fig. 7. Various positions for skeletal suspension wiring. (*From* Bluestone CD, Rosenfeld RM. Surgical atlas of pediatric otolaryngology. Hamilton (Ontario): BC Decker Inc; 2002; with permission.)

When arch bars are used, great care has to be used not to extract teeth with the wires that secure them to the teeth. During mixed dentition, the roots of exposed teeth are resorbing, which makes them vulnerable to avulsion. Also, in children in deciduous and mixed dentition, it is very difficult to apply a stable arch bar owing to the short height of the crowns. An alternative is a Risdon cable, which is basically a narrower arch bar constructed from strands of wire that are fixed to the most posterior dentition (Fig. 8). The original Risdon cable was

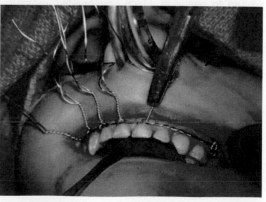

Fig. 8. Application of a Risdon cable for deciduous maxillomandibular fixation.

placed using 2 wires that were tied to the most posterior (distal) molars and brought anteriorly along the teeth and tied together in the midline. Today, it is more typical to start at 1 end, fix the wire to the molar, then attach the twisted wire to each tooth with a circumdental wire (like an arch bar) until it reaches the other end, where it is fixed to the contralateral last molar tooth. The twists of the circumdental wires that fix the cable to each tooth are then used to attach rubber bands for stabilizing the occlusion.

MINIMALLY INVASIVE AND NONOPERATIVE MANAGEMENT

When the bones are stable, particularly when fractures are incomplete, nonoperative management may be possible and desirable because it is associated with fewer complications.[18,19] As long as the patient is able to open and close with approximately normal occlusion, a mechanical soft diet during the healing period may be adequate. Closed reduction of some fractures that are incompletely mobile is another option.

Minimally invasive often refers to the use of endoscopically assisted techniques. These have been used successfully for management of orbital floor fractures, medial orbital fractures, and subcondylar fractures of the mandible. Orbital floor fractures may be approached through the maxillary sinus, but great care must be exercised, because small fragments of bone may be inadvertently advanced into the orbit. Medial orbital fractures may be repaired using endoscopes via the nose; however, in view of the small size of the nasal cavity and ethmoids in small children, this has the potential of being challenging technically. Finally, subcondylar fractures of the mandible are particularly amenable to endoscopically assisted approaches. However, the need to do so should be uncommon in the prepubescent child and likely limited to cases in which conservative measures fail to produce normal occlusion.

FIXATION
Wires

Many modern surgeons forget or never knew that interosseous wire fixation was the mainstay of bone fixation before the introduction of plates and screws for rigid fixation of fractures. It should be emphasized that, although rigid fixation is still recommended, even in the pediatric age group, wire fixation is a reasonable alternative to stabilize mobile fragments, particularly when assisted by the stabilization of the occlusion with arch bars, wires, or splints to limit bone motion. The main

advantage of interosseous wire fixation is that only small drill holes are required for wire placement, thereby making it easier to avoid tooth roots and developing tooth buds.

Plates/Removal

Rigid fixation plates are used in the pediatric population as they are in the adult population, but the locations for placement are more limited owing to the smaller bones and the presence of the tooth buds in both the mandible and maxillae.[20]

Frontal fractures can be repaired using very small plates and screws, but it must be kept in mind that in infants and small children growth may lead to the plates migrating inward, and therefore absorbable plates should be considered. For zygomaticomaxillary and Le Fort fractures, small titanium plates are contoured to the shape of the bones and fixed in place with titanium screws. In the inferior maxillae, great care should be taken to avoid unerupted dentition and tooth roots. Similarly, in the mandible, plates often need to be placed in the biomechanically unfavorable inferior portion of the bone, owing to the presence of the tooth buds. However, this disadvantage is sometimes offset by the overall short stature of the immature bones.

When using nonabsorbable titanium plates, plate removal is commonly recommended in the pediatric population, although this remains controversial. The main reason for advocating removal in the past was the concern about interference with later bone growth, particularly in the prepubescent child. However, this has not been seen in clinical practice. Nonetheless, what has been seen has been bone growth over the titanium plates, thereby incorporating the plates into the developing bone. Although this does not preclude later removal, it certainly does make it more difficult and requires drilling an amount of bone from over the plate, which can sometimes represent a substantial amount of bone loss. For these reasons, many surgeons remove titanium plates and screws from the growing facial bones, particularly the cranium and mandible, 6 months to 1 year after repair.

Absorbable Plates and Screws

As an alternative to titanium plates and screws, biodegradable plates and screws have been developed for use primarily in the pediatric population (although they can be used in adults).[20] These implants are generally made of various (co)polymers of polylactic and polyglycolic acids, although polydioxanone has been used also. The main problems associated with their use include structural weakness compared with titanium, necessitating use of larger implants to accomplish similar fixation, as well as the fact that the greater the stress on the implants, the faster they degrade by hydrolysis. Thus, they seem to offer somewhat less strength for less time when the need for strength might actually be greater. Fortunately, these issues have not seemed to represent a problem in clinical use. Obviously, the use of absorbable hardware obviates the need for reoperation to remove the implants.

COMPLICATIONS
Infection and Malunion

Early complications, such as infection and malunion, are similar to those seen in adults, although less common because of faster bone healing and the potential for compensatory changes with growth, development, and eruption of adult dentition. The likelihood of tooth root injury is greater owing to the lack of space in the bone, and the risk of injury to developing tooth buds is unique to the pediatric population. Unfortunately, tooth root injuries can occur easily from injudicious placement of bone screws. Long-term complications such as growth disturbance are unique to this population.[1,21] The overall complication rate increases with the number and severity of fractures.[18]

Malocclusion

Malocclusion is always a risk when treating maxillary and mandibular fractures, and great care must be taken to ensure that the occlusion is reduced as closely as possible to the premorbid relationship. In addition, any malposition of the facial skeletal bones during repair can result in facial deformities. Imprecise or inadequate reattachment of the medial canthal ligaments can result in persistent and unsightly telecanthus.

Nerve Injury

Nerve injuries are typically a result of the presenting injuries; however, they may also occur as a result of exposure, repair, and particularly screw placement. Great care should be taken to avoid injuring cranial nerve branches during access and repair of maxillofacial fractures. However, for facial nerve injuries, early intervention is recommended, if the possibility of nerve trunk or branch transection is suspected.

Ocular Injury

Ocular injuries are more likely to be owing to the initial trauma; great care must be exercised when operating in and around the orbit to avoid creating any injuries to the globe and/or cornea. In addition,

great care is used to minimize the likelihood of muscle entrapment during repair of orbital fractures. Performing forced duction testing both before and after any intraorbital intervention is recommended. Unfortunately, diplopia may persist even when there is no persistent entrapment after injury to an extraocular muscle, which is believed to be owing to either direct muscle injury or possibly injury to the nerve that supplies the muscle. These are dealt with by ophthalmologists who specialize in the management of problems of the extraocular muscles.

Soft Tissue Injury

Soft tissue injuries and surgical incisions can lead to scarring and contracture that lead to deformities even when the underlying bones are perfectly positioned. Great care must be exercised to avoid trauma to the orbital septum when accessing the orbit, because lid malpositions (ectropion and entropion) can be challenging to repair. Some authors recommend the use of a Frost stitch to stretch the lower lid after surgical access has been performed. Postoperative massage of the lower lid often helps to relax scars in this area and resolve developing malpositions nonsurgically, particularly if the intervention is begun before the problem becomes severe. In young children, scars have a remarkable propensity to improve on their own, so scar revision surgery is usually delayed at least 1 year in most cases to allow nature an opportunity to resolve the problem (of course, dramatic situations might provide exceptions to this recommendation).

Nasal Septal Hematoma

Nasal septal hematomas may complicate nasal trauma. It is important to look for and identify these, because early intervention will minimize the risk of later septal problems that may require challenging reconstructions.

LONG-TERM FOLLOW-UP

Long-term follow-up is typically recommended in children until they have reached skeletal maturity, because growth may be affected by trauma to the developing facial skeleton.[22] Problems that are not obvious immediately after the injury may become more of an issue later on, and secondary surgery may be needed to address such issues.[18]

REFERENCES

1. Maqusi S, Morris DE, Patel PK, et al. Complications of pediatric facial fractures. J Craniofac Surg 2012; 23(4):1023–7.

2. Mathur S, Chopra R. Combating child abuse: The role of a dentist. Oral Health Prev Dent 2013;11(3): 243–50.

3. Thompson LA, Tavares M, Ferguson-Young D, et al. Violence and abuse: core competencies for identification and access to care. Dent Clin North Am 2013; 57(2):281–99.

4. Yang RT, Li Z, Li ZB. Maxillofacial injuries in infants and preschools: a 2.5-year study. J Craniofac Surg 2014;25(3):964–7.

5. Siwani R, Tombers NM, Rieck KL, et al. Comparative analysis of fracture characteristics of the developing mandible: the Mayo Clinic experience. Int J Pediatr Otorhinolaryngol 2014;78:1066–70.

6. Chrcanovic BR, Abreu MH, Freire-Maia B, et al. Facial fractures in children and adolescents: a retrospective study of 3 years in a hospital in Belo Horizonte, Brazil. Dent Traumatol 2010;26(3): 262–70.

7. Thoren H, Iso-Kungas P, Iizuka T, et al. Changing trends in causes and patterns of facial fractures in children. Oral Surg Oral Med Oral Pathol Oral Radiol Endod 2009;107(3):318–24.

8. Morales JL, Skowronski PP, Thaller SR. Management of pediatric maxillary fractures. J Craniofac Surg 2010;21(4):1226–33.

9. Totonchi A, Sweeney WM, Gosain AK. Distinguishing anatomic features of pediatric facial trauma. J Craniofac Surg 2012;23(3):793–8.

10. Steelman R. Rapid physical assessment of the injured child. J Endod 2013;39(3 Suppl):S9–12.

11. Liau JY, Woodlief J, van Aalst JA. Pediatric nasoorbitoethmoid fractures. J Craniofac Surg 2011;22(5): 1834–8.

12. Morris C, Kushner GM, Tiwana PS. Facial skeletal trauma in the growing patient. Oral Maxillofac Surg Clin North Am 2012;24(3):351–64.

13. Stotland MA, Do NK. Pediatric orbital fractures. J Craniofac Surg 2011;22(4):1230–5.

14. Bruckmoser E, Undt G. Management and outcome of condylar fractures in children and adolescents: a review of the literature. Oral Surg Oral Med Oral Pathol Oral Radiol 2012;114(5 Suppl):S86–106.

15. MacLeod SP, Rudd TC. Update on the management of dentoalveolar trauma. Curr Opin Otolaryngol Head Neck Surg 2012;20(4):318–24.

16. Casey RP, Bensadigh BM, Lake MT, et al. Dentoalveolar trauma in the pediatric population. J Craniofac Surg 2010;21(4):1305–9.

17. Roudsari BS, Psoter KJ, Vavilala MS, et al. CT use in hospitalized pediatric trauma patients: 15-year trends in a level I pediatric and adult trauma center. Radiology 2013;267(2):479–86.

18. Rottgers SA, Decesare G, Chao M, et al. Outcomes in pediatric facial fractures: Early follow-up in 177 children and classification scheme. J Craniofac Surg 2011;22(4):1260–5.

19. Meier JD, Tollefson TT. Pediatric facial trauma. Curr Opin Otolaryngol Head Neck Surg 2008;16(6):555–61.

20. Siy RW, Brown RH, Koshy JC, et al. General management considerations in pediatric facial fractures. J Craniofac Surg 2011;22(4):1190–5.

21. Myall RW. Management of mandibular fractures in children. Oral Maxillofac Surg Clin North Am 2009; 21(2):197–201, vi.

22. Goth S, Sawatari Y, Peleg M. Management of pediatric mandible fractures. J Craniofac Surg 2012;23(1): 47–56.

Cleft Lip and Palate

David J. Crockett, MD, Steven L. Goudy, MD*

KEYWORDS

- Cleft lip • Cleft palate • Orofacial clefting • Cleft lip repair • Cleft palate repair • Palatoplasty
- Multidisciplinary care

KEY POINTS

- Cleft lip with or without cleft palate is the most common congenital malformation of the head and neck.
- Each patient should be evaluated for congenital anomalies, developmental delay, neurologic disorders, and psychosocial concerns before surgery.
- A multidisciplinary team is necessary to ensure that every aspect of the child's care is treated.
- The surgeon should be aware of the needs of the cleft patient and be able to educate and assist caretakers as necessary.
- A fundamental understanding by the surgeon of the surgical options for cleft repair is warranted.

OVERVIEW

Cleft lip with or without cleft palate is the most common congenital malformation of the head and neck. The impact on quality of life for the child and the family can be severe, particularly in unsuspecting families. Emotional and psychological needs must be recognized and addressed, in addition to surgical care, for all those involved with the patient. Assessment and treatment of those with cleft lip and/or palate requires a multidisciplinary approach. Access to and evaluation by speech-language pathology, surgery, psychology, psychiatry, social work, audiology, genetics, dentistry, otolaryngology, and pediatric primary care are all recommended by the American Cleft Palate–Craniofacial Association.[1] The recommendation for a team approach allows the child to be able to obtain complete and coordinated care. This article discusses the assessment and treatment recommendations for children born with cleft lip and/or cleft palate. This article focuses on the surgical management and treatment of these special patients.

Incidence and Genetics

Clefts of the lip and/or palate affect approximately 1 in 700 live births.[2] The incidence varies widely depending on geographic origin, racial and ethnic group, environmental exposures, and socioeconomic status. Asian and Native American populations have reported prevalence rates as high as 1 in 500. European populations are approximately 1 in 1000, whereas African populations have a reported prevalence close to 1 in 2500.[2] Clefts of the lip and/or palate can be categorized as syndromic or nonsyndromic. Syndromic clefts are those that occur in association with a recognized pattern of human malformation or syndrome. The cause of a syndromic cleft may be associated with gene transmission, chromosomal aberrations, teratogens, or environmental factors.[3] Identifying an associated syndrome is important, because it

Disclosures: There are no actual or potential conflicts of interest, including employment, consultancies, stock ownership, patent applications/registrations, grants, or other funding.

Department of Otolaryngology – Head and Neck Surgery, Vanderbilt University Medical Center, Vanderbilt University, 1211 Medical Center Drive, Nashville, TN 37232, USA

* Corresponding author.

E-mail address: steven.goudy@vanderbilt.edu

can have prognostic implications that may be helpful to the patient and the family.

Classification

Orofacial clefts include all variations of cleft lip and cleft palate. A variety of classification schemes have been suggested and recommended for typical and atypical orofacial clefts.[4] The features used to initiate the classification of an orofacial cleft include the laterality, completeness, severity (wide vs narrow), and presence of any abnormal tissue. Diminutive orofacial clefts may also be described as microform, occult, or minor.[5] The cleft lip laterality includes unilateral and bilateral. A complete cleft lip extends through the lip and the nasal sill, whereas an incomplete cleft lip extends through the orbicularis oris and skin, but intact lip tissue persists. The cleft alveolus can also be considered complete or only notched. A weblike piece of tissue may extend from the lip's cleft side to the noncleft side at the nasal sill. This abnormal tissue is called a Simonart band and, if present, it is not considered the same as an incomplete cleft.

A cleft palate can be unilateral, when 1 palatal shelf attaches to the nasal septum, or bilateral. The classification scheme introduced by Victor Veau[6] is the most popular system. Clefts of the palate were placed into 4 groups. A group I defect includes a cleft of the soft palate only. Group II clefts exist when the defect involves the soft palate and the hard palate to the incisive foramen (secondary palate). Groups III and IV are unilateral and bilateral defects extending through the entire palate and alveolus, respectively.

PATIENT ASSESSMENT
Multidisciplinary Care

Patients with cleft lip and/or palate may present as early as during the prenatal period. Surgical consultation before birth is becoming more common because of the ability to make the diagnosis on prenatal ultrasonography. Discussion regarding general care issues and surgery can help improve some of the anxiety the expecting mother may be experiencing. After birth, the initial management includes ensuring proper feeding of the neonate and evaluation for other comorbidities. As previously discussed, a multidisciplinary approach should be used in the assessment of the child. The patient should undergo initial evaluations by a pediatrician, geneticist, surgeon, feeding specialist, and social worker. Such services allow immediate education and support for the caretakers and the patient. Future assessments need to be performed by audiology, otolaryngology, dental, maxillofacial, speech-language pathology, and psychosocial practitioners.

Surgical Assessment

Immediately after birth, the surgeon should evaluate and examine the neonate. The various anatomic sites for clefting are assessed, including the upper lip, alveolar arches, nostrils, and primary and secondary palates. These areas should be palpated and inspected under direct visualization. Microform cleft lip and submucous cleft palate can often present with only subtle findings on clinical examination. Particular attention should be given to the nasal characteristics in the setting of a cleft lip. The nasal alar symmetry, tip projection, and alar base position and width should all be assessed. The extent of the clefting can be classified, as described previously. A thorough physical examination is necessary to evaluate for any signs of dysmorphia that may lead to the identification of other congenital anomalies or a syndromic diagnosis.

Regular clinic visits with the patient and caretakers allow the surgeon to provide counsel and guidance before surgery. Feeding and weight gain are important aspects to monitor with each visit. Associated congenital anomalies, developmental delay, and neurologic disorders should also be followed. Any concern for cardiac defects or airway obstruction needs to be identified and evaluated promptly. A multidisciplinary approach is warranted to ensure proper management of all of the needs of the child. The surgeon should be aware of these needs and assist with any referrals to the necessary specialists.

UNILATERAL CLEFT LIP AND NASAL DEFORMITY
Preoperative Planning and Preparation

Before surgical treatment of a unilateral cleft lip, adequate weight should be established, with the child weighing at least 4.5 kg (10 lb). Breast feeding is recommended, when possible, but often this is difficult for the infant. However, pumped breast milk may be taken via bottle feeds with the use of a specialized nipple that controls the flow rate, such as a Haberman or pigeon-type nipple based on an evaluation by speech therapy. Most surgeons prefer an average of 28 g (1 ounce) of weight gain per day beginning 2 after birth.

Adequate management for any cardiopulmonary anomalies should be ensured. If there are any concerns with the ability of the child to tolerate general anesthesia, evaluation by an anesthesiologist before surgery is warranted. The anesthesiologist should be knowledgeable and experienced in pediatric anesthesia.

Consideration must be given to the overall width of the cleft. The presence of a wide cleft may make the repair difficult and place undesirable tension on the closure. Excess tension after lip repair can lead to lip breakdown and scarring. Presurgical devices to improve the success of the repair by narrowing the width of the cleft include lip taping, use of an oral appliance (eg, Latham appliance),[7] and nasoalveolar molding.[8] Surgical options may include performing a 2-staged repair with primary lip adhesion[9] or delaying the repair in order to allow increased growth of the tissues.

Timing of Repair

The surgical repair of the lip is usually performed during the first year of life and may be performed as early as is considered safe for the patient.[1] In utero surgery for cleft lip has been contemplated and attempted because it may potentially provide a scarless repair of the deformity.[10] However, this option must become safer for the fetus and the mother before it can be an acceptable practice. In the 1960s, the general so-called rule over 10 was proposed as criteria for the timing of lip surgery. This rule requires the patient's weight to be more than 10 lbs (4.5 kg), have a hemoglobin more than 10 g, and be more than 10 weeks of age.[11] Millard[12] recommended postponing repair of a unilateral cleft to at least 3 months of age and preferably 4 or 5 months when possible. Many consider that waiting 3 months allows for a safer anesthesia, improved accuracy of the repair, and parental acceptance of the malformation.[13]

Surgical Technique

As mentioned earlier, multiple techniques and options have been described to restore function and anatomic contour to a cleft lip. These options include the straight line closure,[14] geometric lip repair,[15,16] the rotation-advancement technique,[12] and variations on each of these techniques. The ultimate goal is to have a patient with a balanced and symmetric face. The principles of advancement and rotation are common practice in repairing clefts. These principles were first made apparent in the Millard technique. Since Millard's[12] description, a variety of techniques for cleft lip and nasal repair have been described, all with excellent results. Each of these repairs attempts to lengthen the noncleft side by placing a scar at the base of the columella (Millard, geometric) or above the vermilion (straight line). This article provides a detailed description of the Millard rotation advancement, which has provided excellent and reproducible results. However, the various options should be known by the surgeon to allow intraoperative changes because of the unique anatomy that may present with each patient.

Patient positioning
The patient is positioned supine on the operating room bed. Preoperative checklists are performed, correct patient ensured, and the consent is verified. General anesthesia is performed by the anesthesia care team and the patient is intubated with either a standard endotracheal tube or a RAE tube.[17] The tube is taped in the middle of the lower lip on the chin. Tegaderm dressings (3M Health Care, St Paul, MN) are placed to protect both eyes. The surgical bed is typically rotated at least 90° from the anesthesiologist and a shoulder roll is placed. Infraorbital nerve blocks are performed with 0.25% bupivacaine. Intravenous antibiotics are administered. The surgical site is prepared and cleaned with Betadine. The surgical site is then toweled off and draped in a standard fashion.

Procedural design and markings
The incisions are planned and marked using methylene blue or gentian violet on a sharply pointed wooden end of a cotton tip applicator. The markings are similar to those described originally by Millard[12]; however, each patient's malformation is unique and every situation calls for a certain amount of improvisation and artistry by the surgeon (Fig. 1). The peak of Cupid's bow is identified and marked on the noncleft side, followed by marking of the midline of the bow. A mark is placed equidistant from the midline of the Cupid's bow and the peak on the noncleft side. This mark is the point at which the Cupid's bow will be created on the cleft side. On the cleft side, the point corresponding with the new peak is also marked. This point is determined by identifying the end of the white roll and following the white roll laterally until the lip appears to have maximal vermilion height and muscle bulk, usually 1 to 2 mm. Both points

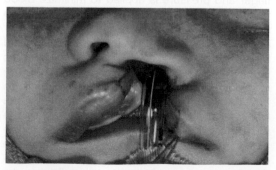

Fig. 1. Preoperative markings in preparation for repair of a unilateral cleft lip.

corresponding with the new Cupid's peak are tattooed at the white roll with either methylene blue or gentian violet using a 27-gauge needle. The tattooed marks are visible subdermally and aid in exact white roll approximation during closure.

The philtral lengths on the cleft and noncleft sides are assessed. A caliper can be used to determine the discrepancy and the amount of necessary rotation of the noncleft flap can be predicted. An incision is marked along the mucocutaneous junction extending from the tattooed Cupid's peak to the medial nasal floor. This mark should not include any mucosa and should attempt to preserve as much skin as possible, depending on the patient's anatomy and the surgeon's artistic eye. Based on the amount of necessary rotation, a curvilinear incision is marked, extending from tattooed Cupid's peak to 1 mm inferior to the subnasale. The arc of rotation should be inferior to the columellar crease and its length should be equal to the philtral height on the noncleft side. This incision usually needs to proceed to the midline of the columella and can proceed up to, but not across, the noncleft philtral ridge. This philtral ridge should be kept in continuity in order to preserve its appearance.

On the cleft side, a similar curvilinear incision is marked along the mucocutaneous junction, extending from the tattooed white roll and then curving to near the alar base superiorly. The advancement flap is marked at a perpendicular angle from the alar base, but there is no need to continue the incision around the alar base, because this may result in an unsightly scar. Markings are then made extending from both tattooed marks perpendicular to the white roll line toward the gingivolabial sulcus. Using 0.5% lidocaine with 1:100,000 epinephrine, the lip, gingivolabial sulcus, pyriform aperture, supraperiosteal maxilla, and nasal septum are injected.

Incisions and flap creation

The lip is grasped between the thumb and index finger and pressure is applied to minimize blood flow from the labial artery. Using a #15 blade scalpel, preferably on a round knife handle for easier mobility, the lateral incision is made and incised down to the labial sulcus, preserving as much of the orbicularis muscle as possible. The incision is extended, as described previously, to the lateral alar base. A back cut is made near the labial sulcus to aid in medial advancement of the lateral lip and to allow improved access to the alar base. Through this incision, the alar base can be released from the premaxilla and orbicularis oris in a supraperiosteal fashion, allowing alar base repositioning superiorly and medially. Using

the scalpel, the edge of the orbicularis muscle is skeletonized from the overlying dermis and underlying mucosa.

The marked incisions are similarly incised medially with a #15 blade scalpel. However, on this side the vermilion mucosa is pedicled on the red lip and can be tailored at the end to assist with providing increased fullness to prevent notching. Careful attention is made to preserve the columellar based skin flap, also known as the c flap, and to separate it from the underlying orbicularis muscle fibers. A back cut is then made in the labial sulcus up to the nasal spine, including the release of the upper labial frenulum. This allows access to release and rotate the orbicularis oris fibers from off the nasal spine in order to provide rotation of the medial lip and lengthening of the lip on the noncleft side. In similar fashion to the contralateral side, the orbicularis muscle is released from the dermis and mucosa of the lip (**Fig. 2**). However, only minimal undermining is performed on the dermal side in order to maintain the philtral dimple.

Closure

Before closure, hemostasis is ensured with the use of needle-tip monopolar electrocautery. The vermilion mucosa is trimmed until the proper amount is left for closure to allow fullness and to prevent notching. The vermilion mucosa most distal from the white roll is closed initially using interrupted 4-0 Vicryl suture, because it is hard to close the mucosa once the orbicularis is approximated. The orbicularis muscle is secured together with a 3-0 Vicryl suture with an RB1 needle in an interrupted fashion, ensuring rotation of the medial lip, advancement of the lateral lip, and proper alignment of the muscle to prevent a whistler deformity. The use of 3-0 Vicryl to approximate the orbicularis oris reduces the likelihood of lip dehiscence. A deep dermal stitch is placed 1 mm from the white roll to approximate the vermilion border using a 5-0 Vicryl suture with a P3 needle. This same suture is placed to inset

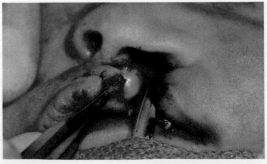

Fig. 2. Intraoperative view of the advancement and rotation flaps during a unilateral cleft lip repair.

the advancement flap from cleft side into the apex of the rotation flap, at the base of the columella. The c flap is advanced laterally and the alar base is advanced medially in order to be approximated using a 4-0 chromic with a G2 needle to form the nasal sill. When closing the nasal floor, the surgeon should ensure that the alar widths on the cleft and noncleft sides are similar. The same suture is used superficially to align the white roll in an interrupted fashion. The red lip is closed using a 4-0 Vicryl with a P3 needle. The gingivolabial sulcus is left to heal by secondary intention. The skin of the philtrum is closed using a 6-0 fast-absorbing suture with a PC1 needle in an interrupted fashion (**Fig. 3**). Surgical glue is then placed over the closed incisions.

Primary rhinoplasty

There are many different approaches to performing a primary cleft rhinoplasty, including using a tunneled incision via the columella and alar base versus a direct marginal incision to free the lower lateral cartilage. Debate continues as to the utility, effectiveness, potential complications, and best practice of performing a primary rhinoplasty. Most cleft surgeons realize that early surgical treatment of the nasal deformity minimizes nasal asymmetries and allows the nose to grow symmetrically.[18]

In order to perform a primary rhinoplasty, further dissection of the lower lateral cartilages must be performed to release the cartilage from the skin soft tissue envelope. This dissection is typically performed through a marginal incision. Surgical scissors are used medially to perform dissection between the medial crura superiorly to the nasal tip. The scissors are again used laterally to dissect the soft tissue envelope off the lower lateral cartilages while using palpation and visualizing the skin until the nasal tip is encountered. The cleft side nasal dome can be repositioned using a lateral crural steal technique; the medial crus is elongated by stealing some additional length from the lateral crus, which is accomplished by passing a full-thickness suture from lateral to

medial through the lower lateral cartilage on the cleft side. This technique provides improved symmetry and projection of the nasal tip. These modifications are often performed using 5-0 PDS suture. Using the same stitch, further sutures can be placed transcutaneously in mattress fashion to further contour the lower lateral cartilage in an attempt to improve symmetry and to more fully define the alar-facial groove. Some investigators advocate the use of tie-over bolsters and/or the use of nasal conformers.[18]

Postprocedural care

During the postoperative period the primary goals include prevention of infection and wound tension, provision of pain relief, and promotion of adequate nutrition. Children are monitored in the hospital for at least 1 night to ensure that they are able to keep themselves hydrated. Arm restraints are used to protect the incision for 2 weeks and are only taken off when the child is in the parents' arms. A 1-week course of oral antibiotics is administered. Pain control with the use of acetaminophen and ibuprofen is recommended. The child is evaluated in clinic at approximately 3 weeks after surgery. The family is counseled to remain vigilant of the child and the healing lip. They are to call or visit the clinic with any concerns.

Potential complications and management

Complications associated with unilateral lip repair include lip dehiscence, vermilion notching, misalignment of the white roll, and orbicularis oris discontinuity.[19] Lip dehiscence is often associated with increased tension of the closure, in the setting of infection, or in children with poor nutritional status. Avoidance of the associated causes is the best prevention. Local wound care is recommended until a secondary repair can be performed. Marking the vermilion more centrally during the repair, where the vermilion is thinner, can lead to the approximation of thinner segments, which may produce notching. For this reason, marking the vermilion slightly more lateral, where there is increased bulk, is recommended to avoid this complication. Mismatch of the white roll is an easily noticeable complication that can be avoided through accurate marking and tattooing before injection of the local anesthetic, followed by careful approximation during the procedure. Prevention of muscle discontinuity begins with adequate muscle dissection and careful suturing of the orbicularis oris. A strong repair also minimizes tension on the closure and prevents other complications. If there is a dehiscence, addressing the muscular tension after healing has occurred allows a successful repair. If a whistler deformity

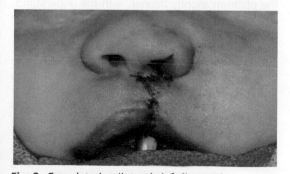

Fig. 3. Completed unilateral cleft lip repair.

(incomplete closure of the orbicularis oris) occurs, then rerepair is indicated.

REPAIR OF BILATERAL CLEFT LIP AND NASAL DEFORMITY
Preoperative Planning and Preparation

The preoperative evaluation and management in patients with a bilateral cleft lip is similar to those in patients with a unilateral malformation. There are different formations of bilateral cleft lip that may affect the position of the premaxilla, such as complete, incomplete, and microform deformities (which may occur in variations on either side of a cleft). As with patients with unilateral cleft lip, the child and the caretakers should be seen in clinic as soon as possible after the birth. After thorough evaluation of the patient, a treatment plan is developed and discussed with the families. Feeding difficulties and poor weight gain must be closely monitored, evaluated, and treated before surgery. Assistance from a multidisciplinary team is helpful in diagnosing and managing other potential cardiac, musculoskeletal, or neurologic disorders.

The commonly discussed treatment options include a bilateral repair in infancy with a delayed columellar lengthening procedure at a later date,[20,21] a 1-stage cleft repair that may or may not include a primary rhinoplasty,[22] and a lip adhesion with a delayed lip repair several months later.[9,23] Infant orthopedics, nasoalveolar molding, and taping of the lip can be considered as an option with any of the techniques described earlier.

The strategies for premaxillary manipulation can be categorized as either active or passive. A passive appliance functions by adding or subtracting material to apply pressure on the maxillary elements to bring the maxillary arches into alignment. Traditional approaches to passive manipulation include performing a lip adhesion and/or lip taping, both of which expand the soft tissue and apply pressure to the premaxilla. More recently Cutting and colleagues[22] advocated a passive technique described as nasoalveolar molding. The main active form of manipulation is the Latham device.[24] This device requires a plate to be pinned in the operating room, followed by active ratcheting of the device to obtain the desired results.[25] Controversy exists regarding the use of presurgical orthopedics, especially active devices, because of concern for midfacial retrusion.[26] However, the seriousness of the effects on maxillary growth continue to be debated.[27]

Timing of Repair

The timeline for repair of a bilateral cleft lip is similar to that of a unilateral cleft lip. The same landmarks and clearances need to be achieved. A bilateral lip is typically repaired at 3 to 5 months of age. Less postoperative nasal obstruction occurs when the child is closer to 5 months of age. The timing of the repair is depends on the selected treatment plan and the use of any presurgical preparations or orthopedics. In the setting of a lip adhesion, the definitive repair is usually performed at 6 to 8 months of age.[9]

Surgical Technique

As discussed earlier, multiple options exist in the treatment of patients with a bilateral cleft lip that produce excellent results, including a bilateral repair in infancy with a delayed columella lengthening procedure at a later date, a 1-stage cleft repair that may or may not include a primary rhinoplasty, and a lip adhesion with a delayed lip repair several months later. Clinicians who advocate lip adhesion suggest that it provides presurgical orthopedics, particularly with a prolabium that is extruding. Columella lengthening at the time of repair with primary rhinoplasty has recently been advocated, although secondary columella lengthening procedures were performed in the past. This article describes the operative steps for completion of a 1-stage cleft repair. Primary rhinoplasty at the time of repair is briefly reviewed.

Patient positioning

The operating setup, anesthesia care, and patient positioning are the same as for unilateral cleft lip. Infraorbital nerve blocks are performed with 0.25% bupivacaine and appropriate antibiotics delivered. Similar preparation and draping are also performed.

Procedural design and markings

A philtrum is designed on the prolabial skin using methylene blue or gentian violet on a sharply pointed wooden stick (Fig. 4). The marking of the newly designed philtrum is narrower at the subnasale than at the inferior aspect. The surgeon must remember that it is recommended to err on making the philtrum slightly thinner, with the understanding that the column will widen with growth. The markings at the base of the columella are usually around 4 mm, whereas the width of the distal flap is usually around 5 mm. The skin lateral to the markings can either be used to create flaps (forked flaps) to assist with future columellar lengthening, or can be de-epithelialized to assist with bulk under the philtrum, or can be discarded.

The lateral lip segments are then evaluated in order to mark the proposed Cupid's peaks on each side. These points are determined by identifying the end of the white roll and following the white

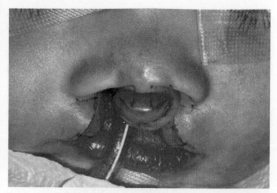

Fig. 4. Preoperative markings in preparation for repair of a bilateral cleft lip.

roll laterally until the lip appears to have sufficient vermilion height and muscle bulk; usually 1 to 2 mm. Both points corresponding with the new Cupid's peaks are tattooed at the white roll with either methylene blue or gentian violet using a 27-gauge needle. The tattooed marks aid in exact white roll approximation during closure. Just above the vermilion-cutaneous junction, 2-mm to 3-mm back cuts paralleling the white roll on each side are marked. These small incisions allow advancement of the white roll flaps to the midline in order to be approximated. Further incisions are marked extending from the tattooed Cupid's peak to the medial alar base, toward the inferior turbinate, following the mucocutaneous junction bilaterally. Advancement flaps perpendicular to the alar base are marked, but do not extend beyond the alar base. These marks should not include any mucosa and should attempt to preserve as much skin as possible. Markings are then made extending from both tattooed marks perpendicular to the white roll line toward the gingivolabial sulcus. Using 0.5% lidocaine with 1:100,000 epinephrine, the lip, gingivolabial sulcus, pyriform aperture, supraperiosteal maxilla, and prolabium are injected.

Incisions and flap creation
The prolabial incisions are made using a #15 blade scalpel through the dermis, along the marked incisions. The incisions can be extended into the nasal septal mucosa in order to assist with nasal floor closure. The tip of the neophiltral flap should not contain mucosa, but should only include skin. The neophiltral flap and both lateral fork flaps are raised from the underlying mucosa, maintaining sufficient tissue depth. A midline wedge of mucosa is removed from the prolabial mucosa. By so doing, as the mucosal edges of the wedged section are approximated, a gingivolabial sulcus can be created on the premaxillary segment (**Fig. 5**).

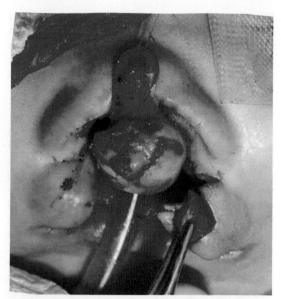

Fig. 5. Intraoperative view during the repair of a bilateral cleft lip. The orbicularis muscle has been isolated on the left, philtral flap is being retracted, and gingival mucosa has been closed.

The lateral lip segments are then incised by grasping the lip between the thumb and index finger while applying pressure to minimize blood flow from the labial artery. Using a #15 blade scalpel, the markings are incised down to the labial sulcus while attempting to skeletonize and preserve as much of the orbicularis muscle as possible. Using the scalpel, the edge of the orbicularis muscle is released from the overlying dermis and underlying mucosa (see **Fig. 5**). Sufficient release is necessary in order to allow the muscle to be approximated in the midline over the premaxilla (usually 3–4 mm). Through the incisions, the alar base can be released in a supraperiosteal fashion from its surrounding attachments to allow for repositioning during closure. In order to allow adequate advancement of the lateral lip segments for a tension-free closure, it is important to completely release muscular and soft tissue attachments from the alar base and lateral pyriform aperture. Also, the gingivolabial sulcus incision can be extended as necessary. Perialar incisions and/or alotomy is unnecessary in most cases. In addition, the markings for the white roll advancement flaps are incised.

Closure
Before closure, hemostasis is ensured with the use of needle-tip monopolar electrocautery. A central gingivolabial sulcus is created by sewing the previously mucosal wedged edges together using a 4-0 Vicryl suture with a P3 needle (see

Fig. 5). This mucosa is advanced superiorly and attached to the premaxilla with the same stitch to assist with maintaining the sulcus during the healing process. Again, using the same suture, the mucosal edges of the red lip segments are approximated in a simple interrupted fashion. Assistance may be required to minimize the tension on the closure until the muscle is approximated. The orbicularis oris muscle is then approximated using a 3-0 Vicryl suture with an RB1 needle (Fig. 6). The superiormost stitch is also adhered to the premaxillary fascia to keep the muscle from drifting inferiorly. Afterward, the remaining portion of the wet lip can be closed with the 4-0 Vicryl suture. The vermilion mucosa is trimmed until the proper amount is left for closure to allow fullness and to prevent notching. A deep dermal stitch is placed to approximate the white roll flaps using a 5-0 Vicryl suture with a P3 needle (see Fig. 6). With the same stitch and in similar fashion, the neophiltrum is approximated to the lateral labial segments. The philtrum is secured with a few superficial interrupted sutures using a 4-0 chromic with a G2 needle. At this point, if the fork flaps are going to be maintained for use in future columellar lengthening, the flaps are trimmed to the necessary size. A further incision may be necessary along the inferior aspect of the flap into the septum to allow rotation of the flap toward the floor of the nasal sill. The previously used chromic suture is used to secure the fork flaps and to close the floor of the nasal sill. The skin of the philtrum is closed with a 6-0 fast-absorbing suture with a PC1 needle in an interrupted fashion (Fig. 7). Surgical glue is then placed over the closed incisions.

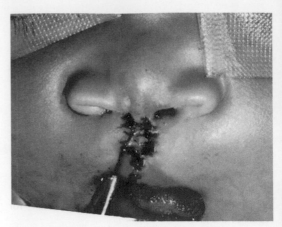

Fig. 7. Completed bilateral cleft lip repair.

Primary rhinoplasty

Similar to unilateral cleft nasal deformity, various techniques have been described to improve the nasal deformity in the setting of bilateral cleft lip repair.[20,28–32] Although multiple techniques can be applied to accomplish this task, the primary goal is to reposition the alar base and position the splayed lower lateral cartilages to form a symmetric nasal tip and upper columella.[21] In order to perform a primary rhinoplasty, further dissection of the lower lateral cartilages must be performed via the columella and alar base or a marginal incision in order to release the cartilage from the skin soft tissue envelope. Sutures can be placed transcutaneously in mattress fashion to contour the lower lateral cartilage in an attempt to improve symmetry and lengthen the columella. As noted previously for unilateral cleft lip nasal deformity, some investigators advocate the use of tie-over bolsters and/or use of nasal conformers.[18]

Postprocedural care

The postoperative care for a patient who has undergone a bilateral cleft repair is the same as for the child who underwent a unilateral repair (as discussed earlier for postprocedural care in a unilateral cleft lip repair).

Potential complications and management

Complications associated with bilateral lip repair include lip dehiscence, creeping of mucosa into the cutaneous lip, misalignment of the white roll, orbicularis oris discontinuity, and poor aesthetic outcome. As mentioned previously, dehiscence and muscle discontinuity are often associated with increased tension on the closure, particularly when the premaxilla erodes through the repair. Infection and poor nutrition leading to inadequate wound healing may also be contributing factors. Poor aesthetic outcomes are difficult to measure

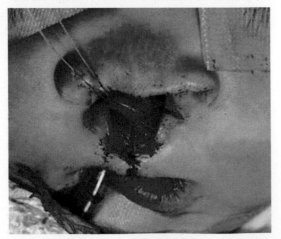

Fig. 6. Intraoperative view during the repair of a bilateral cleft lip. Note the approximation of the orbicularis muscle and the white roll flaps.

objectively but width of the philtrum, width of alar base, and columellar projection are commonly evaluated after surgery.[33,34] An understanding of the fine points of the repair is important in obtaining an acceptable aesthetic appearance of the lip with healing and growth.

REPAIR OF CLEFT PALATE
Preoperative Planning and Preparation

Repair of the cleft palate focuses on the separation of the nasal and the velopharyngeal mechanisms. This repair can determine the outcomes of the child's speech, feeding, and eustachian tube function, and may affect the maxillary growth and dental arch relationship.[35,36] The preoperative evaluation is the same as for a child with only a cleft lip; however, particular attention is paid to ensuring that the caretakers understand proper methods for feeding and caring for the child. Monitoring for adequate weight gain and assessing for associated comorbidities and syndromes are important as well. Cleft palate repair may temporarily cause upper airway obstruction, so any concern for the airway before surgery needs to be addressed.[37,38]

The type of cleft (hard vs soft palate) and the width should be evaluated in order to select a technique to accomplish the goals of repair. As reviewed earlier, many techniques and modifications have been developed over time and successfully used with good outcomes. The type of palatoplasty and associated adjustments that are performed are based on the type of cleft and width of the cleft. Patients diagnosed with a submucous cleft palate can be monitored closely and their palates repaired only if there is evidence of feeding, otologic, or speech problems.[1] The main principles of palatoplasty consist of a tension-free and multilayered closure with repositioning of the velar muscle sling.[39] The 2-flap palatoplasty and the Furlow palatoplasty[40] are reviewed later.

Timing of Repair

In an appropriately developing child, the standard is to repair the palate before 18 months of age and earlier when possible.[1] The timing of repair is a balance between poor speech and language development related to late surgery and potential impairment of maxillary growth related to early surgery. Cleft repair as early as 6 months of age has been shown to enhance speech outcomes and prevent compensatory articulation disorders.[41] The main argument against early palate closure is the possible effect it may have on midfacial growth and need for maxillary surgery.[42] At our institution, cleft palate repair is generally performed around 12 months of age, before any significant speech development. However, patients with Pierre Robin sequence are typically repaired at a later age (14–16 months) to avoid airway obstruction.

Patient Positioning

The positioning is the same for a 2-flap palatoplasty as it is for a Furlow palatoplasty. The patient is placed in a supine position on the operating room bed. Preoperative checklists are performed, correct patient ensured, and the consent is verified. General anesthesia is performed by the anesthesia care team and endotracheal intubated is performed with either a standard endotracheal tube or an RAE tube. The tube is taped in the middle of the lower lip on the chin and secured with an adhesive tape. Tegaderm dressings (3M Health Care, St Paul, MN) are placed to protect both eyes. The surgical bed is typically rotated at least 90° from the anesthesiologist and a shoulder roll is placed. Intravenous antibiotics are administered. The surgical site is then toweled off, draped, and a Dingman mouth retractor is placed in standard fashion to view the surgical site (Fig. 8). The palate is injected with 1% lidocaine with 1:100,000 epinephrine.

Surgical Technique of 2-Flap Palatoplasty

The 2-flap palatoplasty is a widely used technique for complete cleft palate closure. At our institution, this is the preferred technique for most palatal repairs. The procedure is simple and allows easy exposure of the soft palate musculature, which facilitates release of anomalous attachments of the levator veli palatini muscle in order to perform an intravelar veloplasty to reorient the levator sling.

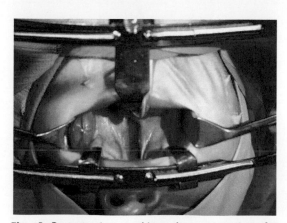

Fig. 8. Preoperative markings in preparation for repair of a cleft palate using a 2-flap palatoplasty technique.

Procedural design and markings

The palate is marked using a standard surgical marker after drying off the mucosal surfaces. Incisions are planned extending from the tip of the uvula medially, along the cleft margin toward the midline of the alveolus. The alveolar ridge is then followed in a curving fashion posteriorly to the end of the alveolus. A small lateral releasing incision is then extended just posterior to the end of the alveolar ridge. Along the cleft margin medially, it is recommended to err the incision toward the side of the oral mucosa by 1 to 2 mm in order to ensure an adequate mucosal flap for a tension-free nasal closure. The contralateral side of the palate is then marked in similar fashion.

Incisions and flap creation

A #15 blade scalpel is used to perform the incisions as marked. A #12 blade scalpel can be used to complete the mucosal incisions along the medial aspect of both uvulae. The palatal flaps are then raised in a subperiosteal manner with assistance of Cottle and Freer elevators. The flaps are elevated until there is complete exposure of the hard-soft palate junction. During this process the greater palatine neurovascular bundle must be identified and preserved (**Fig. 9**). The surrounding foraminal fascia needs to be released in order to have improved mobility of the neurovascular bundle to assist with medial advancement of the flap. A curved scalpel blade and minimal monopolar electrocautery can assist with difficult fibrous adhesions. Injury to the pedicle is to be avoided at all costs, and if this occurs the palate shelf should be sewn back to the adjacent mucosa and the other side completely dissected.

Starting medially, the abnormal levator muscle fiber attachments are released off the posterior aspect of the hard palate and the cleft margin, which is performed with gentle dissection using a Cottle elevator, surgical scissors, and monopolar electrocautery. The nasal mucosa is elevated off the superior aspect of the hard palate and extended into the soft palate. By so doing, the extent of the soft palate musculature is easily identified. The release of the muscle fibers is then extended laterally until the hamulus and the tensor veli palatini muscle are visualized. All soft tissue, musculature, and nasal mucosal lining must be identified and released to allow medial advancement. Advancement of the nasal layer, musculature, and oral layer must be sufficient to allow a tension-free closure. If the nasal layer is unable to be approximated, vomer flaps can be raised to decrease the tension.

Closure

A 4-0 Vicryl with a TF needle is used to close the nasal layer of the uvula in a simple interrupted fashion. The same suture is then used to approximate the miduvula with a mattress stitch in a through-and-through fashion. Interrupted sutures are used to close the nasal mucosal layer anteriorly and posteriorly using a 4-0 Vicryl with a PS-4c needle (**Fig. 10**). The central portion of the nasal layer is closed after muscle approximation to prevent increased tension on that layer. The levator muscle is approximated to create an intravelar veloplasty with a 3-0 Vicryl with an RB1 needle in an interrupted mattress fashion. The closure of the nasal layer is then completed. The oral layer is closed starting at the base of the uvula and proceeding anteriorly using a 4-0 Vicryl with a TF needle in a simple interrupted manner (**Fig. 11**). Once the hard palate is encountered, the dead space between the oral and nasal layers is closed by capturing nasal mucosa using interrupted

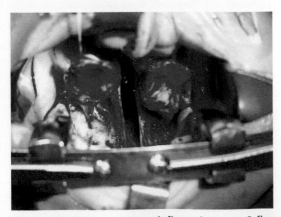

Fig. 9. Raised mucoperiosteal flaps during a 2-flap palatoplasty. Note the intact neurovascular bundle supplying each flap.

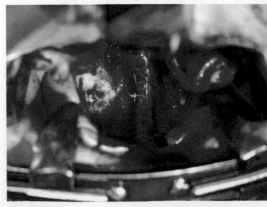

Fig. 10. Closure of the nasal layer during a 2-flap palatoplasty.

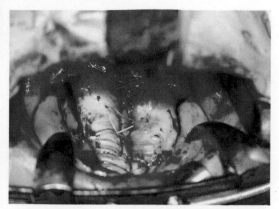

Fig. 11. Completed repair of a cleft palate using a 2-flap palatoplasty technique.

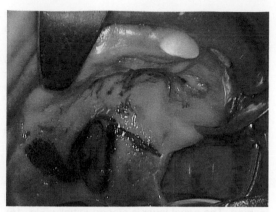

Fig. 12. Preoperative markings in preparation for repair of a cleft palate using the Furlow palatoplasty technique.

horizontal mattress sutures to close the oral layer. At the end of the closure, hemostasis is ensured using monopolar electrocautery. Moist and packed microfibrillar collagen hemostatic agent is placed in the open regions laterally. The stomach is suctioned and a tongue stitch is placed if there is any concern for an obstructed airway. For patients with significantly wide palates (>2 cm), the palate repair can be reinforced with acellular dermal matrix, which is incorporated between the oral and nasal layers as an additional barrier. However, this reinforcement does not replace good surgical technique.

Surgical Technique of Furlow Palatoplasty

The Furlow palatoplasty consists of transposing 2 opposing Z-plasties of the oral and nasal mucosal layers with attached levator muscle in order to reorient the displaced muscle fibers into a more anatomic position. This procedure has been found to lengthen the palate, and both tightens and repositions the levator sling.[43] At our institution, this technique is used primarily for clefts isolated to the velum and submucous clefting. However, the procedure can be combined with other techniques to provide additional closure of clefts that include the hard palate.[44,45]

Procedural design and markings

The incisions are marked with a surgical marker in the same manner as was described by Furlow[40] (1986). The Z-plasty is marked so that on the oral layer, a left posteriorly based myomucosal flap, and a right anteriorly based thick mucosal flap can be raised (Fig. 12). An opposing Z-plasty is created on the nasal layer, such that on the left an anteriorly based nasal mucosal flap and on the right a posteriorly based nasal myomucosal flap are created. The hamulus and eustachian

tubes can be used as guides for the angle of the lateral Z-plasty limbs.

Incisions and flap creation

A #15 blade scalpel is used to perform the incisions through the previously placed markings. The cleft margins are incised along the medial cleft edge. If the operation is being performed on a patient with a submucous cleft, the midline can be divided. Be sure to not extend the lateral limb of the incision through the nasal mucosal layer on the left. On the right, the lateral limb of the incision should extend only until the soft palate musculature is encountered. Using surgical scissors, a posteriorly based myomucosal flap is raised on the left. Further undermining and releasing of the flap laterally can be performed using monopolar electrocautery. After the left-sided myomucosal flap is elevated, the right-sided anteriorly based mucosal flap is raised (Fig. 13). An angled Beaver blade can be helpful, along with surgical scissors,

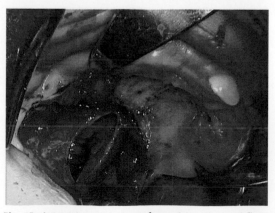

Fig. 13. Intraoperative view after raising the oral flaps during a Furlow palatoplasty.

in the elevation of this flap. An attempt should be made to make a sufficiently thick mucosal flap while leaving the muscle intact.

Once flaps of the oral mucosa have been raised, the cuts for the nasal mucosal layer can be performed. Surgical scissors are used to make the incisions as described earlier and by Furlow[40] (**Fig. 14**). Consider preserving a slight cuff of tissues along the hard palate to assist with closure of the nasal layer.

Closure

A 4-0 Vicryl with a PS-4c needle is used to close the layers and perform the Z-plasties in a standard fashion. The nasal layer is closed initially (**Fig. 15**). Avoid excessive retraction and tension on the flaps. If necessary, further release of the flap segments can be performed using a back cut onto the hard palate. After completion of the nasal layer closure, the left-sided myomucosal flap is rotated into place using 3-0 Vicryl sutures through the levator muscle. The oral layer is then closed in the same fashion as the nasal layer (**Fig. 16**). The uvula is closed with a through-and-through horizontal mattress or interrupted sutures along the incision line. The stomach is suctioned and a tongue stitch is placed if there is any concern for an obstructed airway.

Postprocedural Care

Similar to patients who undergo cleft lip repair, in the postoperative period the primary goals include the prevention of wound complications, provision of pain relief, and promotion of adequate nutrition. Each child is monitored in the hospital for at least 1 night to ensure that there is no airway obstruction and to verify the ability to maintain adequate hydration. If a tongue stitch is placed to ensure airway control, it is removed the following morning.

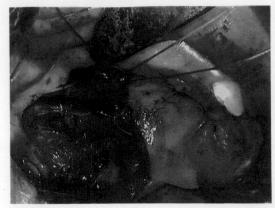

Fig. 15. Closure of the nasal layer during a Furlow palatoplasty.

Arm restraints, to prevent the children from putting their hands in their mouths, are used to protect the palate for 2 weeks. A 1-week course of oral antibiotics is administered. Pain control with the use of acetaminophen and ibuprofen is recommended. The family is counseled to have the child avoid the use of straws and bottle feeding. The child is evaluated in clinic at approximately 3 weeks after surgery. The family is to call or visit the clinic with any concerns.

Potential Complications and Management

Outcomes of success in repairing a cleft palate include complete closure of the oral and nasal layers without a fistula and velopharyngeal competence with speech and feeding. Oronasal fistulas can result in hypernasality, nasal emission, and nasal regurgitation, which typically occur in 10% of patients and usually occur at the junction of the hard and soft palates, but may occur at any point along the surgical lines of closure.

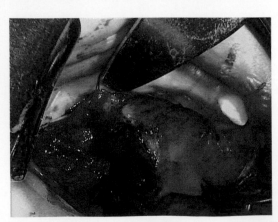

Fig. 14. Intraoperative view after raising the nasal flaps during a Furlow palatoplasty.

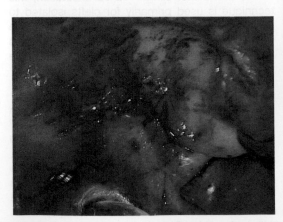

Fig. 16. Completed repair of a cleft palate using a Furlow palatoplasty technique.

Principles of wound closure can assist in preventing this complication, including creating robust flaps, minimizing wound tension, and performing a multilayered closure.[39]

The typical manifestations of velopharyngeal insufficiency, which occur in up to 25% of patients with cleft palate, include hypernasal speech, increased resonance, nasal regurgitation, and nasal emission during phonation.[46] The evaluation of a patient with concern for velopharyngeal insufficiency is best performed by a multispecialty team composed of a speech-language pathologist, otolaryngologist, prosthodontist, and a surgeon trained in velopharyngeal surgery. Multiple surgical and nonsurgical treatment options exist for patients with this condition.[47] A multispecialty team can be helpful in providing patients with the most appropriate treatment of their specific situation.

SUMMARY

Orofacial clefting significantly affects the quality of life of the child involved. The American Cleft Palate – Craniofacial Association recommends a team approach in the management of these patients. Associated congenital anomalies, developmental delay, neurologic disorders, and psychosocial needs should be identified and treated appropriately. A multidisciplinary team can be helpful in ensuring that the child undergoes proper specialty evaluations and in determining the most suitable treatment options. The surgeon should be aware of the needs of the patient and be able to educate and assist the caretakers as necessary. A fundamental understanding of the various options for surgical repair is warranted.

REFERENCES

1. American Cleft Palate-Craniofacial Association. Standards for cleft palate and craniofacial teams. Available at: http://www.acpa-cpf.org/team_care/standards/. Accessed March 31, 2010.
2. Dixon MJ, Marazita ML, Beaty TH, et al. Cleft lip and palate: understanding genetic and environmental influences. Nat Rev Genet 2011;12:167–8.
3. Dyleski RA, Crockett DM. Cleft lip and palate: evaluation and treatment of the primary deformity. In: Bailey BJ, Johnson JT, editors. Head and neck surgery-otolaryngology. 4th edition. Philadelphia: Lippincott Williams & Wilkins; 2006. p. 1317–35.
4. Tessier P. Anatomical classification facial, craniofacial and latero-facial clefts. J Maxillofac Surg 1976;4:69–92.
5. Mulliken JB. Double unilimb z-plastic repair of microform cleft lip. Plast Reconstr Surg 2005;116:1623.
6. Veau V. Bec-de-Liévre; Formes Cliniques–Chirurgie. Avec la collaboration de J Récamier. Paris: Masson et Cie; 1938.
7. Latham RA. Orthopedic advancement of the cleft maxillary segment: a preliminary report. Cleft Palate J 1980;17:227–33.
8. Grayson BH, Cutting CB. Presurgical nasoalveolar orthopedic molding in primary correction on the nose, lip, and alveolus of infants born with unilateral and bilateral clefts. Cleft Palate Craniofac J 2001;38:193–8.
9. Hamilton R, Graham WP, Randall P. The role of the lip adhesion procedure in cleft lip repair. Cleft Palate J 1971;8:1–9.
10. Lorenz HP, Longaker MT. In utero surgery for cleft lip/palate: minimizing the "ripple effect" of scarring. J Craniofac Surg 2003;14:504–11.
11. Wilhelmsen HR, Musgrave RH. Complications of cleft lip surgery. Cleft Palate J 1966;3:223–31.
12. Millard DR Jr. The unilateral deformity. Cleft craft. Boston: Little, Brown; 1976. p. 74.
13. Kapp-Simon KA. Psychological issues in cleft lip and palate. Clin Plast Surg 2004;31:347–52.
14. Thompson JE. An artistic and mathematically accurate method of repairing the defect in cases of harelip. Surg Gynecol Obstet 1912;14:498–504.
15. Tennison CW. The repair of the unilateral cleft lip by the stencil method. Plast Reconstr Surg (1946) 1952;9:115–20.
16. Randall P. A triangular flap operation for the primary repair of unilateral clefts of the lip. Plast Reconstr Surg 1959;23:331–47.
17. Ring WH, Adair JC, Elwyn RA. A new pediatric endotracheal tube. Anesth Analg 1975;54:273–4.
18. Sykes JM. The importance of primary rhinoplasty at the time of initial unilateral cleft repair. Arch Facial Plast Surg 2010;12:53–5.
19. Reinisch JF, Li WY, Urata M. Complications of cleft lip and palate surgery. In: Lossee J, Kirschner RE, editors. Comprehensive cleft care. New York: McGraw-Hill; 2009:chap 29.
20. Millard DR. Closure of bilateral cleft lip and elongation of columella by two operations in infancy. Plast Reconstr Surg 1971;47:324–31.
21. Mulliken JB. Principles and techniques of bilateral complete cleft lip repair. Plast Reconstr Surg 1985; 75:477–87.
22. Cutting C, Grayson B, Brecht L, et al. Presurgical columellar elongation and primary retrograde nasal reconstruction in one-stage bilateral cleft lip and nose repair. Plast Reconstr Surg 1998;101:630–9.
23. Millard DR Jr, Latham R, Xu H, et al. Cleft lip and palate treated by presurgical orthopedics, gingivoperiosteoplasty, and lip adhesion (POPLA) compared with previous lip adhesion method: a preliminary study of serial dental casts. Plast Reconstr Surg 1999;103:1630–44.

24. Millard DR, Latham RA. Improved primary and surgical dental treatment of clefts. Plast Reconstr Surg 1990;86:856.

25. Mulliken JB. Mulliken repair of bilateral cleft lip and nasal deformity. In: Lossee J, Kirschner RE, editors. Comprehensive cleft care. New York: McGraw-Hill; 2009:chap 21.

26. Berkowitz S, Mejia M, Bystrik A. A comparison of the Latham-Millard procedure with those of a conservative treatment approach for dental occlusion and facial aesthetics in unilateral and bilateral complete cleft lip and palate: part I. Dental occlusion. Plast Reconstr Surg 2004;113:1.

27. Chan K, Hayes C, Shusterman S, et al. The effects of active infant orthopedics on occlusal relationships in unilateral complete cleft lip and palate. Cleft Palate Craniofac J 2003;40:511.

28. Tajima S, Maruyama M. Reverse-U incision for secondary repair of cleft lip nose. Plast Reconstr Surg 1977;60:256–61.

29. Trott JA, Mohan N. A preliminary report on one stage open tip rhinoplasty at the time of lip repair in bilateral cleft lip and palate: the Alor Setar experience. Br J Plast Surg 1993;46:215–22.

30. Mulliken JB. Bilateral cleft lip. Clin Plast Surg 2004; 31:209–20.

31. Nakajima T, Yoshimura Y. Secondary correction of bilateral cleft lip nose deformity. J Craniomaxillofac Surg 1990;18:63–7.

32. Pigott RW. Aesthetic considerations related to repair of the bilateral cleft lip nasal deformity. Br J Plast Surg 1988;41:593–607.

33. Ayoub A, Garrahy A, Millett D, et al. Three-dimensional assessment of early surgical outcome in repaired unilateral cleft lip and palate: part 2 lip changes. Cleft Palate Craniofac J 2011;48:578–83.

34. Reddy SG, Reddy RR, Zinser MJ, et al. A comparative study of two different techniques for complete bilateral cleft lip repair using two-dimensional photographic analysis. Plast Reconstr Surg 2013;132:634–42.

35. Mars M, Houston WJ. A preliminary study of facial growth and morphology in unoperated male unilateral cleft lip and palate subjects over 13 years of age. Cleft Palate J 1990;27:7–10.

36. Sommerlad BS. Cleft palate repair. In: Lossee J, Kirschner RE, editors. Comprehensive cleft care. New York: McGraw-Hill; 2009:chap 25.

37. Antony AK, Sloan GM. Airway obstruction following palatoplasty: analysis of 247 consecutive operations. Cleft Palate Craniofac J 2002;39: 145–8.

38. Muntz H, Wilson M, Park A, et al. Sleep disordered breathing and obstructive sleep apnea in the cleft population. Laryngoscope 2008;118:348–53.

39. Allen GC. Cleft palate. In: Goudy SL, Tollefson TT, editors. Complete cleft care. Ahead of publication.

40. Furlow LT. Cleft palate repair by double opposing Z-plasty. Plast Reconstr Surg 1986;78:724–36.

41. Ysunza A, Pamplona M, Mendoza M, et al. Speech outcomes and maxillary growth in patients with unilateral complete cleft lip/palate operated on at 6 versus 12 months of age. Plast Reconstr Surg 1998;102:675–9.

42. Liao YF, Mars M. Hard palate repair timing and facial growth in cleft lip and palate: systematic review. Cleft Palate Craniofac J 2006;43:563–70.

43. Pet MA, Marty-Grames L, Blount-Stahl M, et al. The Furlow palatoplasty for velopharyngeal dysfunction: velopharyngeal changes, speech improvements, and where they intersect. Cleft Palate Craniofac J 2013. [Epub ahead of print].

44. LaRossa D, Hunenko-Jackson O, Kirschner RE, et al. The Childrens Hospital of Philadelphia modification of the Furlow double-opposing Z-palatoplasty: long term speech and growth results. Clin Plast Surg 2004;31:243–50.

45. Furlow LT. Double-opposing Z-plasty palate repair. In: Lossee J, Kirschner RE, editors. Comprehensive cleft care. New York: McGraw-Hill; 2009:chap 23.

46. Woo AS. Velopharyngeal dysfunction. Semin Plast Surg 2012;26:170–7.

47. Ruda JM, Krakovitz P, Rose AS. A review of the evaluation and management of velopharyngeal insufficiency in children. Otolaryngol Clin North Am 2012;45:653–69.

Starting a Cleft Team: A Primer

Randolph B. Capone, MD[a],*, Sydney C. Butts, MD[b], Lamont R. Jones, MD[c]

KEYWORDS

- Cleft lip • Cleft palate • Craniofacial anomaly • Facial plastic surgery • Multidisciplinary cleft team

KEY POINTS

- Care of congenital cleft and craniofacial anomalies is best delivered with multidisciplinary teams led by clinicians with high levels of training and motivation.
- Facial plastic surgeons have the training and expertise to assume leadership positions on multidisciplinary cleft teams.
- Many organizational steps are required to establish a team and to maintain it.
- Formalized parameters have been adopted by the American Cleft Palate-Craniofacial Association for the establishment of teams that describe specialty representation, timing of evaluations, and documentation of clinical activities.
- We present a primer that serves as a guide for developing a team, including the process of needs-assessment, clinician recruitment, and institutional support.

INTRODUCTION

Multidisciplinary, team-based care for patients with congenital cleft and craniofacial anomalies has been a standard format in North America and Europe for more than 70 years.[1–3] Although many teams have been in existence for decades, new teams are encouraged to apply for certification through the American Cleft Palate–Craniofacial Association (ACPA), the largest professional organization representing clinicians that care for patients with orofacial clefts in North America and internationally.[4,5] The ACPA has issued parameters for the establishment and maintenance of cleft and craniofacial teams.[6] Such care requires significant health care resources, because many patients need staged surgery and treatments from infancy until late adolescence.[7–9] Access to expert care must be readily available to prevent treatment delays and their adverse consequences.[9,10]

Otolaryngologists/head and neck surgeons have long provided specialized care for patients with orofacial clefts.[11,12] Over the past few decades, increased interest and expertise in all facets of cleft and craniofacial care have developed among otolaryngologists/head and neck surgeons. Professional societies including the American Academy of Facial Plastic and Reconstructive Surgery (AAFPRS), the American Society of Pediatric Otolaryngology, and the Society for Ear, Nose, and Throat Advances in Children have made the management of cleft and craniofacial anomalies a priority among their members.[13–15] With the efforts of such organizations, greater numbers of facial plastic surgeons and pediatric otolaryngologists are positioned to lead cleft and craniofacial teams and serve local populations in regions where there is a need for this care. Greater domestic participation enhances

a The Department of Otolaryngology - Head and Neck Surgery, Greater Baltimore Cleft Lip and Palate Team, The Johns Hopkins University School of Medicine, 6535 North Charles Street, Suite 220, Baltimore, MD 21204, USA; b The Division of Facial Plastic and Reconstructive Surgery, The Department of Otolaryngology - Head and Neck Surgery, Greater Brooklyn Cleft and Craniofacial Team, The State University of New York, Downstate Medical Center, 450 Clarkson Avenue, Brooklyn, NY 11203, USA; c The Department of Otolaryngology - Head and Neck Surgery, Cleft and Craniofacial Clinic, The Henry Ford Health System, 2799 West Grant Boulevard, Detroit, MI 48202, USA

* Corresponding author. 6535 North Charles Street, Suite 220, Baltimore, MD 21204.
E-mail address: rcapone@jhmi.edu

Facial Plast Surg Clin N Am 22 (2014) 587–591
http://dx.doi.org/10.1016/j.fsc.2014.08.001
1064-7406/14/$ – see front matter © 2014 Elsevier Inc. All rights reserved.

surgeon experience via increased clinical exposure and additional numbers of surgical cases encountered more evenly throughout one's career. This participation also engenders goodwill between the surgeon's institution and the community served.[16]

The Cleft and Craniofacial Subcommittee of the AAFPRS Specialty Surgery Committee makes recommendations for educational and outreach goals related to cleft and craniofacial work. The subcommittee is comprised of surgeons who currently lead US cleft teams domestically and who participate in cleft and craniofacial missions internationally. Many surgeons on the subcommittee are also faculty in residency training programs where comprehensive management of patients with orofacial clefts is emphasized. To assist surgeons interested in starting a cleft team, the subcommittee developed a list of action items believed to be important in the establishment of a cleft team. This article provides surgeons with a guide for assembling a high-quality team, focusing on assessment of clinical need, recruitment of team members, community outreach, and team development.

METHODOLOGY

The authors, who each codirect cleft teams at their home institutions and who are members of the Cleft and Craniofacial Subcommittee of the AAFPRS Specialty Surgery Committee, developed a list of recommendations. The recommendations were circulated to all members of the Subcommittee for feedback and ratification. Current guidelines for multidisciplinary cleft and craniofacial care in the literature served as the basis for many of the recommendations.

RESULTS

A list of 20 recommendations was generated. These recommendations were not ranked in any particular sequence or weighted in order of importance, but were organized into five general categories: (1) surgical training and board certification; (2) identification of clinical need and hospital selection; (3) team format, recruitment, and certification; (4) budget and finance; and (5) marketing.

Surgical Training and Board Certification

Cleft team success relies heavily on clinical ability, surgical skills, and dedication to cleft care. There is no substitute for excellent work. Surgeons should be superbly trained and appropriately board certified (ABFPRS, ABOto). Documentation of appropriate cleft experience (residency, fellowship, and mission caseloads) is a mandatory requirement

to demonstrate proficiency and to obtain surgical privileges for cleft and craniofacial cases. Anyone considering formation of a cleft team should join the ACPA and maintain membership. Attendance at national cleft conferences is advisable. Visits to observe other cleft surgeons are encouraged. It is also important to recognize that it is not essential to start as a team leader; starting as a founding team member is perfectly appropriate.

Identification of Clinical Need and Hospital Selection

The ideal setting for a nascent cleft team is a hospital with a high volume of annual births (>4000), a neonatal intensive care unit (NICU), and the presence of crucial ancillary services including speech-language pathology, nutrition, pediatric dentistry and orthodontics, lactation services, and clinical genetics. The presence of nearby hospitals that do not have a cleft team is helpful for additional referrals.

Cleft team leaders should meet with chairs of clinical departments (pediatrics, plastic surgery, otolaryngology) to discuss the cleft team initiative. These departments are positioned to provide fiscal support, space, and staffing, and also can help identify the optimal physical location for team meetings (clinical examination space and team conference space).

Cleft team leaders should meet with hospital administrators (eg, CEO, director of marketing, director of research, director of development) to explain team goals and how a cleft team can positively impact the community. Meetings with nursing administration should focus on newborn nursery needs, postoperative protocols, and the development of critical pathways and electronic order sets.

Team Format, Recruitment, and Certification

i. Identify and invite a like-minded surgeon to participate equally or to provide mentoring (if someone more experienced). Designate team leaders and codirectors.

ii. Understand and embrace the cleft team concept.[6,8]

iii. Review the ACPA guidelines for a cleft team and make concrete plans to obtain certification within the first 3 to 5 years. The benefits of ACPA certification include listings in the ACPA directory of teams and Web site team locater. Certification also helps significantly with marketing initiatives.

iv. Identify and pick core team members from surgery, orthodontics, speech pathology, social work, pediatrics, genetics, and audiology, and members from related specialties including ophthalmology, oral surgery, and dentistry.

v. Always maintain an attitude of inclusivity with all plastic surgery and oral surgery colleagues.

vi. Meet with your team's key ancillary staff members regularly (eg, speech pathology or audiology) to discuss patient care or interesting new study findings, even if in the early days there are few patients to see. Be careful, however, not to burden them, because they may not share your enthusiasm at first.

vii. Determine a team meeting frequency and format (eg, bimonthly meeting with patient appointments followed by team discussion with care coordination).

viii. Establish clinical goals for your team (eg, a 5-year plan). Such goals as an annual number of new patient encounters and number of surgical cases are very useful. Other goals including publications, additional team member recruitment, and fundraising levels are also recommended.

ix. Develop a patient database and standardize data acquisition. Record patient outcomes. Try to link this database to your team's electronic medical record. Patient outcomes serve as the basis for clinical research.

Budget and Finance

Develop a budget, including such items as educational reference materials, marketing efforts, and team coordinator salary. Costs to support additional needs associated with cleft care including specialty nipples, feeders, and transportation vouchers can be subsidized by the cleft team if there are adequate funds. Fundraising efforts should highlight the costs involved in growing and maintaining a cleft team.

In addition to seeking internal institutional support, identify a list of potential donors (individuals, corporations, foundations) and begin fundraising efforts and grant applications. Multiple fundraising events can be planned that feature members of the cleft team. The recruitment of local figures well known in the community to headline these events is an effective way to increase fundraising success.

Marketing

i. Develop a team name. Create social media accounts. Have the home institution's marketing department create Web pages on the hospital's Web site. Start an independent team Web site and keep content fresh. Develop handouts and a team brochure.

ii. Host simple "meet and greet" events with clinical departments and divisions: NICU, genetics, pediatrics, family medicine, obstetrics and gynecology. Meet their physicians and staff members, hand out brochures, give pertinent contact information and reprints of publications or chapters published by cleft team members.

iii. Be willing to see unrelated consultations and do not expect primary care providers to trust you initially. Revisions, patients with postpalatoplasty velopharyngeal insufficiency, fistulas, and other secondary deformities may make up most initial cases until neonatal referrals become more frequent.

iv. Hold annual team executive meetings to present clinical outcomes and tout academic endeavors. Foster an environment that encourages publishing and presenting. Invite hospital administrators and the team's donors.

v. Strategize marketing plans and be creative. Send the team's cleft coordinator, nurse, or feeding specialist to deliver light food and marketing materials to neighboring NICUs and newborn nurseries. Organize and host a cleft seminar with an invited guest speaker at the home institution, targeting all relevant disciplines in the team's catchment with invitations. Encourage patients, families, and staff to participate in an existing local summer camp for cleft-affected children, or host your own annual team picnic. Identify an energetic team parent (who is happy with their child's outcome) and recruit them to start a local cleft support group, perhaps with the assistance of the team's social worker.

DISCUSSION

The role of the otolaryngologist/head and neck surgeon in cleft and craniofacial teams now routinely includes the reconstructive surgical procedures that patients require throughout the duration of their care. As such, many facial plastic surgeons and pediatric otolaryngologists are poised to assume leadership roles on established cleft and craniofacial teams or to begin new teams. Cleft and craniofacial anomalies represent some of the most prevalent congenital birth defects, yet there may still be areas in which access to multidisciplinary cleft and craniofacial care, the agreed on standard, is suboptimal.[1,2,6,17–20] The availability of surgeons dedicated to the care of these patients should be a high priority for the health care system.

Resident education in otolaryngology/head and neck surgery in the United States includes the management of the care of patients born with congenital craniofacial anomalies, including cleft lip and palate. Additionally, there are an increasing number of fellowships in facial plastic and reconstructive surgery and pediatric otolaryngology that offer strong training in this area, producing individuals skilled in the management of orofacial clefts. On completion of training, all surgeons often face challenges in generating adequate patient referrals, and cleft referrals are no exception. Some providers jettison this part of their practice or alternatively supplement their experience with participation in mission trips abroad. Contemporary management of orofacial clefts, however, ideally warrants homogeneous, year-round experiences. For individuals with serious interest in providing quality cleft care, participation in an established cleft team at a local institution is mandatory.

Many established teams are located at large academic centers with well-established referral patterns. Opportunities to participate with such teams are infrequent because they have little need for additional surgeons given their surgical volumes. The expansion of cleft care in the United States with the formation of additional, high-quality teams is an opportunity for facial plastic surgeons to work with hospitals that possess many of the resources that could support this work, but have never had a clinical leader to spearhead such an initiative. The present work offers guidelines for motivated surgeons who care deeply about practicing cleft care with similarly minded individuals and who desire to provide care commensurate with standards set forth by the ACPA.

SUMMARY

Clinical expertise is the primary qualification for leading a cleft and craniofacial team. Successful teams also implement organizational and outreach strategies to thrive. The establishment of a cleft team at a domestic medical center can provide multiple benefits for the community served, the team's members, the medical center itself, and even the recipients of charity mission work abroad. With diligence, ample forethought, preparation, and networking, surgeons with appropriate cleft training can use the 20 recommendations presented here from the Cleft and Craniofacial Subcommittee of the Specialty Surgery Committee of the American Academy of Facial Plastic and Reconstructive Surgery to develop a local team of experts to provide superlative care to children with congenital facial malformations.

ACKNOWLEDGMENTS

The authors have no conflicts of interest, including financial interests, activities, relationships, or affiliations. No grants or financial support were received for this work. The authors thank Dr S.A. Tatum III and Dr J.M. Sykes for their thoughtful review and constructive comments, and Mrs A.H. Jenne for her administrative assistance.

REFERENCES

1. Long R. Improving outcomes for the patient with cleft lip and palate: The team concept and 70 years of experience in cleft care. The Journal of Lancaster General Hospital 2009;4(2):52–6.
2. Strauss RP. ACPA Team Standards Committee. Cleft palate and craniofacial teams in the United States and Canada: a national survey of team organization and standards of care. Cleft Palate Craniofac J 1998;35(6):473–80.
3. Bill J, Proff P, Bayerlein T, et al. Treatment of patients with cleft lip, alveolus and palate–a short outline of history and current interdisciplinary treatment approaches. J Craniomaxillofac Surg 2006;34(Suppl 2): 17–21.
4. Commision on Approval of Teams. Standards for Approval of Cleft Palate and Craniofacial Teams. Available at: www.acpa-cpf.com. Updated March, 2010. Accessed January 15, 2014.
5. Richman LC. President's perceptions: an historic review of fifty years of the American Cleft Palate-Craniofacial Association. Cleft Palate Craniofac J 1993;30(6):521–7.
6. American Cleft Palate-Craniofacial Association. Parameters for evaluation and treatment of patients with cleft lip/palate or other craniofacial anomalies. Cleft Palate Craniofac J 1993;30(Supp 1):S1–16. revised 2009. Available at: http://www.acpa-cpf. org/uploads/site/Parameters_Rev_2009.pdf. Accessed August 27, 2014.
7. Chuo CB, Searle Y, Jeremy A, et al. The continuing multidisciplinary needs of adult patients with cleft lip and/or palate. Cleft Palate Craniofac J 2008; 45(6):633–8.
8. Capone RB, Sykes JM. The cleft and craniofacial team: the whole is greater than the sum of its parts. Facial Plast Surg 2007;23(2):83–6.
9. New York State Department of Health. Congenital malformations registry summary report: statistical summary of children born in 2005 and diagnosed through 2007. New York: Congenital Malformations Registry, New York State Department of Health Center for Environmental Health, Bureau of Environmental and Occupational Epidemiology; 2008. Available at: http://www.health.ny.gov/diseases/ congenital_malformations/2005/docs/2005_report. pdf. Accessed August 27, 2014.
10. Austin AA, Druschel CM, Tyler MC, et al. Interdisciplinary craniofacial teams compared with individual providers: is orofacial cleft care more comprehensive

and do parents perceive better outcomes? Cleft Palate Craniofac J 2010;47(1):1–8.

11. Smith LK, Gubbels SP, MacArthur CJ, et al. The effect of the palatoplasty method on the frequency of ear tube placement. Arch Otolaryngol Head Neck Surg 2008;134(10):1085–9.

12. Drake AF, Rosenthal LH. Otolaryngologic challenges in cleft/craniofacial care. Cleft Palate Craniofac J 2013;50(6):734–43.

13. Available at: www.aspo.us. Accessed January 15, 2014.

14. Available at: www.sentac.org. Accessed January 15, 2014.

15. Available at: www.aafprs.org. Accessed January 15, 2014.

16. Tolarová MM, Poulton D, Aubert MM, et al. Pacific Craniofacial Team and Cleft Prevention Program. J Calif Dent Assoc 2006;34(10):823–30.

17. Jaju R, Tate AR. The role of pediatric dentistry in multidisciplinary cleft palate teams at advanced pediatric dental residency programs. Pediatr Dent 2009;31(3):188–92.

18. Laub DR Jr, Ajar AH. A survey of multidisciplinary cleft palate and craniofacial team examination formats. J Craniofac Surg 2012;23(4):1002–4.

19. Vargervik K, Oberoi S, Hoffman WY. Team care for the patient with cleft: UCSF protocols and outcomes. J Craniofac Surg 2009;20(Suppl 2):1668–71.

20. Wellens W, Vander Poorten V. Keys to a successful cleft lip and palate team. B-ENT 2006;2(Suppl 4):3–10.

Surgical Speech Disorders

Tianjie Shen, MD[a], Kathleen C.Y. Sie, MD[b,c],*

KEYWORDS

- Ankyloglossia • Frenotomy • Frenuloplasty • Velopharyngeal insufficiency
- Velopharyngeal dysfunction • Pharyngoplasty • Furlow palatoplasty

KEY POINTS

- Frenotomy is a common procedure treating ankyloglossia in infants with thin frenulum.
- The incision needs to be carried posteriorly until the tongue is sufficiently released before closing with interrupted sutures.
- Complete clinical history, including speech, communication, swallowing, airway, and sleep symptoms, is important in velopharyngeal insufficiency management.
- A team using a standardized approach should evaluate the patient and perceptual speech assessment should be conducted by a qualified speech pathologist to provide speech differential diagnosis.
- Furlow palatoplasty can optimize the levator veli palatini (LVP) muscular function and increase the length of the palate, and sphincter pharyngoplasty is best suited for patients with transverse orientation of LVP and poor lateral wall movement.

OVERVIEW

Speech is one of the main forms of communication. Speech production is a complex motor activity that requires generation of air pressure (respiratory control), vocal function (phonation), articulation, motor planning, and velopharyngeal (VP) function. Coordination of these components is needed to produce intelligible speech.[1,2] Most speech delays, such as dysfluency, articulation errors, and childhood apraxia of speech, are treated with speech therapy. However, 2 conditions, ankyloglossia and VP dysfunction (VPD), may require surgical intervention for their associated speech symptoms. This article discusses the surgical management of ankyloglossia and VPD.

ANKYLOGLOSSIA

There are several important structures required for correct articulation. The most important active articulator is the tongue. Ankyloglossia is a condition associated with a shortened lingual frenulum that restricts movement of the tongue tip. The clinical phenotypes vary from mild abnormalities to complete ankyloglossia in which the tongue is fused to the floor of the mouth (**Fig. 1**).

Symptoms of ankyloglossia may include breastfeeding difficulties, speech disorders, or problems with deglutition and dentition. Any of these symptoms may be an indication for surgical management. During infancy breastfeeding may be the most salient symptom. Ankyloglossia in infants is associated with a 25% to 60% incidence of difficulties with breastfeeding, including failure to thrive and maternal breast pain. Studies have shown that, for every day of maternal pain during the initial 3 weeks of breastfeeding, there is a 10% to 26% risk of cessation of breastfeeding.[3]

Speech production is another common indication for surgery. The effect of ankyloglossia on speech has been a subject of debate. Some children with tongue-tie are able to develop normal speech without treatment, whereas others have articulation difficulties. The speech problems associated with ankyloglossia are typically the

[a] Department of Otolaryngology Head and Neck Surgery, Kaiser San Francisco, 4131 Geary Boulevard, San Francisco, CA 94118, USA; [b] Department of Otolaryngology-Head and Neck Surgery, University of Washington, 1959 Pacific Avenue Northeast, Seattle, WA 98195, USA; [c] Division of Pediatric Otolaryngology, Childhood Communication Center, Seattle Children's Hospital, 4800 Sand Point Way Northeast, Seattle, WA 98105, USA
* Corresponding author. Division of Pediatric Otolaryngology, Childhood Communication Center, Seattle Children's Hospital, 4800 Sand Point Way Northeast, Seattle, WA 98105.
E-mail addresses: kathysie@uw.edu; kathleen.sie@seattlechildrens.org

Facial Plast Surg Clin N Am 22 (2014) 593–609
http://dx.doi.org/10.1016/j.fsc.2014.07.010
1064-7406/14/$ – see front matter © 2014 Elsevier Inc. All rights reserved.

facialplastic.theclinics.com

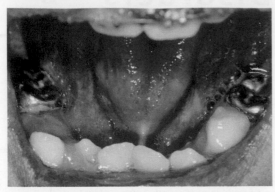

Fig. 1. Ankyloglossia with thick frenulum that requires frenuloplasty. (*From* Anatomy & Physiology for Speech, Language, and Hearing by J. A. Seikel, D. King, & D. Drumright, 2010, 4E. Copyright © 2010 Delmar Learning, a part of Cengage Learning, Inc. Reproduced with permission.)

production of lingual dental sounds (such as t, d) and sibilants (such as z, s, th). Up to one-half of young children with ankyloglossia referred for otolaryngology evaluation have articulation difficulties.[4] The 2 main surgical approaches are frenotomy and frenuloplasty.

FRENOTOMY

The most common treatment of ankyloglossia in infants is frenotomy by incising a few millimeters into the lingual frenulum when it is thin. Frenotomy can be performed at the bedside or in the clinic with or without topical anesthesia. In general, the discomfort associated with release of thin frenulum is very brief. If desired, oral sucrose solution may be given a few minutes before the procedure to provide short-term analgesia.

The infant is positioned directly in front of the surgeon. Fingers or a groove retractor is placed on either side of the frenulum, and the ventral surface of the tongue is exposed. A hemostat is used to clamp the frenulum in order to reduce bleeding. Iris scissors are used to divide the frenulum. Care is taken to avoid injury to the submandibular ducts. Two or more sequential cuts may be needed to accomplish a complete release. The incision does not require sutures. Feeding is allowed immediately after the procedure. Bleeding is generally scant and controlled with pressure or breastfeeding. Complications associated with this procedure are usually negligible.

FRENULOPLASTY

In older children, frenuloplasty with sutures is generally performed to allow a more complete release. Local anesthesia in clinic may be considered for cooperative older children. If surgery is deferred until the child is more than 1 year old or the frenulum is thick, general anesthesia is normally preferred. When general anesthesia is used, intermittent mask ventilation is usually sufficient. Local anesthetic with epinephrine can be infiltrated at the surgical site to improve hemostasis and postprocedure pain. The tongue is retracted superiorly with a groove retractor or a penetrating clamp to expose the frenulum. The frenulum is sharply divided in a horizontal fashion to the level of ventral tongue. This division creates a diamond-shaped defect. The incision needs to be carried posteriorly until the tongue is sufficiently released to allow protrusion. Hemostasis is obtained with electrical cautery. The defect is then closed in a vertical fashion with interrupted absorbable sutures. For more severe ankyloglossia, Z-plasty reconstruction of the floor of the mouth may be considered. Prophylactic antibiotics are not prescribed because infection is rare.

VPD

VPD results in failure of the VP port to close appropriately during speech production. It is characterized by hypernasal resonance and nasal air emissions. VPD includes VP incompetence, VP mislearning, and VP insufficiency (VPI).

VP incompetence is caused by poor motor speech function despite adequate anatomy. Patients with VP incompetence are likely to improve with speech therapy. VP mislearning includes disordered speech behaviors such as compensatory misarticulations in spite of normal VP anatomy and function. VPI is caused by incomplete closure of the VP port during speech production.

Cleft palate is the most common congenital anomaly associated with VPI.[5] Unrepaired cleft palate predictably results in VPI. Speech production is the main indication for cleft palate repair. Patients who undergo cleft palate repair remain at risk for developing VPI, particularly if the misaligned soft palate musculature is not addressed, resulting in a situation similar to submucous cleft palate. The estimated frequency of VPI after cleft palate repair ranges from 10% to 40%.[5–7] Increased palatal cleft width may be associated with a higher risk of VPI after palate repair.[6]

Submucous cleft palate can also cause VPI. Submucous cleft palate is defined by the presence of bifid uvula, a bony notch at the caudal edge of the hard palate, and a translucent zone in the midline of the soft palate caused by the sagittal orientation of the LVP muscles. The abnormal insertion of levator palatini muscles may be associated with inadequate elevation of the soft palate during speech, which results in incomplete VP closure. The estimated frequency of VPI in patients with submucous cleft palate is around 25%.[8] Speech symptoms are the main indicators for repair of submucous cleft palate.

VP ANATOMY AND PHYSIOLOGY

It is important to understand the normal anatomy and physiology of VP closure when treating patients with VPD. The soft palate and pharyngeal muscle play an important role in normal speech production. Complete VP closure is required to direct the airflow to oral articulation muscles during production of nonnasal sounds.

The 5 major muscles that comprise the palatal apparatus are levator veli palatini (LVP), tensor veli palatini (TVP), palatoglossus, palatopharyngeus (PP), and muscularis uvulae. Other muscles,

including the salpingopharyngeus and superior pharyngeal constrictors (SPC), also contribute to the lateral and posterior pharyngeal wall movements (**Fig. 2**).

The LVP muscle is one of the most important muscles for VP closure. It originates from the eustachian tube and inserts into the midline palatal aponeurosis at an oblique angle. The fibers of LVP muscles create a dynamic sling in order to suspend the velum from the skull base. Its force of contraction pulls the velum both posteriorly and laterally.

The TVP muscle originates from the medial pterygoid palate and the lateral eustachian tube. It inserts into the palatal aponeurosis and the horizontal plate of the palatine bone. Its contraction tenses the palate. Because TVP is an important muscle in equilibrating the middle ear pressure, patients with VPD frequently have eustachian

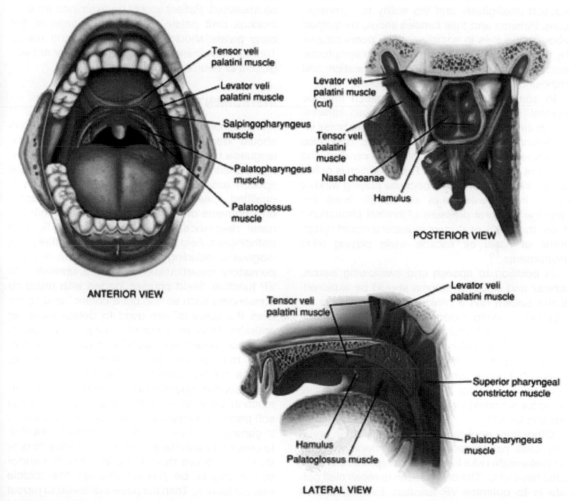

Fig. 2. Muscles of the VP mechanism: the 5 major muscles that comprise the palatal apparatus are LVP, TVP, palatoglossus, PP, and uvulae. (*From* David LJ. The basics of velopharyngeal function: a brief review for the practicing clinician. Perspect Speech Sci Orofac Disord 2012;22:28; with permission.)

tube dysfunction caused by the abnormal insertion of TVP.

The PP muscle originates from the velum and inserts into the thyroid cartilage. It defines the posterior tonsillar pillar. Contraction of PP and SPC muscles pulls the lateral pharyngeal wall medially. The SPC muscle forms a hemisphincter that is closely associated with the PP muscle at the VP isthmus. Its contraction pulls the lateral and posterior pharyngeal walls both medially and anteriorly.

PATIENT ASSESSMENT

The initial patient evaluation starts with complete clinical history, focusing on speech and communication. Information about a child's ability to communicate in the setting of school and home can be acquired through family members. Important areas of discussion include the degree of speech intelligibility and the ability to communicate. Patients and their families should be queried about difficulties in socializing with peers caused by the speech issue. Other nonspeech symptoms, such as nasal regurgitation, nasal congestion, and rhinosinusitis, should also be discussed.

In some older patients, the speech may be normal. However, the ability to sustain intraoral pressure for activities like playing wind or brass instruments is compromised. Patients may also describe difficulties in blowing out candles and may not be able to whistle. This condition is called stress VP incompetence, because playing wind or brass instruments takes up to 30 times the average intraoral pressure of normal phonation.[9] More than 30% of student musicians report symptoms of nasal air escape while playing wind instruments.[10]

In addition to speech and swallowing issues, airway and sleep symptoms should be explored. If the patient has a clinical history equivocal for obstructive sleep apnea, an overnight sleep study may help to determine the severity of the sleep problems. The patients and their families should understand that the VPI management might make obstructive symptoms worse. Medical intervention or surgical management of obstructive symptoms should be addressed before the intervention for VPI.

Other important medical history, such as previous cleft palate repair or adenoidectomy, may also elucidate risks for VPI. All unrepaired cleft palates have VPD. The main reason to repair cleft palate is to optimize VP function. Even after cleft palate repair, these patients remain at risk for postoperative VPI. Adenoidectomy has also been associated with the development of VPI, especially in patients with unrecognized submucous cleft palate. The incidence of speech alteration after adenoidectomy has been reported to be 1 in 1200.

The medical history may also help identify previously undiagnosed syndromes. The most common genetic syndrome associated with VPD is 22q11.2 deletion or velocardiofacial syndrome (VCFS), which is associated with deletion or duplication of a variable portion of the long arm of chromosome 22. Patients with VCFS often have palatal abnormalities, heart defects, characteristic facial appearance, and learning disabilities. It has been estimated that 75% of patients with VCFS have some degree of VPD.[11,12]

A compete head and neck examination should be a part of the initial physical assessment. Intraoral examination provides information on the LVP muscle movement, tonsil size, palate function, tongue mobility, dentition, and occlusion. The status of both primary and secondary palate should be assessed. Patient should be examined for submucous cleft palate. The caudal margin of the bony palate should be palpated for the notch. Tongue movement should be checked for ankyloglossia or neuromuscular disorder.

INSTRUMENTAL ASSESSMENT

The diagnosis of VPI can be difficult. Surgeons should ideally collaborate with skilled speech-language pathologists when assessing and managing children with speech disorders. Perceptual speech assessment should be conducted by a qualified speech-language pathologist, focusing on judgments of articulation, speech intelligibility, nasal resonance, and nasal emission. Speech pathologists help to provide speech differential diagnosis, including speech mislearning or compensatory misarticulations that are unrelated to VP function. Short phrases loaded with pressure consonants such as "Go get a cookie" and "Suzy sees the scissors" are used to detect nasal air emission. In the presence of hyponasal resonance, nasal consonants such as "Mama made some mittens" may become nonnasalized. For example, "Mama" would sound more like "Baba."

Nasoendoscopy is regularly used to assess VP function by examining the nasal aspect of the soft palate and pharynx during speech production. In general, children more than 3 years old are able to cooperate with the examination. In order to provide a bird's-eye view of the VP port, the endoscope should be passed through the middle meatus (**Box 1**). Then the patient is asked to repeat oral and nasal loaded speech samples to assess VP function. During nasoendoscopy, the presence of a Passavant ridge and the size of the adenoid

Box 1
Pediatric Voice Outcome Survey

1. In general, how would you say your child's speaking voice is?
   - Excellent
   - Good
   - Adequate
   - Poor or inadequate
   - My child has no voice

The following items ask about activities that your child might do in a given day.

2. To what extent does your child's voice limit his or her ability to be understood in a noisy area?
   - Limited a lot
   - Limited a little
   - Not limited at all

3. During the past 2 weeks, to what extent has your child's voice interfered with his or her normal social activities or with his or her school?
   - Not at all
   - Slightly
   - Moderately
   - Quite a bit
   - Extremely

4. Do you find your child straining to speak because of his or her voice problem?
   - Not at all
   - A little bit
   - Moderately
   - Quite a bit
   - Extremely

pad can be observed. The presence of a notch or a groove on the nasal surface of the palate is an indication for the sagittal orientation of the LVP musculature, as in a submucous cleft palate. Nasoendoscopy helps to verify the presence of VPI, to assess the status of LVP musculature, and to characterize the degree of lateral pharyngeal wall and palatal motions.

The estimation of the degree of VP closure is important to optimize surgical outcome (**Fig. 3**). A universal, standardized reporting system for VP function was proposed.[13,14] The lateral wall and palatal movement during the nasoendoscopy can be classified using the International Working Group Scale as described by Golding-Kushner and colleagues. This scale has good intrarater and inter-rater reliability.[15] For lateral wall movement, 0 indicates no movement, and 0.5 means movement to the midline. For palatal movement, 0 signifies no movement, and 1.0 indicates movement to the posterior pharyngeal wall. The posterior wall movement is described with the same scale from 0 to 1.0, with 1.0 signifying the movement to meet the soft palate.[14]

After initial nasoendoscopy to determine the VP port closure, videofluoroscopy may be helpful to determine the surgical approach. During the videofluoroscopy, barium drops are placed into the nose, then the anterior-posterior and lateral images are recorded. The speech pathologist at our institution rates the lateral wall motion on the anterior-posterior projection. The lateral view can show the level of attempted palatal closure. In addition to anatomic information, videofluoroscopy also helps to diagnose abnormal speech patterns, such as tongue backing instead of active palate elevation.

Information provided by nasoendoscopy and videofluoroscopy can be complementary. Sometimes videofluoroscopy may show adequate VP closure on lateral images, but patients with clinical VPI may have nasoendoscopy evidence of VP gap.[16] The correlation in findings of these two examinations has been shown to be between 70% and 75%.[17] The information from both nasoendoscopy and videofluoroscopy can be used to plan the surgical approach. If patients have persistent VPI after speech surgery, instrumental assessment is repeated.

Nonvisualizing assessments include nasometry. Nasometry is designed to measure the aerodynamic characteristics of VP function. The ratio of nasal to oral energy during the production of oral and nasal loaded speech samples is reported as a nasalance score. Increased nasal energy results in a higher nasalance score. It may be useful in assessing the degrees of improvement after the VPI surgery.

Another indirect evaluation of VP function is to measure the extent of nasal airflow during speech with pressure-flow device.[18] Measurements are obtained during the production of high-pressure oral consonants with repeated words or blowing tasks for younger children. There is normally no nasal airflow during the production of nonnasal phonemes. The presence of nasal airflow produces detectable changes in intraoral pressures. VP orifice area can be calculated in millimeters squared.[19]

A combination of these assessments can define the extent of VPI in order to guide the type of

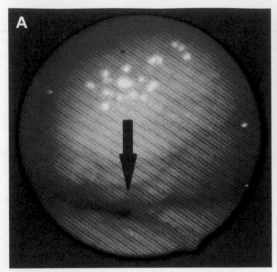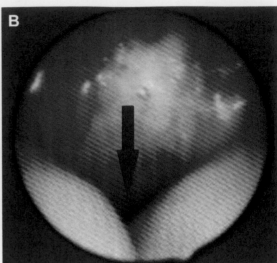

Fig. 3. Nasoendoscopy provides a bird's-eye view of the VP port. (*A*) Small VP gap and prominent adenoid pad. (*B*) Deep dorsal palatal notch (*arrow*). The presence of a notch on the nasal surface of the palate is an indication for the sagittal orientation of the LVP musculature.

intervention needed to correct it. The clinical variables, perceptual speech assessment, and instrumental assessments can help to optimize speech outcomes and minimize risks.

QUALITY-OF-LIFE EVALUATION TOOLS

Several tools have been described to provide voice-related quality of life (VRQOL) measures in the pediatric population. The Pediatric Voice Outcome Survey (PVOS) is a 4-item instrument designed to measure VRQOL. It has been validated to measure functional outcomes of the surgical intervention for VPI.[20] It can be easily administered to determine the overall functional outcome (see **Box 1**).

The VPI Quality-of-Life instrument (VPIQL) provides a condition-specific measure. Although it was developed to evaluate the many ways that VPI affects children's lives, its 48-item questionnaire may make this instrument too burdensome for clinical use. The VPI Effects on Life Outcomes (VELO) is a 23-item instrument that was condensed from the VPIQL (**Fig. 4**). It has 6 domains: speech limitation, swallowing problems, situational difficulty, emotional impact, perception by others, and caregiver impact. It has been shown to provide excellent internal consistency, reliable discriminant validity, and good correlation with the Pediatric Quality of Life inventory (PedsQL™).[21,22]

Although both nasal endoscopy and perceptual speech analysis are essential in assessing patients with VPI, perceptual speech analysis results have a better correlation with quality of life (QOL) in young children, whereas nasoendoscopy may be better in older children.[22]

MANAGEMENT

Speech therapy should be considered for patients with non–VP-related speech disorders such as VP mislearning. Patients with VPI are most likely to benefit from physical intervention such as obturator or speech surgery. Here this article focuses on surgical management to correct the structure of the VP port.

Pierre Franco, a sixteenth-century surgeon, noticed that plugging the cleft palate with cotton resulted in more intelligible speech. Later surgeons such as Passavant (1862) designed different procedures to restore a competent VP mechanism. Passavant designed an early pharyngoplasty with a posterior pharyngeal flap. Sphincter pharyngoplasty was first introduced by Hynes in 1950 and was further modified by other surgeons.

During the last century, the widespread use of flexible nasoendoscopy significantly improved VPI diagnosis. The movement of pharyngeal walls and palate can be measured objectively. Traditional techniques have consequently been modified to produce optimal results.[2,23,24] Numerous surgical procedures, such as Furlow double Z-plasty palatoplasty, sphincter pharyngoplasty, and pharyngeal flap, have been advocated.

SURGICAL TECHNIQUES

There are several surgical techniques to correct VPI. These surgical interventions are intended to

A

In the past **four weeks**, how much of a **problem** has your child had with (circle one for each question):

	Never	Almost Never	Sometimes	Often	Almost Always
Speech Limitations (problems with...)					
1. Air comes out his or her nose when talking	0	1	2	3	4
2. Runs out of breath when talking	0	1	2	3	4
3. Difficulty speaking in long sentences	0	1	2	3	4
4. Speech is too weak	0	1	2	3	4
5. Difficulty being understood when in a hurry	0	1	2	3	4
6. Speech gets worse toward the end of the day	0	1	2	3	4
7. Speech sounds different than other kids	0	1	2	3	4
Swallowing Problems (problems with...)					
8. Liquids come from the nose while drinking	0	1	2	3	4
9. Solid food comes from the nose while eating	0	1	2	3	4
10. Others make fun of my child when food or liquids escape through the nose	0	1	2	3	4
Situational Difficulty (problems with...)					
11. Speech is difficult for strangers to understand	0	1	2	3	4
12. Speech is difficult for friends to understand	0	1	2	3	4
13. Speech is difficult for family to understand	0	1	2	3	4
14. Difficulty being understood when not speaking face to face, eg, as in a car	0	1	2	3	4
15. Difficulty being understood on the phone	0	1	2	3	4
Emotional Impact (problems with...)					
16. Teased because of speech	0	1	2	3	4
17. Child gets sad because of speech	0	1	2	3	4
18. Gets frustrated or gives up when he or she is not understood	0	1	2	3	4
19. Is shy or withdrawn because of speech	0	1	2	3	4
Perception by Others (problems with...)					
20. Treated as if he or she is not very bright because of speech	0	1	2	3	4
21. Others ignore my child because of his or her speech	0	1	2	3	4
22. Others do not like to talk on the phone with my child because of his or her speech	0	1	2	3	4
23. Family or friends tend to speak for my child	0	1	2	3	4
Caregiver Impact (problems with...)					
24. I am worried or concerned about my child's speech	0	1	2	3	4
25. I find it difficult to understand my child	0	1	2	3	4
26. My child's speech problem slows me down or inconveniences me	0	1	2	3	4

Fig. 4. (*A*) The VELO: parental report for children. (*B*) VELO: youth report.

improve VP function and minimize hypernasal resonance.[25] Surgical options can be divided into 3 categories: palatal, pharyngeal, and palatopharyngeal procedures based on the goal of the surgeries.

Palatal procedures include veloplasty, palatal push back, palate rerepair, and double opposing Z-plasty. The goal of palatal procedures is to increase the length of the palate in order to contribute to the VP closure. These procedures can optimize the muscular palate function with a low risk of airway obstruction.[26] Furlow double opposing Z-plasty is a procedure that is particularly well

B

In the past **four weeks**, how much of a **problem** has this been for you (circle one answer for each question):

	Never	Almost Never	Sometimes	Often	Almost Always
Talking (problems with...)					
1. Air comes out my nose when I talk	0	1	2	3	4
2. I run out of breath when I talk	0	1	2	3	4
3. It is hard talking in long sentences	0	1	2	3	4
4. My speech is too weak	0	1	2	3	4
5. I have trouble being understood when I'm in a hurry	0	1	2	3	4
6. My speech gets worse toward the end of the day	0	1	2	3	4
7. My speech sounds different than other kids	0	1	2	3	4
Swallowing (problems with...)					
8. Liquids come out my nose while drinking	0	1	2	3	4
9. Food comes out my nose while eating	0	1	2	3	4
10. Others make fun of me when food or liquids come out my nose	0	1	2	3	4
Times when I have trouble (problems with...)					
11. My speech is hard for strangers to understand	0	1	2	3	4
12. My speech is hard for friends to understand	0	1	2	3	4
13. My speech is hard for family to understand	0	1	2	3	4
14. I have trouble being understood when others can't see my face, for example, in a car	0	1	2	3	4
15. I have trouble being understood on the phone	0	1	2	3	4
How I feel (problems with...)					
16. I am teased because of how I talk	0	1	2	3	4
17. I get sad because of how I talk	0	1	2	3	4
18. I get frustrated or give up when I am not understood	0	1	2	3	4
19. I am shy because of how I talk	0	1	2	3	4
How others feel about me (problems with...)					
20. I am treated like I am not smart because of how I talk	0	1	2	3	4
21. Others ignore me because of how I talk	0	1	2	3	4
22. Others do not like to talk on the phone with me because of how I talk	0	1	2	3	4
23. My family or friends tend to talk for me	0	1	2	3	4

Fig. 4. (continued)

suited for patients with abnormal orientation of the LVP. Furlow Z-plasty not only helps to reposition the LVP but also increases the length and thickness of the velum.

Pharyngeal procedures include pharyngoplasty, such as lateral pharyngeal myomucosal flaps. There are many variations of pharyngoplasty described in the literature.[27–30] The most popular procedure involves the creation of 2 superiorly based lateral pharyngeal myomucosal flaps that are rotated to the level of the VP to create a narrowed single, central port. The sphincter pharyngoplasty is best suited for patients with poor lateral wall movement. The term sphincter remains controversial, because there is no clear evidence that the muscle in the flaps develops sphincteric function. Other techniques that can be included in the category of pharyngoplasty are pharyngeal augmentation and injections. There are attempts in the literature to compare outcomes using randomized controlled prospective studies. However, these studies failed to show significant differences, partially because of the small sample sizes with inadequate statistical power.[29,31]

Palatopharyngeal procedures involve attachment of the pharyngeal constrictor muscles to the velum to create 2 lateral ports. One example of a palatopharyngeal procedure is the posterior pharyngeal flap. It was initially designed for the management of cleft palate. The superiorly based pharyngeal flap was later described for the surgical treatment of postpalatoplasty VPI. The pharyngeal flap is best suited for patients with large VP defects but adequate lateral pharyngeal motion. This procedure is appealing to many surgeons because the width of the flap may be modified to the size of the VP port insufficiency to achieve a successful result. For some surgeons, it is the workhorse of VPI management.

HOW WE DO IT

We have established the Seattle Protocol to systematize VPI management at Seattle Children's Hospital.[2] The goal of our protocol is to standardize our description of speech and VP function with instrumental assessment. In addition, this protocol helps to guide our selection for surgical procedures (**Fig. 5**).

Patients undergo standardized perceptual speech analysis in order to provide speech differential diagnosis. After the perceptual speech assessment, the instrumental assessment is used to determine the pattern and the degree of VP closure. Nasoendoscopy is performed by an otolaryngologist and a speech pathologist. The position of LVP and degree of VP closure are recorded by applying the International Working Group Scale (**Fig. 6**).[13,32] If the patient has obstructive sleep apnea, we usually prefer to perform tonsillectomy and adenoidectomy before speech surgery.

The selection criteria for the surgical options are based on the instrumental assessment (**Fig. 7**). If the patient has a notch on the dorsal surface of palate suggesting sagittal orientation of LVP, we recommend Furlow palatoplasty to reorient the LVP. Studies showed that in patients with VPI caused by the LVP sagittal orientation, the restoration of the normal LVP position has a high success rate.[33–35] In addition to restoring LVP position, Furlow palatoplasty also increases the palatal length. Patients with submucosal cleft palate and previously repaired cleft palate are frequently candidates for Furlow palatoplasty. For patients with small VP gaps, the success rate with Furlow palatoplasty can be higher than 90%.

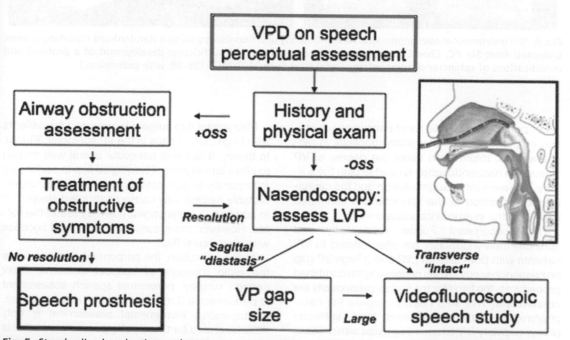

Fig. 5. Standardized evaluation and assessment protocol for patients with VPI at Seattle Children's Hospital.

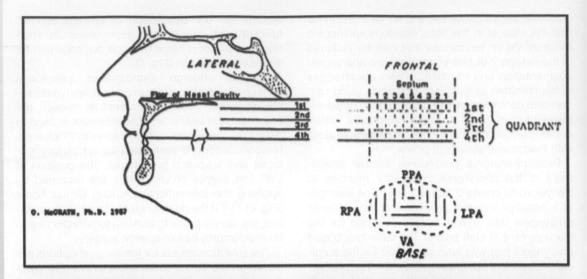

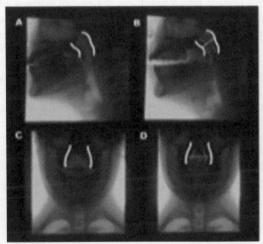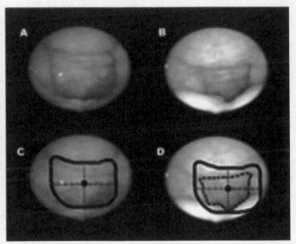

Fig. 6. VPI instrumental assessments with nasoendoscopy and fluoroscopy using a standardized reporting system. (*Adapted from* Sie KC, Chen E. Management of velopharyngeal insufficiency: development of a protocol and modifications of sphincter pharyngoplasty. Facial Plast Surg 2007;23(2):128–39; with permission.)

For patients with evidence of transverse orientation of LVP, the sphincter pharyngoplasty is recommended. Information about the degree of VP closure on nasoendoscopy is used to plan the surgery. The amount of augmentation and the cephalocaudal position of the sphincter are estimated based on the instrumental assessments.

The concomitant Furlow palatoplasty and sphincter pharyngoplasty are often offered to VPI patients with both sagittal LVP and a large VP gap on nasoendoscopy. When performing the combined procedures, the flaps for the Furlow palatoplasty are created first. This step helps to expose the nasopharynx for better visualization. Next, sphincter pharyngoplasty is performed as usual with mucosa closure, and the palatal flaps are closed.

Pharyngeal flap surgery is indicated for patients with large central gaps in the VP sphincter (**Fig. 8**). In theory, it requires adequate lateral wall motion to close lateral ports. Pharyngeal flap is performed infrequently in our institution, because its unpredictable healing may cause obstructed sleep.[27,28] In addition, the pharyngeal flap may tether the palate. However, many surgeons have good success with pharyngeal flap.

At our institution, the perceptual assessment is the main measure of surgical outcome. After speech surgery, perceptual speech assessment is performed at 3 months, and annually thereafter. Postoperative instrumental assessment is only recommended for those patients who have clinical evidence of VPI.

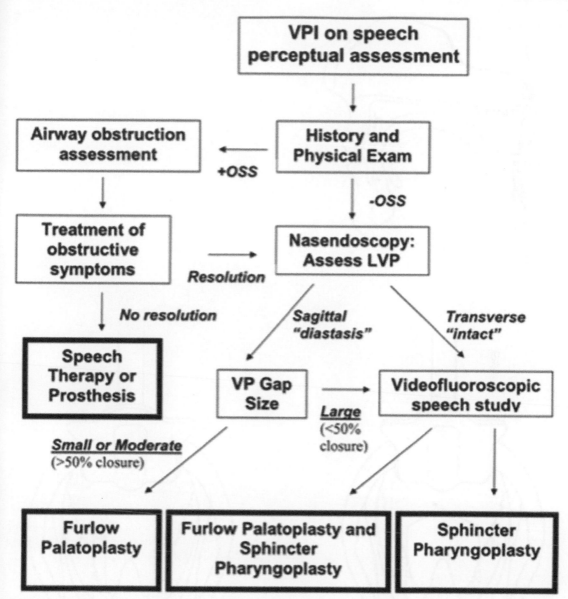

Fig. 7. Standardized VPI management protocol at Seattle Children's Hospital. OSS, obstructive sleep symptoms. (*From* Sie KC, Chen E. Management of velopharyngeal insufficiency: development of a protocol and modifications of sphincter pharyngoplasty. Facial Plast Surg 2007;23(2):128–39; with permission.)

FURLOW PALATOPLASTY

This surgical technique was initially described by Dr Leonard Furlow (**Fig. 9**).[36] A Dingman retractor is used for optimal exposure. After infiltrating the muscular palate with local anesthetic, the oral Z-plasty is created first before the opposing Z-plasty is created on the nasal surface. The soft palate is split into two halves from midline passing through the zona pellucida. We usually do not include the uvula in the flaps for speech surgery.

After the oral incisions are made, the posteriorly based myomucosal flap is dissected posteriorly and laterally. The LVP muscle is separated from the nasal mucosa along the medial margin. The muscle is then elevated from the nasal mucosa. The TVP muscular aponeuroses are divided until the muscle bundles can easily be reoriented into the transverse position. The angle of the posteriorly based oral myomucosal flap is typically 60°. The anteriorly based oral mucosal flap on the contralateral side is elevated from underlying muscle.

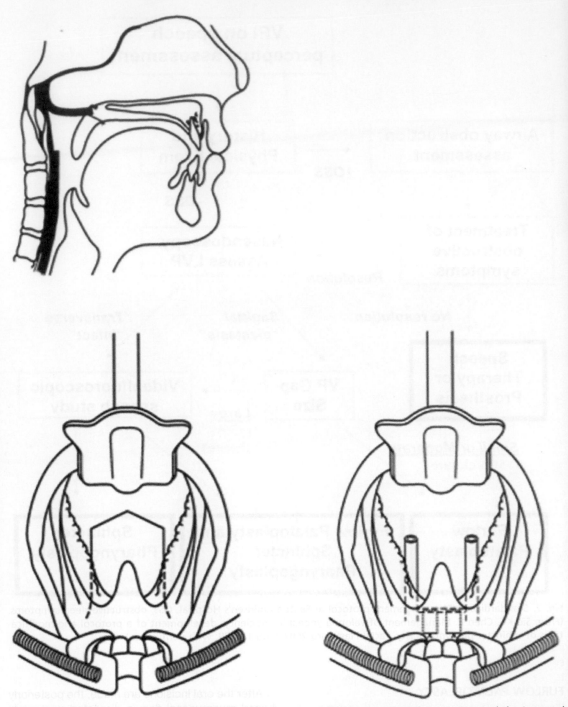

Fig. 8. Line drawings of superiorly based posterior pharyngeal flap in the sagittal projection and the intraoral exposure.

The anteriorly based nasal mucosa flap is created by incising the mucosa from the base of the nasal surface of the uvula toward the eustachian orifice. Care should be taken to leave an adequate rim of mucosa at the nasal mucosa–only incision. On the contralateral side, the lateral limb of the posteriorly based nasal myomucosal flap is also cut toward the eustachian orifice. This incision frees the flap with its muscle to swing across the midline. Lateral dissection may be performed to minimize tension on closure.

The nasal Z-plasty is closed first with knots tightened to the nasal surface. The oral Z-plasty is closed next with interrupted sutures. The double

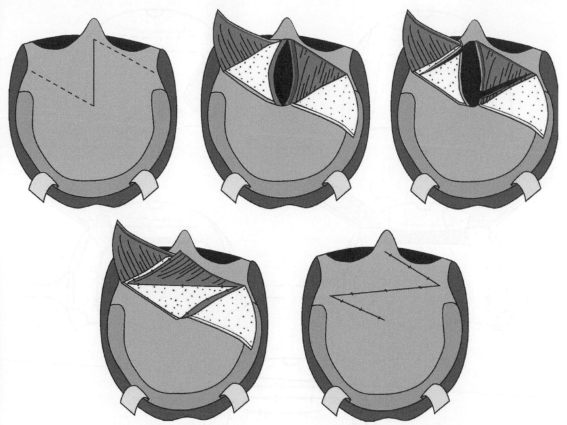

Fig. 9. Line drawings of double opposing Z-plasty for repair of intact palate and sagittal levator veli palatini.

Z-plasties transpose the LVP muscle toward the midline bilaterally. Both myomucosal flaps are overlapping each other posteriorly.

SPHINCTER PHARYNGOPLASTY

A Dingman mouth retractor is used for optimal exposure (**Fig. 10**). Before making incisions in the pharynx, the surgeon needs to look for aberrant pulsations that suggest medially displaced internal carotid arteries, which are often associated with velocardiofacial syndrome. Local anesthetic is injected submucosally in areas of flaps and incisions. A permanent suture is placed at the uvula to retract the soft palate into the nasopharynx. The oropharynx can be visualized well, including the interior aspect of adenoid pad. Sutures may be used to retract the posterior tonsillar pillars laterally.

The surgeon then designs 2 laterally and superiorly based myomucosal flaps that contain fibers of the constrictor and palatopharyngeus muscles. The mucosal incisions are marked out. The size of the sphincter is determined by the width, length, and position of the flaps. The use of both constrictor and PP muscles is appropriate for patients with large VP gaps requiring large, bulky sphincter reconstruction. For patients with smaller VP gaps, surgeons can use the flaps with primarily the constrictor muscles.

To prepare the recipient bed along the posterior pharyngeal wall, a small transverse strip of mucosa is excised between the medial limbs of the two flaps. The position of the mucosal removal determines the cephalocaudal position of the sphincter. The sphincter ideally is placed at the cephalocaudal level of attempted palatal closure as shown on videofluoroscopy. In general, the mucosa is excised 1 to 2 mm inferior to the caudal margin of the adenoid bed to accommodate mucosal sutures. The width of the mucosa strip is usually between 5 and 10 mm.

The superiorly based flaps are then transposed 90°. All mucosal edges need to be approximated and closed with absorbable sutures. Careful approximation of the mucosal edges is important in promoting reliable healing. At the end, the donor sites after the transposition of the flaps should also be closed with absorbable sutures.

The important factors that may influence the size of the sphincter include the length and the width of the flaps, the relationship of these flaps, and the

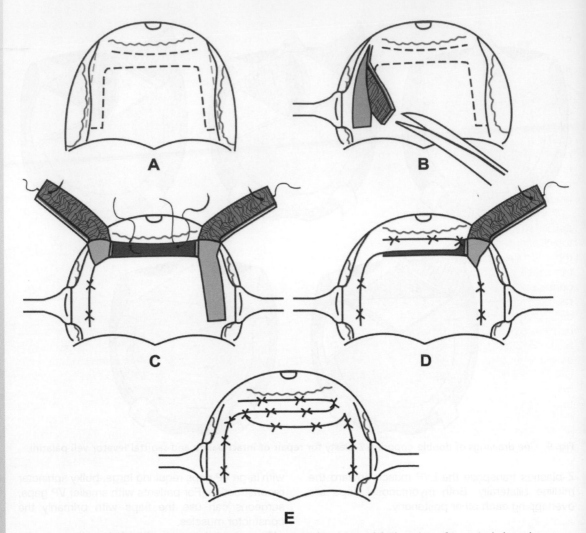

Fig. 10. Sphincter pharyngoplasty. (*A*) Placement of mucosal incisions. (*B*) Elevation of superiorly based myomucosal flaps. (*C*) Both flaps have been elevated and the right donor site closed. Note placement of sutures at the superior aspect of the recipient site. (*D*) transposition of the myomucosal flaps. (*E*) Closure of all mucosal incisions. (*From* Chiu L, Sie KC. Sphincter pharyngoplasty for management of velopharyngeal insufficiency. Operative Techniques in Otolaryngology 2009;20(4):263–7; with permission.)

size of the excised mucosal strip. The main benefit of the sphincter pharyngoplasty comes from the augmentation of the superior posterior pharyngeal wall. The sphincter typically is not dynamic.[37] Surgeons can modify these factors to tailor the procedure for patients with various VP gaps.

COMPLICATIONS AND AVOIDANCES

The complications of speech surgery include unacceptable nasal resonance, bleeding, fistula, or persistent VPI. From reviewing the outcomes at our institution, we learned that the VPI resolution rate was close to 65% after sphincter pharyngoplasty. Thirteen percent of patients with small VP

developed hyponasal resonance after surgery. This result emphasizes the importance of modifying the design of the flaps in sphincter pharyngoplasty in patients with small VP gaps to avoid airway obstruction and hyponasal resonance.

Persistent VPI after Furlow palatoplasty can be managed by sphincter pharyngoplasty to provide augmentation of superior posterior pharyngeal wall. If the patient continues to have persistent VPI after sphincter pharyngoplasty, the most likely cause of failure is either inadequate augmentation or placement of the sphincter inferior to the level of palatal closure. In these cases, revision sphincter pharyngoplasty to augment or reposition the sphincter more superiorly may be considered.

Upper airway obstruction from speech surgeries often manifests as sleep disordered breathing.[26] There is increased incidence of obstructive sleep apnea and increased apnea hypopnea index after sphincter pharyngoplasty. For patients with obstructive sleep symptoms after speech surgery, a trial of nasal steroids can be used initially. For symptoms that persist for more than 3 months after the surgery, an overnight polysomnogram is recommended to define the degree of the obstruction. Continuous positive airway pressure should be considered, although compliance can be challenging among pediatric patients.

The most common causes of obstructive sleep apnea after sphincter pharyngoplasty are adenotonsillar hypertrophy and VP stenosis. Tonsillectomy can be accomplished without compromising the speech outcome. Adenoidectomy can also be considered, although care is required to minimize recurrent VPI. Revision sphincter pharyngoplasty can be performed when the obstruction is at the nasopharyngeal level because of an excessively bulky sphincter or VP stenosis. The stenosis is typically related to lateral scar bands at the level of the velopharynx. The relaxing incisions are made from medial to lateral (ie, from the edge of the sphincter toward the lateral pharyngeal wall). It is performed through a transoral approach at the lateral aspects of the sphincter. After a widened VP inlet is created with appropriate dimensions, the mucosal edges are approximated. The procedure is simple and has an easy postoperative recovery. The release of VP stenosis usually does not compromise speech outcome. Nevertheless, repeat sleep study and perceptual speech analysis are recommended 3 months after the revision surgery.

MEASURING OUTCOMES

The definition for successful outcome after speech surgery has been characterized as no need for further surgery, decrease of hypernasal resonance, improvement of VPI severity, and elimination of nasal air escape during speech. Determining a child's QOL gives a more general assessment of day-to-day ability to communicate. In our institution, the VELO is the QOL instrument used to evaluate the surgical outcome in addition to perceptual speech analysis.

Successful management of VPI can be highly variable, from 20% to 90%, partially because of the variability in defining success. The outcomes with the speech surgery can be affected by many factors, including the patient selection, presence of syndrome, dimension of the nasopharynx, or history of cleft palate. In few studies, the VP gap size can be used to predict the speech outcome

reliably.[6,38] On the contrary, syndrome diagnosis does not have a statistically significant impact on speech outcome.[39]

Concurrent palatoplasty and sphincter pharyngoplasty has been shown to provide good speech outcome in the literature.[35,40,41] In one study, the speech improvement was greater in the combined procedure compared with sphincter pharyngoplasty alone, but no differences were observed between the pharyngeal flap and the combined procedure. There were also no differences in complications among these surgical interventions. In addition, the combined procedure had a lower revision rate than either sphincter pharyngoplasty or pharyngeal flap.[35]

RECENT TRENDS AND CONTROVERSIES

One emerging surgical option for treatment of patients with VPI is the augmentation of the posterior pharyngeal wall with implants. The implantation causes anterior displacement of the posterior pharyngeal wall, which allows adequate VP closure. Both autologous and nonautologous implant materials are discussed in the literature. Implant materials include cartilage, fat, fascia, paraffin, silicone, acellular dermis, injectable calcium hydroxyapatite, and dextranomer with hyaluronic acid. Injection pharyngoplasty with calcium hydroxyapatite has been shown to be a useful adjunct in the treatment of patients with mild VPI. Efficacy and safety have been shown more than 24 months after injection.[42,43]

Patients with chromosome 22q11 deletion present special challenges for many surgeons. VPI following adenoidectomy has been shown to have a strong association with 22q11 deletion.[11] Many surgeons think that patients with the 22q11 deletion syndrome and VPI tend to have residual VPI following speech surgery, possibly caused by a hypodynamic velopharynx. One retrospective study showed that superiorly based pharyngeal flap resulted in a significant speech improvement for treatment of VPI in patients with 22q11 deletion.[44] To compare outcomes of various speech surgical procedures for patients with 22q11 deletion, a systematic review analyzed 27 studies. Overall, 83% of patients had understandable speech. There was no significant difference in speech outcomes between patients who underwent a fat injection, Furlow palatoplasty, intravelar veloplasty, pharyngeal flap, or sphincter pharyngoplasty. More patients who underwent a palatoplasty needed further surgery than who underwent a pharyngoplasty. Thus, these investigators favor pharyngoplasty for patients with 22q11 and VPD.[12,45]

SUMMARY

In order to achieve the best treatment outcomes for patients with VPI, the patients should be evaluated by a team using a standardized approach. It is important for surgeons to work with an experienced speech pathologist in order to provide an accurate diagnosis for disorders of speech. The clinical evaluation including a detailed perceptual and instrumental speech assessment with nasoendoscopy can be essential in characterizing the VP function. The standardized clinical assessment should guide the treatment recommendations and surgical approaches. Surgeons should try to develop a treatment protocol that can be tailored to address each patient's specific defect.

ACKNOWLEDGMENTS

We gratefully acknowledge Eden Palmer, the photographer at Seattle Children's Hospital, for her assistance with the figures.

REFERENCES

1. Kleppe SA, Katayama KM, Shipley KG, et al. The speech and language characteristics of children with Prader-Willi syndrome. J Speech Hear Disord 1990;55(2):300–9.

2. Sie KC. Cleft palate speech and velopharyngeal insufficiency: surgical approach. B-Ent 2006;2(Suppl 4):85–94.

3. Schwartz K, D'Arcy HJ, Gillespie B, et al. Factors associated with weaning in the first 3 months postpartum. J Fam Pract 2002;51(5):439–44.

4. Messner AH, Lalakea ML. The effect of ankyloglossia on speech in children. Otolaryngol Head Neck Surg 2002;127(6):539–45.

5. Ysunza A, Pamplona MC, Molina F, et al. Surgery for speech in cleft palate patients. Int J Pediatr Otorhinolaryngol 2004;68(12):1499–505.

6. Lam DJ, Chiu LL, Sie KC, et al. Impact of cleft width in clefts of secondary palate on the risk of velopharyngeal insufficiency. Arch Facial Plast Surg 2012;14(5):360–4.

7. Marrinan EM, LaBrie RA, Mulliken JB. Velopharyngeal function in nonsyndromic cleft palate: relevance of surgical technique, age at repair, and cleft type. Cleft Palate Craniofac J 1998;35(2):95–100.

8. Garcia Velasco M, Ysunza A, Hernandez X, et al. Diagnosis and treatment of submucous cleft palate: a review of 108 cases. Cleft Palate J 1988;25(2):171–3.

9. Sell D, Harding A, Grunwell P. GOS.SP.ASS.'98: an assessment for speech disorders associated with cleft palate and/or velopharyngeal dysfunction (revised). Int J Lang Commun Disord 1999;34(1):17–33.

10. Malick D, Moon J, Canady J. Stress velopharyngeal incompetence: prevalence, treatment, and management practices. Cleft Palate Craniofac J 2007;44(4):424–33.

11. Perkins JA, Sie K, Gray S. Presence of 22q11 deletion in postadenoidectomy velopharyngeal insufficiency. Arch Otolaryngol Head Neck Surg 2000;126(5):645–8.

12. Spruijt NE, Widdershoven JC, Breugem CC, et al. Velopharyngeal dysfunction and 22q11.2 deletion syndrome: a longitudinal study of functional outcome and preoperative prognostic factors. Cleft Palate Craniofac J 2012;49(4):447–55.

13. Golding-Kushner KJ, Argamaso RV, Cotton RT, et al. Standardization for the reporting of nasopharyngoscopy and multiview videofluoroscopy: a report from an International Working Group. Cleft Palate J 1990;27(4):337–47 [discussion: 347–8].

14. Tieu DD, Gerber ME, Milczuk HA, et al. Generation of consensus in the application of a rating scale to nasendoscopic assessment of velopharyngeal function. Arch Otolaryngol Head Neck Surg 2012;138(10):923–8.

15. Yoon PJ, Starr JR, Perkins JA, et al. Interrater and intrarater reliability in the evaluation of velopharyngeal insufficiency within a single institution. Arch Otolaryngol Head Neck Surg 2006;132(9):947–51.

16. Warren DW, Dalston RM, Mayo R. Hypernasality in the presence of "adequate" velopharyngeal closure. Cleft Palate Craniofac J 1993;30(2):150–4.

17. Karling J, Henningsson G, Larson O, et al. Comparison between two types of pharyngeal flap with regard to configuration at rest and function and speech outcome. Cleft Palate Craniofac J 1999;36(2):154–65.

18. Kummer AW. Disorders of resonance and airflow secondary to cleft palate and/or velopharyngeal dysfunction. Semin Speech Lang 2011;32(2):141–9.

19. Losken A, Williams JK, Burstein FD, et al. An outcome evaluation of sphincter pharyngoplasty for the management of velopharyngeal insufficiency. Plast Reconstr Surg 2003;112(7):1755–61.

20. Boseley ME, Hartnick CJ. Assessing the outcome of surgery to correct velopharyngeal insufficiency with the pediatric voice outcomes survey. Int J Pediatr Otorhinolaryngol 2004;68(11):1429–33.

21. Skirko JR, Weaver EM, Perkins J, et al. Modification and evaluation of a velopharyngeal insufficiency quality-of-life instrument. Arch Otolaryngol Head Neck Surg 2012;138(10):929–35.

22. Skirko JR, Weaver EM, Perkins JA, et al. Validity and responsiveness of VELO: a velopharyngeal insufficiency quality of life measure. Otolaryngol Head Neck Surg 2013;149(2):304–11.

23. LaRossa D, Jackson OH, Kirschner RE, et al. The Children's Hospital of Philadelphia modification of the Furlow double-opposing z-palatoplasty: long-term

speech and growth results. Clin Plast Surg 2004;31(2): 243–9.

24. Sie KC, Chen EY. Management of velopharyngeal insufficiency: development of a protocol and modifications of sphincter pharyngoplasty. Facial Plast Surg 2007;23(2):128–39.

25. Sommerlad BC, Fenn C, Harland K, et al. Submucous cleft palate: a grading system and review of 40 consecutive submucous cleft palate repairs. Cleft Palate Craniofac J 2004;41(2):114–23.

26. Huang MH, Riski JE, Cohen SR, et al. An anatomic evaluation of the Furlow double opposing Z-plasty technique of cleft palate repair. Ann Acad Med Singapore 1999;28(5):672–6.

27. Orticochea M. Construction of a dynamic muscle sphincter in cleft palates. Plast Reconstr Surg 1968;41(4):323–7.

28. Gray SD, Pinborough-Zimmerman J, Catten M. Posterior wall augmentation for treatment of velopharyngeal insufficiency. Otolaryngol Head Neck Surg 1999;121(1):107–12.

29. Ysunza A, Pamplona C, Ramirez E, et al. Velopharyngeal surgery: a prospective randomized study of pharyngeal flaps and sphincter pharyngoplasties. Plast Reconstr Surg 2002;110(6):1401–7.

30. Huskie CF, Jackson IT. The sphincter pharyngoplasty–a new approach to the speech problems of velopharyngeal incompetence. Br J Disord Commun 1977;12(1):31–5.

31. Abyholm F, D'Antonio L, Davidson Ward SL, et al. Pharyngeal flap and sphincterplasty for velopharyngeal insufficiency have equal outcome at 1 year postoperatively: results of a randomized trial. Cleft Palate Craniofac J 2005;42(5):501–11.

32. Sie KC, Starr JR, Bloom DC, et al. Multicenter interrater and intrarater reliability in the endoscopic evaluation of velopharyngeal insufficiency. Arch Otolaryngol Head Neck Surg 2008;134(7):757–63.

33. Dailey SA, Karnell MP, Karnell LH, et al. Comparison of resonance outcomes after pharyngeal flap and Furlow double-opposing z-plasty for surgical management of velopharyngeal incompetence. Cleft Palate Craniofac J 2006;43(1):38–43.

34. Wojcicki P, Wojcicka K. Prospective evaluation of the outcome of velopharyngeal insufficiency therapy after pharyngeal flap, a sphincter pharyngoplasty, a double Z-plasty and simultaneous Orticochea and Furlow operations. J Plast Reconstr Aesthet Surg 2011;64(4):459–61.

35. Bohm LA, Padgitt N, Tibesar RJ, et al. Outcomes of combined Furlow palatoplasty and sphincter pharyngoplasty for velopharyngeal insufficiency. Otolaryngol Head Neck Surg 2014;150(2):216–21.

36. Furlow LT Jr. Cleft palate repair by double opposing Z-plasty. Plast Reconstr Surg 1986;78:724.

37. Ysunza A, Pamplona MC. Velopharyngeal function after two different types of pharyngoplasty. Int J Pediatr Otorhinolaryngol 2006;70(6):1031–7.

38. Deren O, Ayhan M, Tuncel A, et al. The correction of velopharyngeal insufficiency by Furlow palatoplasty in patients older than 3 years undergoing Veau-Wardill-Kilner palatoplasty: a prospective clinical study. Plast Reconstr Surg 2005;116(1):85–93 [discussion: 94–6].

39. de Buys Roessingh AS, Herzog G, Cherpillod J, et al. Speech prognosis and need of pharyngeal flap for non syndromic vs syndromic Pierre Robin Sequence. J Pediatr Surg 2008;43(4):668–74.

40. Nadjmi N, Van Erum R, De Bodt M, et al. Two-stage palatoplasty using a modified Furlow procedure. Int J Oral Maxillofac Surg 2013;42(5):551–8.

41. Li CH, Shi JY, Zheng Q, et al. The Children's Hospital of Philadelphia modification of the Furlow double-opposing Z-Palatoplasty: 30-year experience and long-term speech outcomes. Plast Reconstr Surg 2014;133(3):429e–31e.

42. Sipp JA, Ashland J, Hartnick CJ. Injection pharyngoplasty with calcium hydroxyapatite for treatment of velopalatal insufficiency. Arch Otolaryngol Head Neck Surg 2008;134(3):268–71.

43. Brigger MT, Ashland JE, Hartnick CJ. Injection pharyngoplasty with calcium hydroxylapatite for velopharyngeal insufficiency: patient selection and technique. Arch Otolaryngol Head Neck Surg 2010;136(7):666–70.

44. Filip C, Matzen M, Aukner R, et al. Superiorly based pharyngeal flap for treatment of velopharyngeal insufficiency in patients with 22q11.2 deletion syndrome. J Craniofac Surg 2013;24(2):501–4.

45. Spruijt NE, Reijmanhinze J, Hens G, et al. In search of the optimal surgical treatment for velopharyngeal dysfunction in 22q11.2 deletion syndrome: a systematic review. PLoS One 2012;7(3):e34332.

Pediatric Esthetic Otoplasty

Noah Benjamin Sands, MD, FRCSC[a,b], Peter A. Adamson, MD, FRCSC[a,b,*]

KEYWORDS

- Otoplasty • Esthetic ear surgery • Auricular deformity • Prominauris • Cartilage suturing

KEY POINTS

- Otoplasty is a thinking-surgeon's operation, much like rhinoplasty, that requires assiduous planning and execution.
- Meticulous attention to detail is required during initial patient evaluation, including less commonly appreciated features such as asymmetries, cartilaginous contours, and abnormalities of the scapha and lobule.
- Suture techniques provide a more predictably natural auricular contour compared with cartilage-cutting otoplasty but potentially at the expense of diminished stability of the correction over time.
- Conchal setback sutures should be placed before antihelical contouring, because much of the medialization desired can be achieved in this manner, while obviating over-tightening the antihelical sutures.
- A single triangular fossa–temporalis fascia suture can help address persistent overprojection of the superior pole.

INTRODUCTION/OVERVIEW

Auricular deformities in children are a frequent source of ridicule and ruthless taunting by peers, beginning at an early age.[1] "Bat ears," "elephant ears," "Dumbo ears," and "donkey ears" are only some of the unflattering names heard in association. As such, cosmetic ear problems, none more common than protruding ears, or *prominauris*, frequently impose developmental psychological problems on young children, including behavioral disturbances such as aggression and petulant behavior, social phobias, neurosis, and feelings of insecurity.[2] Such issues may impact social development and persist in later stages of life. One particular study demonstrated that 40% of adolescents with problem behaviors had auricular deformities.[3] Adults with auricular deformities frequently continue to suffer from varying levels of insecurity and may contemplate corrective surgery for years while attempting to hide their ears with camouflaging hairstyles. Thankfully, there are techniques today that allow for correction of these deformities with minimal pain and require limited time away from school and extracurricular activities.

Surgical techniques for correction of auricular deformities have evolved considerably over time. The expansive history is detailed in other works of the senior author.[1,4] Despite inventive and varied contributions to esthetic correction of the malformed auricle by surgeons over the last century, modern-day "cartilage-sparing" techniques have only evolved since the 1960s. Notable

The authors have no conflicts of interest or disclosures.
[a] Division of Facial Plastic and Reconstructive Surgery, Department of Otolaryngology – Head and Neck Surgery, University of Toronto, Toronto General Hospital, R. Fraser Elliott Building, 190 Elizabeth Street, 3rd Floor, Room 3S-438, Toronto, Ontario M5G 2C4, Canada; [b] Adamson Associates Cosmetic Facial Surgery, 150 Bloor Street West, M110, Toronto, Ontario M5S 2X9, Canada
* Corresponding author. Adamson Associates Cosmetic Facial Surgery, 150 Bloor Street West, M110, Toronto, Ontario M5S 2X9, Canada.
E-mail address: paa@dradamson.com

facialplastic.theclinics.com

contributions include those of Mustarde[5] and Furnas,[6] who influenced the shift in philosophy away from cartilage-cutting otoplasty techniques. The more aggressive excisional techniques can result in contour irregularities, auricular instability, and an operated appearance. It should be noted that cartilage-cutting techniques are still more commonly applied in certain parts of the world such as Europe.[7] Cartilage-sparing surgery involves reshaping techniques using sutures; these have been largely adopted in North America. These more conservative techniques, which attempt to re-create and strengthen the antihelical fold by folding scaphal cartilage using permanent transcartilaginous sutures (Mustarde), and setback the concha using tacking sutures to the mastoid periosteum (Furnas), provide a more predictably natural auricular contour. They also help eliminate unsightly cartilage ridging, which commonly results from resection techniques. These advantages are, arguably, at the expense of diminished stability of the correction over the long term.

Furnas later described additional suture methods, including fossa triangularis–temporalis fascia sutures to medialize a protruding superior crus and lobule-mastoid sutures to medialize a prominent cauda helicus.[8] Webster[9] is credited with assimilation of many of these available techniques to provide a comprehensive approach to otoplasty, including posterior skin and soft tissue excision, circumspect conchal resection, anterior cartilage scoring, and application of suture techniques as described.[6] The senior author's current philosophy and approach to pediatric otoplasty have largely evolved as an adaptation of the historical techniques already mentioned, principally relying on suture techniques with adjunctive cartilage scoring or shaving performed in rare cases as required. The authors' most updated methodology is shared in this article.

CLINICAL ASSESSMENT

As is the case with all facial plastic surgical procedures, pediatric otoplasty requires meticulous attention to detail including careful patient evaluation during consultation and astute preoperative planning to optimize outcomes. The surgeon must have an appreciation for facial esthetics, which is expected of the facial plastic surgeon but, naturally, less of a focal point for the pediatric Otolaryngologist. Extensive knowledge of ear anatomy and a firm understanding of the rationale for the various techniques applied are required.

As of the 1990s, nearly two-thirds of the senior author's otoplasty cases had been performed on the pediatric age group, with 50% of patients falling between the ages of 5 and 9 years of age.[10] Since that time, most cases have been performed on adults, many of them revisions, which reflect the author's transition to a mostly noninsured private practice.

In general, the multimodal peaks in demand for otoplasty coincide with early school years, adolescence, and early adulthood, when social pressures reach their pinnacle.[1] Patients should be considered for otoplasty no earlier than age 5 when the auricle's size and strength approximates its mature form but remains pliable and elastic. These features diminish with age, necessitating more aggressive treatment in older patients. Five is also the approximate age when children begin to notice abnormalities in others, and teasing may begin. As this also happens to be a key childhood stage of social growth and identity development through interaction with peers, surgical correction at this stage is almost a way of "protecting" children from senseless bullying.[11]

During the initial patient evaluation, it is extremely important to elicit both the child's and their parents' specific concerns about their ears. Needless to say, young children will often be unable to voice specific cosmetic concerns and are more likely to share their general distress imposed by their esthetic disadvantage. In other instances, the decision to proceed to surgical consultation might be solely the parents' initiative, with the best interest of their child in mind. Parents should be asked about school performance, self-esteem, and potential bullying and teasing within the classroom. A medical history should be elicited, including associated medical conditions and fitness for surgery, developmental history, allergies, and medications. As the inheritance of auricular deformities is autosomal-dominant with variable penetrance, and close to 60% of otoplasty patients have a family history,[11] an extended family history of auricular deformities and associated syndromes should be investigated. Potential familial concerns, such as bleeding tendencies, pathologic scar formation, and potential anesthetic concerns such as pseudocholinesterase deficiency, should be elucidated.

On physical examination, each ear must be examined in isolation and in relation to each other. Although both ears tend to share similar characteristics, they are not infrequently affected to varying degrees by deformities, and in some instances, only one ear is affected. Asymmetries in contour, projection, and size must be noted and brought to the attention of the parents, as some of these elements may be difficult or impossible to correct. The individual anatomic features of the auricle should be noted and recorded in a systematic way, effectively taking note of each anatomic constituent in an orderly fashion. In the authors' practice an itemized template is used to be as comprehensive as possible. Although more obvious and common deformities, such as a deficient antihelix or superior crus, are likely to be apparent to the surgeon at first glance, secondary deformities such as excessive vertical height of the concha wall, excessive angulation between the triangular fossa and squamosal of the temporal bone, or unfurling of the helical rim require more focused inspection to be noted. The mastoid prominence should be examined, because it is occasionally hyperpneumatized and may contribute to lateral displacement of the auricle. Unlike in older adults, the lobule is less commonly redundant or elongated, but may be outstanding. Cartilaginous contours should be inspected for prominence of the tragus or antitragus and for the presence of a Darwinian tubercle. If missed on consultation, these issues are unlikely to be addressed at the time of surgery and may result in either undercorrection of the auricle or overcompensation in other parameters.

During the evaluation, measurement of auricular protrusion from the temporal bone is mandatory, and each side should be measured and compared at 3 points: (1) the most cephalic aspect of the helical rim (ideal = 10–12 mm from the temporal bone), (2) the most laterally prominent part of the rim (generally at the midpoint of the helix, ideally 16–18 mm), and (3) caudally at the intertragal incisura (ideal = approximately 20 mm). The helical rim should be roughly 2 to 5 mm lateral to the antihelical ridge on the frontal view. The auriculocephalic angle should measure from 25° to 35° and typically exceeds 40° in prominauris cases. The conchal-mastoid angle should be between 45° and 90°, whereas the chonchal-scaphal angle should measure less than 90°.

The auricular cartilage should be evaluated for its pliability and density by manually simulating correction of the deformities. This approach also helps instill confidence in the patient/parents by demonstrating to them a general sense of the expected result. For instance, the antihelix can be re-created by applying gentle posterior pressure on the helical rim. Pressure with a cotton-tip applicator applied at the concha bowl can simulate conchal setback sutures. Greater strength in the cartilage and its tendency to recoil may confer a higher risk of unfurling following suture correction and necessitate adjunctive scoring or weakening of the cartilage. Anticipated redundancy in posterior soft tissue and skin can be gauged through this process as well. Depending on the age, disposition, and degree of cooperation of the child, these elements may be hard to elucidate during

consultation and can only be appreciated once under sedation at the time of surgery. Although most school-age children will be sufficiently collaborative, those that are uncooperative can potentially be poor candidates for otoplasty considering the postoperative care involved.

Finally, standard preoperative photography should be performed, including frontal view, both lateral views (with close-ups), and a posterior view. A birds-eye (cranio-caudal) view can also be used to demonstrate lateral projection. If applicable, hair should be held out of the way with a concentric elastic band. Photography is later repeated at 6 and 12 months postoperatively.

SURGICAL GOALS

Much like rhinoplasty, otoplasty is a thinking-surgeon's operation that requires detailed planning and execution, frequently involving the orchestration of a combination of techniques to achieve desired results. It also commands recognition of the balance and harmony among the various elements of the auricle and the interplay between these elements, in addition to the relationship to the face, in contributing to the overall esthetics. It is an operation with no predefined steps but rather a compendium of employable techniques. Otoplasty has to be adapted and tailored on a case-by-case basis. Although the pathway is certain to vary, the desired endpoint is generally a shared theme, namely, the achievement of a natural, unoperated, and durable postoperative appearance. This natural appearance is constituted by gracefully arcing curvatures to the helical and antihelical contours and the absence of any obvious interaural asymmetries to the observer. Similar to the nose, the auricles are not commonly considered to be hallmarks of facial beauty; however, they can certainly detract from an otherwise beautiful face if these objectives are not met, and a "normal" appearance is not obtained.

More specific goals should include the following[1]: (1) precise anatomic defects and contour abnormalities should be corrected, most commonly an unfurled antihelix and a high conchal wall; (2) auriculocephalic angles and distances should fall within normal limits, as detailed earlier; (3) the helical rim should project slightly more lateral than the antihelix, at least down to the level of the midauricle, to avoid a "stuck-on" appearance; (4) the posterior sulcus should be maintained (facilitated by avoiding incision placement directly in the furrow and by trimming only the redundant soft tissue), (5) interaural "approximate symmetry" should be coveted, and the lateral protrusion of the helices should be within 3 mm of one another at the 3 points of measurement; (6) both the anterior and the posterior surfaces should be devoid of sharp notches, edges, creases, and unfavorable scars; and (7) the superior and inferior poles should be aligned with the concha. A "no-frills" set of guidelines for the otoplastic surgeon has been proposed by McDowell and elaborated by Mallen.[3] These guidelines include absence of protrusion in the upper one-third (although slight residual protrusion of the lower two-third is permissible), helix visible to mid ear, smooth helix, postauricular sulcus preservation, appropriate auriculocephalic distances, and symmetry.

The senior author uses a postauricular approach and relies primarily on cartilage-sparing techniques to help achieve these goals consistently. Again analogous to rhinoplasty, a logical stepwise progression through the case is used. The exercise is anatomic, with constant attention to the combination of deformities. With respect to suturing, some degree of trial and error is at play. This process typically begins with conchal setback sutures through which most of the medialization desired can be achieved and proceeds to antihelical contouring. As a general rule, slight overcorrection is required because cartilage memory and elastic recoil will result in as much as 40% loss of correction, especially in the upper one-third.[12] Particularly in the early postoperative period, slight overcorrection is likely to be perceived by patients and their families as a successful outcome, and undercorrection is likely to be perceived as a surgical failure. Even in the setting of a unilateral deformity, bilateral surgery is often advantageous if there is even minimal deformity because it can account for the overcorrection-recoil cycle and help achieve a balanced outcome from the very outset.

SURGICAL TECHNIQUE
Preparation and Incision

The goals of the operation should be reviewed briefly with the patient before the induction of anesthesia. The senior author usually prefers general anesthesia for young children, but adolescents and young adults can elect for local anesthesia or conscious sedation if preferred. Preoperative marking is occasionally indicated at the level of the lobule if slated for reduction or to highlight previous scars requiring revision.

The patient is positioned in slight reverse Trendelenberg position. A conservative amount of hair may be trimmed around the auricle superiorly. Circumferential autoclave tape is used to keep the hair out of the operative field. Both ears are prepared and draped simultaneously and should be visible at all times for the purpose of comparison on the fly. The more involved auricle is selected first for correction. A measured amount of postauricular skin for excision should be measured and marked before distortion with local anesthesia. This redundancy created by the conchal setback is usually in the 10-mm to 12-mm range. The auricular and mastoid soft tissues are widely infiltrated with equal parts lidocaine 1% with 1:100,000 epinephrine and bupivacaine 0.5% with 1:200,000 epinephrine. If placed in the appropriate supraperichondrial plane, the injection will provide some hydrodissection.

Postauricular Skin Excision

An eccentric fusiform excision based around (but not incised within) the postauricular sulcus is made (**Fig. 1**). Greater extension is made onto the posterior concha than onto the mastoid. In this way, forces acting on the medialized cartilage are distanced from the soft tissue closure, which can help prevent wound complications and suture extrusion. This incision placement also allows for adequate cartilage exposure and placement of sutures. Furthermore, an anterior bias will allow the incision to fall back into the sulcus as the ear is set closer to the skull, rather than falling into visible postauricular skin. The ends of incision should be kept at least 1 cm away from the superior and inferior edges for camouflage. Skin and soft tissue excision (usually 10–12 mm at its widest point) is performed en bloc down to the level of the perichondrium/periosteum, encompassing a variable amount of mastoid soft tissue to allow for later retro-displacement. More soft tissue is excised superiorly, because this is where the most correction is desired, and to avoid the neurovascular bundles at the inferior pole. Wide undermining is then performed. Frequently a superolateral releasing incision is made 1 cm from the superior apex of the ellipse, resulting in a "Y" or "T" shape. This releasing incision will aid exposure for Mustarde suture placement. Hemostasis is achieved with bipolar electrocautery.

Incisionless Otoplasty

Following a more global trend in virtually all surgical fields, a relatively recent innovation in otoplasty has been the introduction of "minimally invasive" techniques, such as endoscopic and incisionless otoplasty, first introduced by Fritsch in 1995.[13] Although there was merit in this procedure when simply correcting an unfurled antihelix, the original description of this approach could not be used to address conchal protrusion or excess and did not address auricular abnormalities found in

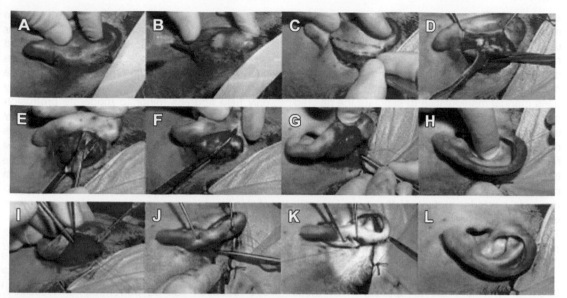

Fig. 1. Sequence of the authors' preferred otoplasty technique. (*A, B*) Marking and local infiltration; (*C, D*) excision of skin and soft tissue down to periosteum; (*E*) wide skin undermining; (*F*) releasing incision; (*G, H*) conchal setback suture; (*I*) Mustarde suture; (*J, K*) skin closure; and (*L*) final intraoperative appearance.

association with prominent ears. However, this innovative thinking prompted a more recent iteration of the technique, which addresses some of these issues.[14,15] The advantages to an incisionless approach are maintenance of the auricular structure with little risk of contour irregularities, no visible scars or potential for wound complications, lower risk of hematoma and postoperative infection, and presumably quicker healing. Bulky dressings may also be avoided.

Conchal Setback

The senior author prefers to establish the approximate position of the concha by creating the desired conchal-mastoid angle before the application of antihelical contour sutures. Much, if not all, of the desired reduction in lateral projection can be achieved with the concha setback sutures alone. This order of steps also obviates the temptation to overtighten the antihelical sutures, which can result in an overfolded, unattractive scapha. As a rule, the author uses 3 individual Furnas-type 4-0 polyethylene terephthalate (Mersilene; Ethicon, Somerville, NJ, USA) horizontal mattress sutures to appose the conchal bowl to the mastoid periosteum (see **Fig. 1**). The advantage of a braided, nonabsorbable polyester suture material is its ease of handling, permanence, knot security, and biocompatibility. Polypropylene (Prolene; Ethicon) is a reasonable alternative but may stretch and offer less knot stability over time. The sutures are roughly positioned at the superior (cymba concha),

inferior (cavum concha), and middle aspect of the bowl, in that order. The sutures can be placed closer to the external auditory canal on the conchal floor if less correction is desired, or closer to the vertical conchal wall/antihelix if more significant correction is warranted. Each suture is placed through the scaphal cartilage including both layers of the perichondrium, without catching the dermis of the anterior skin, and through a substantial bite of the mastoid periosteum to ensure stability. The sutures are clamped and left untied until each of the 3 is placed in satisfactory position. The sutures are tightened in the order of placement. This order of placement helps avoid overcorrection of the mid one-third and potential telephone ear deformity. The vector of correction is superoposterior to prevent advancement of the anterior concha into the meatus. Occasionally, it may be advisable to reduce an excessively deep conchal bowl by cartilage-island shave excision of the ponticulus, triangular, or conchal eminences, allowing for further retrodisplacement of the overdeveloped cartilage into the deepened sulcus. In such cases, if the excess is not trimmed, contact points with the mastoid will prevent adequate medialization of the concha bowl.

Antihelix Repositioning

Generally, less antihelical correction is required than initially anticipated, once the conchal setback sutures have been placed. Correction of antihelical unfurling is achieved through the precise application of 2 or 3 Mustarde-type horizontal mattress sutures (4-0 Mersilene). Although widely used elsewhere, the senior author does not use methylene blue dye, needle fixation, or temporary suture placement before the application of the permanent sutures. In place of these tools, the author uses manual manipulation to simulate the desired correction and guide the exact placement of the sutures. External pressure is applied on the anterior surface by either the index finger pad or the fingernail, supporting the helix with the thumb of the same nondominant hand. Once the scapho-conchal entry and exit points are visualized on the bare posterior surface of the auricular cartilage, the sutures are accurately positioned (see **Fig. 1**). Tissue trauma is also minimized using this approach. Sutures are applied using a 4-mm 6-mm bite through cartilage and anterior perichondrium. As performed for the conchal setback sutures, a specific order of application of these sutures is maintained; namely, the most superior suture is placed first, extending from superior scapha to the fossa triangularis, to set the superior and inferior crura into position. Next, the most inferior suture is applied near the lower aspect of the antihelix. Finally, midlevel intervening sutures are applied on an as-needed basis. The result of these sutures should be a smooth, natural, gentle curvature of the antihelix. Once positioned, they are tied in the same order they are placed. Although classically these sutures are described as being a set distance apart from one another,[16] the author advocates suture placement on a customized basis to achieve the best contour possible. Once the Furnas-type and Mustarde-type sutures have been tied on both sides, measurements of lateral projection should again be undertaken to ensure symmetry. As mentioned, the auriculocephalic correction at the midauricle, the most projected point, should measure 15-mm to 18 mm intraoperatively, slightly more than desired, to allow for postoperative loss of correction.

Supplementary Maneuvers

Additional sutures may be placed as necessary to correct remaining deformities or asymmetries. Occasionally, the superior pole maintains a slight laterally projected appearance, refractory to already positioned sutures. To address this, a single triangular fossa–temporalis fascia suture can be placed, this acting in a similar manner to the conchal setback sutures applied more caudally. It is very important to provide adequate correction in this area. In a review of 62 of the author's cases, only 8 patients (13%) required such sutures.[10] If lateral projection persists in the lower one-third,

an additional conchal-mastoid suture can be placed in the cavum concha. Persistent lobular protrusion, frequently related to a lateralized cauda helix which drags the lobule,[17] is often adequately addressed with a single cavum concha to mastoid mattress suture. This technique may only help address minor to moderate protrusion in the coronal plane, according to a study by Sadick and colleagues.[18] The authors of this article further describe a fillet technique of the lobule, by releasing the posterior ligamentous attachments of the lobule to the concha bowl and antihelix, and resuspension of the posterior flap of skin to address more severe protrusion in either the coronal or the axial plane. Although the senior author of this article has not experimented with this technique, it appears to have sound anatomic reasoning and should be considered.

Beyond repositioning, additional lobule soft tissue reduction can be performed as necessary. Scoring and rasping of cartilage on the anterior surface is rarely required in pediatric cases, aside from older teenagers with unusually stiff auricular cartilage. One needs to use meticulous technique and minimize trauma to minimize contour irregularities that can ensue.

A different school of thought is illustrated by Raunig,[19] who relied primarily on abrasion of the anterior surface of the antihelical cartilage, using a diamond-coated file, to encourage biomechanical remodeling with resultant strengthening of the antihelix. This modification of the cartilage-sparing approach of Weerda and Siegert[20] had been applied in a case series of greater than 194 ears (both pediatric and adult) with isolated hypoplasia of the antihelix, without any resultant deformity. Only a limited number of patients required adjunctive suturing; however, at least 6 weeks of postoperative taping was required.

Closure and Dressing

Although skin closure and dressing application are frequently an afterthought for various surgical procedures, this should not be the case with otoplasty. Haphazard application of the dressing may contribute to disastrous results after this operation, including distortion, infection, ischemia, and chondritis. Following completion of the techniques applied during otoplasty, and once the conchal bowl and antihelix are in favorable positions, the tissues are liberally irrigated with either a clindamycin or a bacitracin solution before closure. The posterior incision is closed with interrupted, intradermal 4-0 chromic gut sutures. No tension should be encountered because the skin edges are approximated. No epidermal layer of closure is applied, to allow for egress of any accumulated blood; this also helps eliminate the need for drains, facilitating outpatient care. Bolsters of soft cotton soaked in equal parts mineral oil and peroxide are applied on both surfaces of the auricles, contouring them around the folds. Soft Kerlix fluff followed by cling is firmly, not tightly, applied transversely and coronally as a mastoid dressing. This dressing is taped extensively to keep it bound and secure. Pressure points must be avoided as they can contribute to focal skin necrosis.

LESS COMMON TECHNIQUES
Helix

The helical rim can be occasionally unfurled in much the same way as the antihelix. The treatment for this condition follows similar principles, but in reverse order of importance. The mainstay of treatment is scoring of the lateral aspect of the helix followed by adjunctive placement of mattress sutures applied from scapha to helix along the extent of the arc. A through-and-through bolster should be secured for approximately 7 days to provide additional "memory."

Darwinian tubercles are easily approached via direct incision, camouflaged in the curl of the helix, followed by excision of the cartilage protuberance, frequently along with a small fusiform wedge of skin to aid in redrapage. Closure is performed using 5-0 Nylon placed in a running fashion (Fig. 2).

Schaphal Excess

Excess scaphal cartilage tends to accompany a generally oversized auricle including the helical rim and, in such cases, excision of a segment of

scapha can be performed at once with reduction of the helical rim. Although a variety of excisional techniques have been proposed, each of these should be avoided unless the deformity is significant, because troublesome scarring may result. When necessary, the authors' preferred approach involves the excision of a crescent-shaped portion of scaphal cartilage, adjacent to the helix, with a stair-step rectangular extension of the crescent onto the helix, allowing for reduction in both height and width of the auricle (Fig. 3). This step at the junction of the helical rim and scapha breaks up the incision, facilitating scar camouflage while decreasing the incidence of scar contracture across the rim. The incisions are carried through the anterior skin and cartilage only, without violating the posterior skin. Preservation of the posterior skin, and corresponding arterial perforators, helps preserve the predominant blood supply to the auricle. Surrounding skin is undermined to facilitate redrapage. The arch is then reconstituted by approximating the cut ends of the cartilage with 4-0 Polyglactin (Vicryl; Ethicon) or 4-0 PDS (polydioxanone; Ethicon). Frequently, a Burow triangle needs to be excised from the intact posterior skin.

Redundant Lobule

Although a large, dependent lobule (referred to as "lobule-chalasis"[17]) is more of a feature in middle-aged adults, through loss of elasticity and tissue ptosis, a congenitally large lobule in a child can be readily addressed using a simple crescentic excision of skin and soft tissue at the free edge of the lobule or lobules (Fig. 4). This excision of skin and soft tissue is performed by carefully

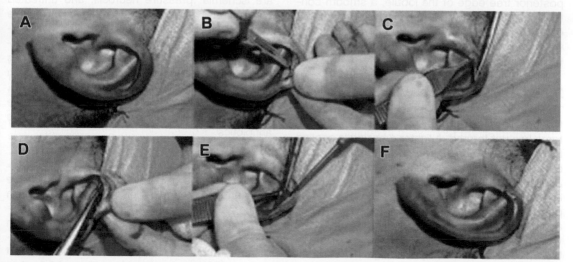

Fig. 2. Excision of excess helical cartilage. (*A*) Skin ellipse marked; (*B, C*) fusiform skin excision; (*D*) cutaneous undermining; (*E*) excision of prominent cartilage; and (*F*) final intraoperative appearance.

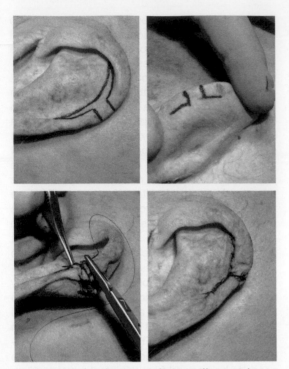

Fig. 3. Scaphal reduction technique illustrated on a cadaver. Excision of a crescent-shaped portion of scaphal cartilage, adjacent to the helix, with a stair-step rectangular extension onto the helix, allows for reduction in both height and width the auricle.

marking the lobule with corresponding anterior and posterior lines and trimming the excess tissue in a curvilinear manner with curved tissue scissors. Although other lobule reduction techniques have been proposed by authors, including Tanzer,[21] this technique allows for a concealed scar on the posterior free edge of the lobule, a smooth contour, and the ability to gauge the exact amount of tissue trimming required. The incision is closed with running 5-0 Nylon. Sutures are removed on postoperative day 6.

Postoperative Care

The senior author always removes the dressing on the first postoperative day to ensure that a hematoma has not formed. A lighter dressing is applied following inspection of the incisions and is worn for an additional 3 days. Older children and young adults may opt to simply wear a sports headband instead of having a second dressing applied. All patients are instructed to wear the headband day and night for 2 weeks, then nightly for 2 additional weeks. Patients should be instructed to avoid contact sports or physical play that might lead to accidental trauma in the surgical area. Approximately one-half of cases of loss of correction requiring

revision surgery are related to auricular trauma in the early postoperative period.[10] Patients are given general education regarding cleansing and application of antibacterial ointment over the incisions following dressing removal.

Early Complications

Early hematoma is a concerning complication that, if left untreated, can progress to infectious chondritis and subsequent necrosis. The most feared result of this is a cauliflower ear deformity. Causes of hematoma formation are improper plane of dissection, inadequate hemostasis before closure, poor protection of the auricle with a dressing, and postoperative trauma. The incidence is approximately 3%, and pain is often the presenting feature.[11] Any report of extreme or asymmetric pain should be followed by prompt evaluation and management. A bent ear and pressure necrosis are other scenarios that may cause unilateral pain. If found, a hematoma is evacuated by releasing sutures and milking out the clotted blood. Active bleeding is quite rare. The incision is then loosely closed over a passive Penrose drain. A fresh dressing should be applied and the patient prescribed a course of broad-spectrum antibiotics.

Infection

The risk of infection is minimized by the use of aseptic operative technique and antibiotic irrigation before closure. Overall, it is fairly uncommon. It typically presents in the first postoperative week with symptoms of pain and associated focal erythema. Purulence may also be visible or expressed from the wound. Precursors to infection are ischemia, pressure necrosis, and untreated hematoma. Treatment of infection is by simple incision and drainage, wound irrigation with clindamycin or gentamycin solution, and postoperative antistaphylococcus and antipseudomonas antibiotics (oral or intravenous depending on age and severity). In cases of severe chondritis, devitalized tissue should be debrided and the patient admitted and maintained on intravenous antibiotics.

Skin and Cartilage Necrosis

Skin necrosis is exceedingly rare and would be attributable to technical error, including violation of the subdermal plexus during surgical dissection, excessive use of cautery, application of an overly compressive dressing causing compartment syndrome, and placement over a bent ear. Management is similar to that of infection, with the addition of possible skin grafting or flap

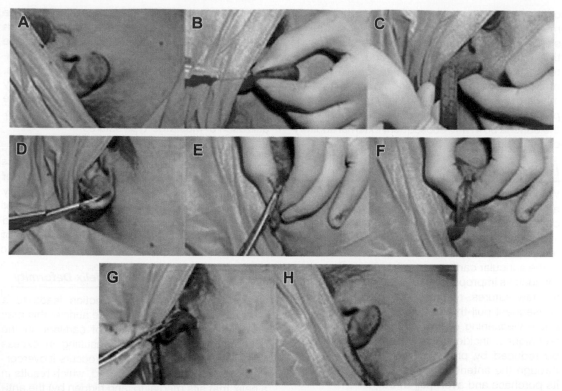

Fig. 4. Lobule reduction. (*A*) Symmetric anterior and posterior marking of preferred lobule margin; (*B, C*) local infiltration and measuring; (*D*) eccentric excision of redundant skin and soft tissue; (*E, F*) further excision of fatty tissue to facilitate closure; and (*G, H*) skin suturing and final intraoperative appearance.

advancement to cover exposed cartilage. Necrotic tissue must be debrided before coverage.

LATE COMPLICATIONS
Patient Dissatisfaction

Perhaps the most common complication is patient dissatisfaction (3%–17% with cartilage-sparing techniques[1]). Preoperative dialogue with the patient and family must establish realistic expectations. Like rhinoplasty, considerable improvement, not perfection, is the goal. Asymmetries in lateral projection within 2 to 3 mm are within normal range and often exist preoperatively. It is the authors' experience that slight overcorrection is more accepted than slight undercorrection. If the remaining deformity can be corrected surgically, then revision can be undertaken when appropriate. Correction is not always possible, or worth the risk of potentially making matters worse, which must be gently communicated to patients and their family.

Suture Complications

Various complications can occur with cartilage-sparing techniques, including suture complications. Unlike resorbable sutures, which are a common source of inflammation and stitch abscess formation in the short term, permanent sutures more frequently cause delayed, indolent infections and foreign-body granulomas. The reported incidence of this complication is 4.6% to 15%[1] with cartilage suturing techniques alone, and slightly higher if adjunctive excisional techniques are used. In these settings, the offending suture, which may be eroding or extruding partially through the skin, should be removed. The procedure is curative, provided any associated infection is properly managed. Consideration should be given to delaying the removal of the offending suture if it is early in the postoperative period and the correction is likely still reliant on the suture itself, rather than scar tissue, which may secure the position after several months. This is particularly true of Mustarde-type sutures at the superior pole. In general, monofilament sutures, while less reactive, have a greater tendency toward slippage, which could negatively affect the cosmetic result. It is for this reason that despite carrying a higher risk of infection, the authors prefer braided sutures for otoplasty. If scaphoconchal sutures are placed too far apart transversely relative to the antihelical fold, they may result in a "bow-string" appearance, or tenting underneath the skin. This situation is made worse if excessive postauricular skin excision is performed, resulting in a tense skin closure that thins out the suture coverage. Dermal flap techniques (involving de-epithelialization instead of skin excision) have been proposed to help mitigate this problem.[22] Finally, improper suture placement can cause anterior displacement of the concha bowl and subsequent external auditory canal occlusion.

Loss of Correction

With suture techniques, slight overcorrection is advisable to account for the expected loss of correction, the incidence of which is 6.5% to 12%[4] and is more a feature of cartilage-sparing techniques. It may be inherent to the elastic recoil of the auricular cartilage or, related to technical error such as improper suture location or placement, too few sutures, resulting in excess tension and subsequent pull-through of the sutures, or inadequate weakening of the cartilage with adjunctive techniques. Incidence of this complication may be reduced by proper placement of the suture through the anterior perichondrium to strengthen its purchase and avert pull-through.

Pathologic Scarring

Hypertrophic scarring or keloid formation may occur, particularly following postauricular incision. Patients at risk are younger or darkly pigmented or those with either a personal or family history. Pathologic scarring occurs almost exclusively in Asians, Africans, and Scandinavians. Preventive modalities include avoidance of excessive wound tension and careful surveillance for infection. Such scars are treated as they are in other locations.

Hypesthesia

Sensory disturbances are quite rare following otoplasty and, in cases where postoperative hypoesthesia occurs, it usually resolves spontaneously over several months. Instructions should be given to patients in subzero climates during the winter months to cover their ears when outside for prolonged periods to help avoid frostbite. Patients may be at increased risk of frostbite following otoplasty because of disruption in blood supply and/or transient sensory changes.

ESTHETIC COMPLICATIONS
Telephone Ear Deformity and Reverse Telephone Ear Deformity

Telephone-ear deformity occurs because of overcorrection in the mid-third, such as overzealous conchal setback or excessive skin removal in the mid-portion of the auricle. A relative protrusion is seen at the superior and inferior poles. Reverse telephone ear deformity occurs in the opposing scenario, in which prominence in the mid-third persists, and the superior and inferior poles are relatively overcorrected; this tends to occur in the absence of conchal setback sutures when indicated, or overutilization of Mustarde-type sutures.

Vertical Post-deformity

Vertical postdeformity refers to a unique type of exaggerated vertical scaphal folding caused by Mustarde-type sutures placed in a vertical, rather than oblique, fashion. Prevention can be achieved by placement of sutures along the natural arc of the antihelix.

Overcorrection and Hidden Helix Deformity

Overcorrection of lateral projection leads to a "stuck down" appearance of the auricle; this may occur if excessive reduction of cartilage in the concha bowl is performed, resulting in excess flattening. More commonly, this occurs if overcorrection of the antihelix is applied, which results in a helix that sits medial to (and hidden by) the antihelix on frontal view. This problem can be circumvented by initial placement of conchal setback sutures to avoid overtightening the antihelical sutures.

Antihelix Creasing and Puckering

Mustarde sutures that are too closely placed will cause notches or creases to form within the antihelix, rather than the desired gentle curvature. Similarly, overly large bites of more than 6 mm may cause puckering within the scapha.

Tragal Prominence

Tragal prominence occurs when a considerable degree of conchal setback is attempted without adequate excision of postauricular soft tissue to accommodate the conchal retrodisplacement. Thus, persistent postauricular soft tissue exerts anterior and outward counterpressure on the concha that is transmitted to the tragus, increasing its prominence.

Auricular Ridges

Cartilage-cutting techniques tend to destabilize the auricular cartilage. Changes in tensional forces with healing over time predispose to visible step deformities and ridging in patients subjected to these techniques. Therefore, cutting techniques are confined to finely feathered abrasions or scoring of the anterior antihelical surface only in the rare instance of markedly stiff cartilage. In this way, visible contour irregularities are avoided.

Interaural Asymmetry

Precise replication of both the sites for suture placement and the vectors of pull for each conchomastoid suture is critical to maintaining interaural symmetry. Frequent reevaluation and comparisons of both ears throughout the procedure will increase the probability of attaining a natural and consistent result. Final suture knot tightening should be postponed until the surgeon is assured of precise and correct suture placement. As discussed earlier, when prominauris is present only unilaterally, the patient should be advised of the possibility of achieving greater balance if both ears are operated on despite the relative normalcy of the uninvolved side.

SUMMARY

Otoplasty is generally considered to be a quick and painless procedure, but the experienced and knowledgeable surgeon recognizes the complexity of the operation and is mindful of its potential pitfalls. The vast number of known otoplasty methods is a testament to the complexity and level of difficulty involved with this procedure. Cartilage-sparing techniques, while offering a more predictable and natural result, attempt to counter the natural spring of auricular cartilage using sutures, which is a challenging proposition. Comprehensive and detail-oriented planning is required to optimize surgical outcomes, the importance of which cannot be overemphasized. In the authors' experience, a graduated, suture-based approach to correction of the auricle, beginning with conservative skin excision and conchal setback, followed by antihelical contouring and completed with adjunctive refinements, yields exceedingly reproducible outcomes and a high degree of patient satisfaction. It is hoped that the surgical pearls highlighted here can be of use to otoplasty surgeons in their current and future practice.

REFERENCES

1. Adamson PA, Litner JA. Aesthetic otoplasty. Shelton (CT): People's Medical Publishing House; 2011.
2. Becker OJ. Surgical correction of the abnormally protruding ear. Arch Otolaryngol 1949;50(5): 541–60. illust.
3. Adamson JE, Horton CE, Crawford HH. The growth pattern of the external ear. Plast Reconstr Surg 1965;36(4):466–70.
4. Adamson PA, McShane DP, Feldman RI. Otoplasty: an update. J Otolaryngol 1987;16(4):258–62.
5. Mustarde JC. The correction of prominent ears using simple mattress sutures. Br J Plast Surg 1963;16: 170–8.
6. Furnas DW. Correction of prominent ears by concha-mastoid sutures. Plast Reconstr Surg 1968;42(3): 189–93.
7. Adamson PA, Litner JA. Otoplasty technique. Facial Plast Surg Clin North Am 2006;14(2):79–87, v.
8. Furnas DW. Correction of prominent ears with multiple sutures. Clin Plast Surg 1978;5(3):491–5.
9. Webster GV. The tail of the helix as a key to otoplasty. Plast Reconstr Surg 1969;44:455–61.
10. Adamson PA, McGraw BL, Tropper GJ. Otoplasty: critical review of clinical results. Laryngoscope 1991;101(8):883–8.
11. Adamson P, Doud Galli SK, Chen T. Otoplasty. In: Flint PW, Haughey BH, Lund VJ, et al, editors. Cummings Otolaryngology - head and neck surgery. Philadelphia: Mosby Elsevior; 2010. p. 475–80.
12. Adamson PA, Strecker HD. Otoplasty techniques. Facial Plast Surg 1995;11(4):284–300.
13. Fritsch MH. Incisionless otoplasty. Laryngoscope 1995;105(5 Pt 3 Suppl 70):1–11.
14. Fritsch MH. Incisionless otoplasty. Facial Plast Surg 2004;20(4):267–70.
15. Fritsch MH. Incisionless otoplasty with conchal bowl recession. HNO 2012;60(10):856–61 [in German].
16. Bull TR. Otoplasty: Mustardé technique. Facial Plast Surg 1994;10(3):267–76.
17. Siegert R. Correction of the lobule. Facial Plast Surg 2004;20(4):293–8.
18. Sadick H, Artinger VM, Haubner F, et al. Correcting the lobule in otoplasty using the fillet technique. JAMA Facial Plast Surg 2014;16(1):49–54.
19. Raunig H. Antihelix plasty without modeling sutures. Arch Facial Plast Surg 2005;7(5):334–41.
20. Weerda H, Siegert R. Complications of otoplasty and their treatment. Laryngorhinootologie 1994; 73(7):394–9 [in German].
21. Tanzer RC. Deformities of the auricle: congenital deformities. In: Saunders W, editor. Reconstructive plastic surgery. Philadelphia: WB Saunders; 1977. p. 1671–719.
22. Basat SO, Askeroğlu U, Aksan T, et al. New otoplasty approach: a laterally based postauricular dermal flap as an addition to mustarde and furnas to prevent suture extrusion and recurrence. Aesthetic Plast Surg 2014;38(1):83–9.

Microtia Reconstruction
Autologous Rib and Alloplast Techniques

Jonathan A. Cabin, MD[a], Michael Bassiri-Tehrani, MD[a],
Anthony P. Sclafani, MD[b,*], Thomas Romo III, MD[c]

KEYWORDS

- Microtia • Rib graft • Medpor • Porous polyethylene • Auricular deformity

KEY POINTS

- Microtia, or abnormal external ear development, is a relatively rare congenital condition that is more common in certain ethnic groups, in men, and in the right ear.
- Given the complex structure of the ear and the difficulty in creating the anatomic environment for a neo-appendage, reconstruction of the auricle has always been a unique and challenging problem.
- There is no universal consensus on grading microtia. The most common nomenclature is the Weerda classification, which involves classifying the microtic ear on scale of grade 1 (small with normal features) to grade 3 (mass of deformed tissue).
- Autogenous rib reconstruction involves at least 2 stages (typically more), is generally a more durable reconstruction, and is less prone to infection.
- Alloplastic porous high-density polyethylene reconstruction typically involves 2 stages, is generally more aesthetic, involves less morbidity, and can be done at a younger age.

 Videos of microtia reconstruction accompany this article at http://www.facialplastic.theclinics.com/

OVERVIEW

Microtia, or abnormal external ear development, occurs in 1 in 4000 to 10,000 births. It has a higher incidence in Asian, Hispanic, and Native American populations, with some studies citing a statistically significant increased risk in children of multiparous mothers. There is also a higher risk in males versus females, and microtia more commonly affects the right ear.[1]

Embryologically, microtia is caused by malformation of the 6 hillocks that eventually join to form the auricle. During the sixth week of gestation, these hillocks form from the first and second branchial arches, eventually developing into the helix, lobule, tragus, and antihelix.[2] The concha and external auditory meatus are formed by the first branchial groove and, as such, can be affected independently of the other structures.

Reconstruction of the auricle is a unique and challenging problem faced by surgeons today. The complex structure of the ear, along with the inherent difficulty of placing a framework within a tight skin pocket, leads to a spectrum of results among the varying surgeons who have performed

Disclosure Statement: No disclosures.
[a] Otolaryngology – Head & Neck Surgery, New York Eye & Ear Infirmary of Mount Sinai, 310 East 14th Street, New York, NY 10003, USA; [b] Division of Facial Plastic & Reconstructive Surgery, Otolaryngology – Head & Neck Surgery, New York Eye & Ear Infirmary of Mount Sinai, Icahn School of Medicine at Mount Sinai, 310 East 14th Street, New York, NY 10003, USA; [c] Division of Facial Plastic & Reconstructive Surgery, Lenox Hill Hospital, 135A East 74th Street, New York, NY 10021, USA
* Corresponding author.
E-mail address: asclafani@nyee.edu

these procedures. Over the years, methods of treatment have evolved, with techniques becoming more refined, but the core concepts remain the same. In general, there are 2 potential reconstructive options: autogenous rib cartilage and alloplastic implantation.

HISTORICAL PERSPECTIVE

Reports of ear reconstruction attempts date back to the sixteenth century, with the first documented successful reconstruction reported by Johann Friedrich Dieffenbach in the mid-nineteenth century, using a folded mastoid flap to repair a traumatic defect. Pierce discussed the use of a cartilage graft in 1930, with Gilles first describing attempted microtia reconstruction with donor cartilage from a patient's mother in 1937. From this point forward, cartilage grafts (both human and bovine) gained favor; however, it was quickly noted that these grafts tended to soften and sag over time, with some ultimately resorbing or being rejected.

In 1943, Peer developed a technique whereby the auricle was prefabricated using costal cartilage fragments, which were fitted to a mold and stored in the abdomen for future implantation. There were issues surrounding the need for multiple operations, and that the structural integrity of the molded fragments could not withstand the deforming force of a tight skin pocket.[3] Tanzer described the subcutaneous placement of an autogenous cartilage graft framework in 1959.

The history of alloplastic auricular reconstruction is more recent. The use of alloplastic implantation for auricular reconstruction was initially attempted in the 1960s using silicone implants, but this reconstruction technique was fraught with complications, with a high incidence of implant failure, especially related to minor trauma or abrasions.[4,5] In 1990, Shanbhag and colleagues[6] first wrote of the feasibility of using porous high-density polyethylene (PHDPE) in a baboon animal model. Wellisz and colleagues,[7,8] in 1992, described the use of a prefabricated alloplastic implant for microtia reconstruction in humans, constructed from PHDPE, subsequently marketed in the United States under the trade name of Medpor PHDPE (Stryker, Kalamazoo, MI). This material proved to have many properties that are ideal for auricular reconstruction, and continues to be the alloplastic microtia reconstruction material of choice.

PATIENT ASSESSMENT

The grading of microtia suffers from the disagreement on a universally accepted standardized scale (**Table 1**). The most commonly referenced scale was originally described by Weerda and later refined by Aguilar. The Weerda classification is based on the severity of auricular deformity: grade I describes a small ear with normal features, grade II describes a rudimentary auricle with some recognizable components, and grade III refers to a mass of deformed tissue. The Nagata grading is based according to vestigial structures rather than a scale.[9]

Brent[10] uses 2 general categories to describe microtia: classical and atypical. Classical is used to describe a vestige resembling a "sausage-shaped

---

Table 1
Classification schemes

	Classical			Atypical	
Brent	Remnant vestige ("sausage-shaped appendage") Relatively normal lobule			All other types, including anotia, conchal remnants, vestiges with pits and grooves	
	Lobule Type	Conchal Type		Small Conchal Type	Anotia
Nagata	Remnant ear: + Lobule − Concha − Acoustic meatus − Tragus	Some: Lobule Concha Acoustic meatus Tragus Incisura tragus		Remnant ear: + Lobule + Small indent for concha	Complete absence of an auricle
	Grade I	Grade II			Grade III
Weerda/ Aguilar	Small ear: normal features	Rudimentary auricle: some recognizable components			Mass of deformed tissue

appendage" with a relatively normal lobule that is misplaced. The atypical category represents all other types, including anotia, microtias with conchal remnants, and vestiges with furrows, pits, or grooves.[11]

Nagata[12–14] also developed a grading system for microtia, consisting of the following categories: lobule type, concha type, small concha type, and anotia. Lobule type is a remnant of an ear with a lobule but no concha, acoustic meatus, or tragus. Concha type has some lobule, concha, acoustic meatus, tragus, and incisura tragica. Small concha type is a remnant ear and lobule with a small indent for a concha. Finally, anotia is the complete absence of an auricle.

Regardless of the system used to describe microtia, a surgeon must be mindful of other hypoplastic features of the face and temporal bone when planning reconstruction. Ultimately, symmetry is the goal.

Microtia is frequently associated with conductive hearing loss (CHL), with rates of concordant CHL upward of 90%. Sensorineural hearing loss is also seen, but at a much lower rate (~15%). It is therefore critical to assess the extent of the external auditory canal development and the child's hearing status. Children with bilateral CHL need to be fitted with a bone-conducting hearing aid from a young age to ensure normal cognitive development. Abnormalities associated with microtia include cleft lip/palate, microphthalmia, anophthalmia, cardiac defects, abnormal limb development, renal malformation, holoprosencephaly, and facial nerve dysfunction. Overt facial nerve dysfunction has been reported in as many as 15% of patients with microtia.

Associated anomalies occur in approximately 50% of cases and are most frequently in the regions arising from the first or second embryologic branchial arches. Craniofacial microsomia is a spectrum of malformations that affect these arches, and includes malformations such as Goldenhar syndrome, hemifacial microsomia, and oculoauricular vertebral dysplasia.[15]

Microtia is more common in the setting of Goldenhar and Treacher Collins syndromes, among other, rarer syndromes. With this in mind, all newborns with a microtic ear should be fully assessed for concurrent congenital abnormalities.[1]

Potential otologic surgery for atresia should be investigated. If aural atresia surgery is pursued, it is typically done after completed auricular reconstruction to preserve the blood supply for the reconstruction and aesthetic positioning of the neoauricle.[16] A thorough physical examination should be performed with attention to facial development and animation, ear symmetry, and dental occlusion. Further otologic evaluation with an audiogram and high-resolution temporal bone computed tomography (CT) scan are indicated before surgery. The CT temporal bone provides important information regarding the status of the middle ear, ossicles, and course of the facial nerve, all critical when weighing the benefits of, or planning, otologic surgery. A lateralized facial nerve will be at risk of injury during otologic drill-out surgery for an atresia repair. Alternative measures, such as bone-anchored hearing aide (BAHA) placement, should be considered in this situation. Family history of genetic disorders should be elicited, and if appropriate, genetic testing should be initiated.[17]

Timing of surgery plays an important role in reconstructive options. The age for optimal reconstruction varies depending on the particular surgical option.

In autogenous cartilage reconstruction, limitations in available rib cartilage must be balanced with potential psychological sequelae to a child with an auricular deformity. This has led to a general consensus that an appropriate window of rib reconstruction is between the ages of 7 and 10 years old. The Brent technique allows for the option for rib reconstruction as early as age 5, but the ideal age is still 7. The greater cartilage demands of the Nagata procedure require a larger chest circumference (at least 60 cm), which roughly correlates to an age of 10 for reconstruction. This limitation may be a factor for an anxious family or a child suffering psychological distress.

In comparison with autologous rib cartilage reconstruction, the indications for PHDPE reconstruction are narrower. PHDPE is indicated only in patients with Weerda second-degree and third-degree dysplasias, and in patients with failed autogenous rib reconstructions. PHDPE reconstruction can be done at an earlier age, as there is no need for donor rib to be a certain size. The patient should be at least 5 to 6 years old, as this is when the contralateral (normal) ear is approximately 85% of its normal, adult size. From a social perspective, this age also happens to coincide with the commencement of school, where the risk of ridicule and ostracism suddenly becomes higher.[1]

Of equal importance is the number of stages of reconstruction a patient or family is willing to endure, as cartilage reconstructive options require a commitment to a greater number of surgeries than alloplastic reconstruction. It is also wise to consider the inherent maturity of the child, factoring in the child's age and his or her observed behavior. Older children obviously have a greater understanding of what reconstruction entails and tend to be more engaged in the postoperative course. Familial concerns can be allayed with discussions and reassurance that the long-term benefits of a proper reconstruction ultimately outweigh the negatives of expedited surgery.[18]

CURRENT PRACTICE
Autogenous Cartilage

Rib reconstruction is the oldest method of microtia repair, and is touted by its proponents to be both the most stable in response to trauma, as well as more resistant to infection, when compared with alloplastic reconstruction. Essentially, rib reconstruction first involves carving and assembling a framework of costal cartilage with carefully placed sutures, and inserting this sculpted framework within a skin pocket in an aesthetically appropriate position. The later stages refine the appearance of the framework by introducing finer details, as well as elevating the framework away from the scalp.

The current era of the rib reconstruction has been credited to Tanzer. Other subsequent surgeons have contributed modifications and alterations to his technique, most notably Brent and Nagata. Regardless of specific technique, all reconstructive surgeries using rib cartilage adhere to the same general principles of tissue handling and skin redraping. The spectrum of techniques differs in terms of surgical timing, patient selection, and stage number.

Controversy continues to exist in terms of autogenous reconstruction itself, particularly between the Brent and Nagata techniques, the 2 most popular methods using costal cartilage. Both techniques borrow from Tanzer's original description, but have their own advantages and disadvantages. Although the Nagata operation has fewer stages, and reconstruction has been demonstrated to be more consistent, this technique requires more cartilage, and thus can be performed only at an older age. The Brent operation emphasizes limited cartilage harvesting, along with minimization of the chest wall deformity. The reduced cartilage demand for this procedure means that children can begin surgery at a younger age, potentially limiting psychological sequelae at school.

To this effect, surgical planning is critical to all reconstructive efforts in the ear. Accurate assessment as to the structures present helps to guide incision design and framework crafting. Miscalculations will result in the suboptimal appearance of the reconstructed ear. The numerous modifications described in Nagata's papers illustrate how attention to detail is necessary for creating a fabricated ear that is realistic and cosmetically appropriate; for example, although much of the Nagata procedure is the same for all 3, alterations in incisions and framework fabrication need to be customized to a patient's preoperative microtia type.

Brent technique

The Brent technique is a 3-stage to 4-stage procedure using autogenous rib cartilage, and is recognized among various rib reconstructive techniques for its durability. As of 1999, Brent had reported more than 70 reconstructed ears that had survived major trauma. In addition to blunt trauma, there are reports of graft survival after a bee sting and, in another, a dog bite. As a result, patients can resume normal activities after reconstruction.[10,19] The Brent technique also requires less costal cartilage, so it limits chest wall deformity and allows patients to be younger at time of first procedure.

Preoperative evaluation involves template formation using translucent x-ray film for proper placement and alignment of the future framework in the skin pocket using the contralateral ear as a reference point. The template is made using either the patient's unaffected ear, or in cases of bilateral microtia, a parent's ear. This template is sterilized and used during surgery.

The designed framework is made several millimeters smaller than the unaffected ear to account for skin thickness. The framework axis should be roughly parallel to the nasal profile and have the same distance from the lateral canthus as the contralateral side. The microtia vestige is drawn into the template so intraoperatively the template can be placed in the correct position without using other facial reference points.[10] Positioning of the construct can be much more difficult in the patient with facial asymmetry.

First stage Rib from the contralateral side is harvested, as its configuration allows the most efficient use of cartilage. Fabrication is undertaken using the synchondrosis of the 6th and 7th ribs.

An incision approximately 4 cm in length is marked (**Fig. 1**) and local anesthetic is injected 2 cm above the costal margin. A subperiosteal dissection begins at the inferior boarder of the costal cartilage and progresses posterolateral until the eighth rib is encountered (**Fig. 2**). The ribs are dissected to the osseocartilaginous junction laterally using Freer and Doyen rib elevators to carefully separate the cartilage from the intact deep perichondrium. Next, the synchondrosis usually found between ribs 6 and 7 is exposed. The connection between these ribs provides a large enough piece of cartilage to form the base of the framework. The previously made template is placed over the

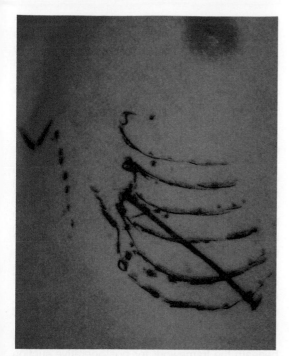

Fig. 1. A skin incision is made 2 cm above the lower costal border.

synchondrosis to plan the ideal area of the rib cartilage to harvest, which is then done with the superficial perichondrium intact. A malleable retractor is placed before harvest to protect the pleura and cartilage is cut out (**Fig. 3**).[2] Approximately 8 cm of eighth rib is needed for reconstruction. The eighth rib is also harvested for the creation of the helix (**Fig. 4**).

It is important to preserve an intact rim of the superior margin of the sixth rib to prevent chest wall deformity. Maintaining even a minimal rim will anchor the rib to the sternum, preventing chest flair and distortion, something that can become more apparent as the patient grows.

The wound bed is flooded with saline and a Valsalva maneuver is performed to assess for pneumothorax. Bubbles indicate the location of pleural violations. To repair any pleural tears, a soft, red rubber catheter is placed through the pleural rent and a 4-0 chromic purse-string suture is placed around the edges. Suction is applied to the catheter as it is withdrawn and the suture tied. Additional cartilage is banked either under the chest incision or in the scalp for future framework projection in a later stage. Next, the muscle, subcutaneous dermis, and skin of the chest incision are closed in a layered fashion with a suction drain placed over the muscle closure.

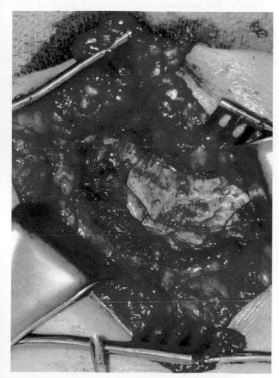

Fig. 2. Seventh rib, with synchondrosis with the sixth and eighth ribs, is exposed.

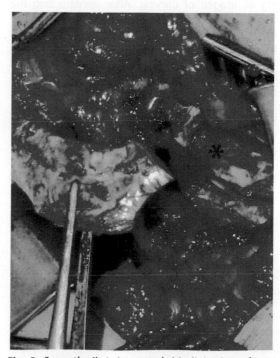

Fig. 3. Seventh rib is harvested. Medial edge of seventh rib (*asterisk*).

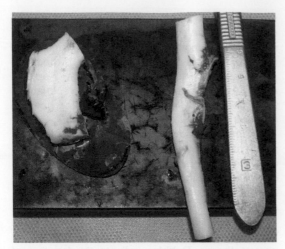

Fig. 4. Seventh rib, along with synchondrosis with sixth rib, is seen on the radiograph template. Approximately 8 cm of the eighth rib is harvested.

The cartilage framework is addressed next. Gentle tissue handling is essential during this stage. The cartilage is living tissue that must be kept moist. Perichondrium should be left intact when possible. Power tools are not used so as to avoid thermal damage to tissue. Use of foreign materials, such as permanent suture, is limited to prevent extrusion.

The framework base is fabricated by carving the sixth and seventh ribs. Sharp blades are used during all stages of carving. After constructing the base shape of the ear, the eighth rib is thinned longitudinally, allowing it to be wrapped around this base and secured judiciously by clear nylon sutures (**Fig. 5**, Video 1). Exaggerating helical height in this step is important to give the appearance of additional auricular projection.[10]

Details are carved into the framework after the helix is affixed (Videos 2 and 3). Carving is done with #11 and #15 scalpels, initially at the inferior aspect of the framework to create an antitragus.

A 5-mm gouge is then used for scooping out cartilage in the areas of antihelix to give it definition. The limit of gouging is the medial perichondrium, which needs to remain intact. In general, over-contouring is needed, as postoperative form is not as conspicuous as the underlying framework (**Figs. 6** and **7**).[2]

The skin pocket for the framework is also created in this first stage (Video 4). An incision is made via a small incision anterior to the microtia vestige. Remnant cartilage is dissected and discarded. Meticulous technique is used to ensure subdermal plexus is intact and the skin remains viable. Posterior dissection over the mastoid allows the skin to drape neatly over the framework. If not operated on before, the untouched skin pocket will have good skin elasticity.

Hemostasis is achieved and the framework is introduced into the pocket. Evaluating skin tension is essential for prevention of breakdown. Epinephrine is avoided so that blanching can be reliably used to indicate tension.

Before closure, infusion catheters are placed beneath the framework for postoperative suction drainage (**Fig. 8**). These are connected to vacuum test tubes in the recovery period. These suction drains have greatly reduced postoperative complications of cartilage exposure, infection, and hematoma compared with earlier mattress suturing.

Finally, the auricular contours are packed with Vaseline gauze, adding external pressure to aid in contouring and tight skin redraping. A loose overlying dressing of fluffed gauze is placed over the reconstructed site to protect it from trauma.[10]

Second stage In the second stage, the earlobe is transposed into its proper position. Transposition can be undertaken approximately 6 to 8 weeks after the initial surgery as an outpatient, or either combined with the stage 1 framework placement (**Fig. 9**) or the stage 3 framework elevation. Usually the lobule is situated too high and anterior. Thus,

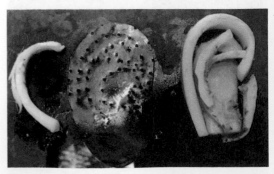

Fig. 5. Harvested cartilage is carved. Eighth rib is split longitudinally to serve as the helix. Auricular base is carved from ribs 6 and 7. Excised cartilage is saved.

Fig. 6. The final auricular framework (*right*), template (*center*), and cartilage to be banked and used during elevation (*left*).

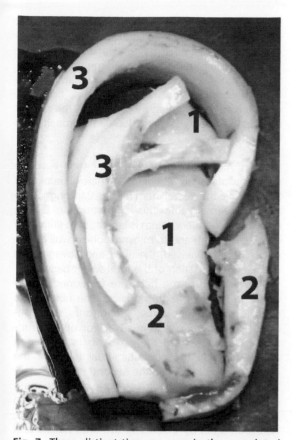

Fig. 7. Three distinct tiers are seen in the completed framework. The fossa triangularis and conchal bowl are the lowest (1), the lower antihelix, antitragus, and the cartilage cantilevered off the base to serve as the tragus, are slightly higher (2). Finally, the helical rim (resting on the lateral base of the scaphoid fossa) and the upper antihelix (additional cartilage sutured on to the carved antihelical base) project most laterally (3).

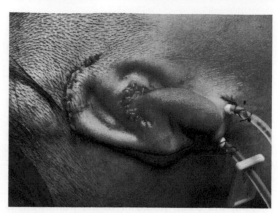

Fig. 8. Suction drains placed deep to the framework help coapt the skin to the auricular contours. Banked cartilage is placed superior to the upper helical incision, through which the framework was placed. The incision superior to the untransposed lobule was used to excise malformed microtia remnant cartilage.

rotation inferiorly will reposition it appropriately. Soft tissue of the lobule can be thinned superiorly, leaving fullness inferiorly. An inverted-V incision is made around the lobule, leaving an inferior pedicle (see Video 4). The helical rim of the framework is incised inferiorly to accommodate the newly rotated lobule on both sides. It is crucial to leave the framework intact during repositioning, as exposure of cartilage risks infection and extrusion. Xeroform dressings are applied to protect the closed incision lines, and the repositioned lobule is wrapped loosely with gauze again to minimize pressure or trauma.[2]

Lobule transposition may be staged to avoid scarring that would inhibit circulation to the framework and restrict elasticity during stage 1. Additionally, it may be more favorable to transpose the lobule once the framework is in proper position, so that its position can be aesthetically optimized.

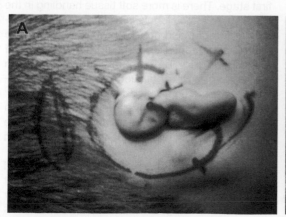

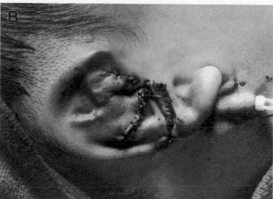

Fig. 9. Placement of auricular framework and simultaneous z-plasty lobule transposition. (*A*) Preoperative views. (*B*) Postoperative view.

Third stage The framework is elevated from the mastoid, creating a more natural-appearing ear capable of supporting eyeglasses and hearing aids. This step was neglected or delayed by some in the past, but doing so neglected the psychological impact of the reconstruction.

An incision is placed from the anterior crus and is extended superior to the auricle until reaching the area of the antitragus inferiorly. The lobule may need to be repositioned after framework elevation from the mastoid. If repositioning is anticipated, the incision should extend inferiorly to include the lobule.[2]

Next, the scalp posterior to the framework is undermined extensively. The banked portion of rib from stage 1 is wedged between framework and the mastoid bone. This is then covered with an occipitalis fascia turnover flap. The turnover flap is then covered with a split-thickness skin graft obtained from a donor site of the surgeon's preference. The turnover flap allows for adequate coverage for safe healing, and minimizing infection and extrusion. The skin graft is sutured and then secured with a Xeroform bolster in the postauricular sulcus. The bolster is removed after 5 days.

Fourth stage The tragus is constructed using a composite graft from the contralateral concha cymba of the unaffected ear. An incision is placed in the reconstructed ear where the posterior border of the tragus is anticipated. Skin flaps are undermined anteriorly and cartilage is inserted and sutured to the skin. Bolsters are applied again, creating the pretragal sulcus. A small skin graft is placed for coverage of the newly extended concha. The cartilage donor site of the contralateral ear is closed primarily.[2]

Adequate projection of the affected ear is often not achieved when compared with the unaffected ear. Therefore, otoplasty of the unaffected ear can be performed simultaneously during the fourth stage for maximal symmetry.

This fourth stage also can be included in the stage 1 reconstruction. In that situation, a rib cartilage graft is cantilevered off the inferior aspect of the original framework superiorly, simulating a tragus.[9,19]

Nagata technique

The Nagata technique begins in a fashion similar to the Brent technique. All preoperative assessments are the same, except Nagata categorizes microtia differently and technically uses ipsilateral rib cartilage for reconstruction. In essence, the Nagata technique combines the framework construct, placement, lobule transposition, and tragal reconstruction into the first stage of the procedure. The subsequent second stage is performed for elevation.

Its most obvious advantage is having fewer stages. It is a more challenging technique and requires knowledge of the nuances of auricular anatomy.

Preoperative analysis, measurements, and planning of framework placement are the same as the Brent technique. Incision planning is, however, customized to the category of microtia the patient has, as it also serves as the lobule transposition in the first stage.

Stage 1 Auricular framework fabrication is made using ipsilateral rib cartilage. An incision is placed 2 cm above the costal margin. Ribs 6 through 9 are harvested en block for this reconstruction. During rib harvest, perichondrium is left intact to stimulate cartilage growth and to minimize chest wall deformity. Once harvested, the sixth and seventh ribs are used for creation of the framework base.

The helix and crus helix are fashioned out of cartilage from the eighth rib, and the ninth rib is used for the superior crus, inferior crus, and antihelix. Residual cartilage is saved for other structures. Cartilage from the sixth rib is harvested and banked in the subcutaneous tissue of the chest incision for use in the second stage.

Construction of the framework requires more carving than the Brent technique. There is an emphasis on the helical crus, intertragal notch, and antitragus by extending the crus helicis and fixing it to the undersurface of the base frame.

The reconstructed frame has 4 different levels. From bottom up, they are the cymba and cavum conchae, crus helicis, fossa triangularis and scapha, and helix/antihelix/tragus/antitragus.[20]

Components of the framework are secured together using wire sutures. The loops of the wire are embedded into the cartilage by making small incisions with a scalpel, thus limiting chance of extrusion.

Lobule transposition is also performed during the first stage. There is more soft tissue handling in the initial stage as the lobule is dissected. The reconstructed tragus and concha have a deeper, more natural appearance as a result, but perfusion of the earlobe may be compromised. There is an increased chance of tissue necrosis with the Nagata reconstruction, which can be as high as 14%.[9]

Skin incisions for the lobule separate it into 3 skin flaps: the posterior and anterior skin flap of the lobule and the skin flap of the tragus. Skin is then undermined just below the subdermal plexus.[20]

Skin incisions for the lobule transposition are all modifications of the original Tanzer method that have allowed for more skin to be available for framework coverage. The Tanzer V incision starts from the mastoid and carries to the posterior portion of the lobule or remnant cartilage, with its most inferior point being at the lobule-mastoid junction. This V has been extended into a deeper more inferiorly placed W incision, with a subcutaneous pedicle to preserve perfusion. Location of the anterior incision is changed based on the Nagata classification system. In situations such as small lobule type microtia, the incision will be placed behind the indentation of the concha, and remnant cartilage will be removed. In conchal type microtia, only the upper portion of the native cartilage will be removed.[12,13,21]

During the lobule transposition, mastoid and posterior auricular flaps are raised, with a subcutaneous pedicle left intact. The blood supply of this pedicle has been controversial; however, one study analyzing the vascular supply during pedicle dissection demonstrated that perforators do exist and likely augment the blood supply to the skin flaps. These vessels were thought to derive from the posterior auricular artery based on location, but were not confirmed during the study.[22]

Once adequate undermining is achieved, the previously constructed framework is introduced into the skin pocket centered at the subcutaneous pedicle and the flaps are closed with the lobule in its newly transposed position. In conchal-type microtia, the framework insertion is quicker, as there is no inferior or tragal portion to insert.[20]

Stage 2 Stage 2 consists of elevating the framework off of the mastoid. This stage is usually performed 6 months after the first. The portion of banked sixth rib is retrieved. Before placement, the banked cartilage is shaved to a semilunar shape with an approximate thickness of 1 cm. An incision is made approximately 3 to 5 mm away from the edge of the framework in the mastoid skin following the shape of the helix from its insertion extending to inferior to the lobule. The framework is then elevated off of the mastoid and the previously carved semilunar cartilage is wedged between the framework and the mastoid and secured in place with nylon suture. The elevation and exposed portion of the mastoid is then covered with a temporoparietal fascia flap that is passed under a subcutaneous tunnel. This vascularized coverage will again prevent infection and extrusion. Superficially, the temporoparietal fascia (TPF) flap is covered with a skin graft that is bolstered in place.[9,20,23]

Complications

Potential complications for all autogenous costal cartilage reconstructions are similar. Donor site complications include pneumothorax, atelectasis, and scarring. Pneumothorax is avoided by careful dissection of rib cartilage and leaving perichondrium behind. After harvest, it is imperative to check for any air leak from the chest cavity by filling the wound with saline and performing a Valsalva maneuver. The presence of air bubbles indicates violation and requires repair. A red rubber catheter should be inserted into the defect and pleura and muscle should be closed over the defect in a purse-string fashion during positive-pressure ventilation while withdrawing the catheter. The less ominous possibility of atelectasis can be prevented by preoperative education and respiratory therapy as well as adequate postoperative pain control to prevent splinting.[20]

Auricular complications of hematoma and infection of framework are rare now that suction drains have become standard. Still, skin necrosis remains a possibility. Assessment of the skin pocket postoperatively for excess tension is needed to prevent necrosis and exposure of the framework. Appropriate undermining in the correct plane will prevent disruptions in perfusion. The Nagata technique has evolved over the years to create skin incisions that will maximize viable skin for the implant pocket. Skin shortage and scarring are troublesome problems in previously operated ears.

Usually, the TPF is used for salvage coverage of extruded grafts. In the Nagata technique, this flap is used upfront and is no longer available for salvage surgery.

Alloplastic Reconstruction

The other main option for auricular reconstruction with alloplastic grafts is PHDPE (Medpor; Stryker). PHDPE has several qualities that make it the ideal alloplastic material for total auricular reconstruction: it is a stable, inert substance that easily integrates with human tissue due to its porosity (average pore size of approximately 150 μm); it is thermoplastic, which allows it to mold and contour to its surroundings; and is associated with minimal foreign body reaction in the host. Compared with autogenous cartilage, it can be performed on a patient of a younger age, decreases operative time, and eliminates the morbidity of rib cartilage harvesting. It also has less resorption potential than rib, is less susceptible to operator ability, and tends to be more aesthetically accurate given its standardized and precise manufacturing process. For total auricular reconstruction, surgeons use a 2-stage approach that involves placing PHDPE under a TPF flap and covering it with full-thickness skin grafts.[7,8,24]

Planning

Before undergoing PHDPE auricular reconstruction, the patient must be evaluated for functioning superficial temporal artery and venous system to ensure viability of TPF grafting. Magnetic resonance imaging angiography, CT angiography, or even direct angiography has been used in cases of abnormal or difficult anatomy, and when the patient has had previous surgery, likely disrupting the normal anatomic configuration. A Doppler stethoscope is typically used to mark anterior and posterior superficial branches of superficial temporal artery at the time of surgery. In addition to anatomic planning, the surgeon should ensure that the patient is psychologically capable of understanding the surgery and its limitations, as well as aftercare and postsurgical restrictions.[25]

Procedural approach

In PHDPE auricular reconstruction, there are generally 2 surgical stages: stage 1 involves placement and coverage of the implant and stage 2 involves lobule transposition. This 2-stage procedure is described in the following paragraphs. Some investigators have described a 3-stage procedure, with an extra initial stage that involves the placement of a soft tissue expansion device in the area of the mastoid. The second stage of this modified procedure begins with the removal of this device, with the extra skin negating the need for skin grafting, with a subsequent and final stage involving the interposition of the lobule.

Stage 1

Preparation The surgical area is shaved and the entire face and neck are prepped in the usual fashion. An exposed radiograph template is used to trace the borders of the normal/contralateral ear (**Fig. 10**). As previously mentioned, this normal template can be obtained from a parent if the child does not have an anatomically normal contralateral ear. Although this template outlines the precise dimensions of the child's normal ear, after obtaining it, the template must be scaled down

to account for the soft tissue bulk that will eventually surround the PHDPE framework and, together, will create the ultimate auricular shape and size.

The patient is placed in the supine position, with the head flat and turned approximately 30° toward the contralateral side, as this provides greatest access to the area of concern and comfort to the surgeon.

The surgical field must be marked with a permanent black marker to carefully approximate the aesthetic positioning of the ear. The anterior helix should be approximately 6 cm from the lateral canthus and positioned at a 20-degree angle from a vertical line.

After marking aesthetic positioning of the auricle, using a Doppler stethoscope and a red marker, the anterior and posterior branches of the superficial temporal artery are traced to the height of the parietal scalp in preparation for TPF flap elevation. Using a green marker, the approximate course of the frontal branch of the facial nerve is marked as a line midway between the lateral eyebrow and the hair-bearing temporal skin.

Finally, a "Y"-shaped incision is marked, with the inferior aspect of the tail of the "Y" ending just superior to the position of the intended helix. The goal is to place the scalp incisions where they do not cross arterial junctions, while keeping these incisions perpendicular to hair growth (**Fig. 11**).

Initial local anesthesia The area of intended flap elevation (typically 10 cm superior to the intended helix and 5 cm posterior to the intended helical rim) is injected with 0.5% lidocaine and 1:200,000

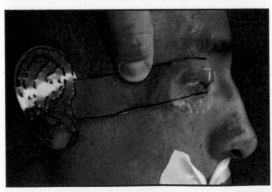

Fig. 10. Template created from contralateral "good" ear using radiograph film. A second, smaller template can be made to allow for the added bulk of fascia and skin.

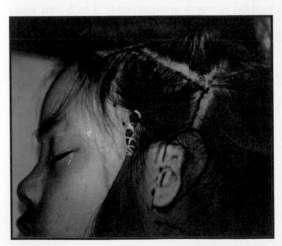

Fig. 11. Y-incision for scalp flaps outlined with indelible marker. This indicates the intraoperative outlining course of superficial temporal artery. The blood vessel's path is indicated with a red marking from scalp downward, ending superior to the position of the intended helix ear.

The resultant full implant is then placed into the inferior aspect of the temporal flap, marked as such before the procedure. A back-cut is made along the incision, to allow the implant to lateralize and project more naturally from the temporal bone.

A Hemovac drain (Zimmer Inc, Roodeport, South Africa) is placed at the level of, and posterior to, the helix. This drain, together with the implant, is placed into the created pocket.

The PHDPE framework is sutured to the post-auricular mastoid fascia using a 3-0 Prolene, and the drain is sutured in place using a 5-0 fast-absorbing gut.

At this point, the lower portion of the implant is covered with skin, comprising approximately the inferior two-thirds of the total implant.

Harvest and rotation of the TPF flap After measuring the correct TPF flap size for implant coverage, the flap is harvested and rotated down, ensuring complete coverage of the implant and the drain. The TPF flap is sutured into to the postauricular mastoid fascia using 5-0 chromic

sutures, ensuring secure placement and elimination of dead space around the implant. During this process, it is critical to ensure that the superficial temporal vessels are not kinked due to the flap placement (**Figs. 13 and 14**).

Final closure The drain is brought out the inferior portion of the incision and sutured into place using a 4-0 nylon suture. A 10-French bulb suction drain is placed in the surgical field, and the scalp flaps are closed over it. Once covered by the scalp flaps, the drain is sutured to the skin using 3-0 Prolene suture. The scalp flaps are then closed with alternating staples and 4-0 Prolene sutures.

After closure of the scalp flaps, native temporal skin is used to cover the lower two-thirds of the flap, and the upper one-third of the flap is covered with the full-thickness skin graft (harvested in typical fashion) (**Figs. 15 and 16**).

Stage 2 The second stage of the PHDPE microtia repair is generally performed approximately 3 months after the initial procedure, and involves the transposition of the lobule.

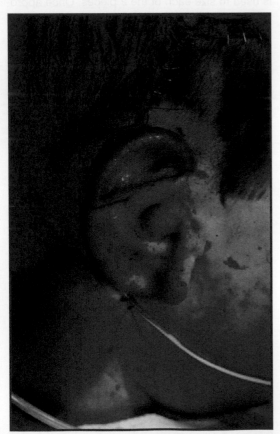

Fig. 15. The upper one-third of the framework and TPF combination is covered with full-thickness skin grafts harvested from original skin.

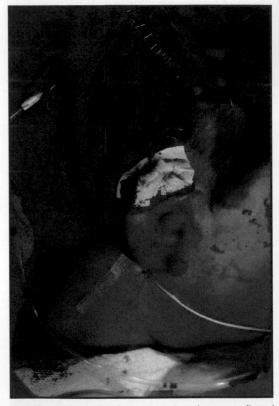

Fig. 16. The temporal scalp is closed over a fluted drain (shown exiting the skin to the left). The Hemovac draining the framework is brought through a skin incision below the auricle (bottom of the photo).

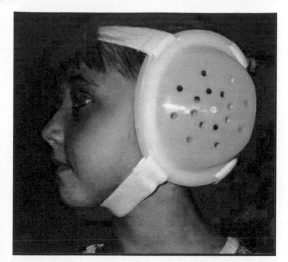

Fig. 17. A firm plastic cup dressing with Velcro straps is worn over the auricle day and night for 2 weeks.

To rotate the lobule into a cosmetically appropriate position, an inferior pedicle must be used. The fatty (inferior) portion of the auricular vestige is incised and rotated posteriorly, and sutured into place.

During the second stage of the repair, other fine-tuning can be achieved, including tragus creation (typically based on the superior portion of the vestige), deepening of the conchal bowl, and/or scalp scar revision. If indicated, a BAHA also can be placed at this time.

Postprocedural care After the first stage of auricular reconstruction, the patient must avoid any pressure on the reconstruction, and is instructed to use a firm, plastic ear cup over the reconstructed ear 24 hours per day for at least 2 weeks (**Fig. 17**). The reconstructed auricle is kept clean and dry for 2 weeks, with frequent applications

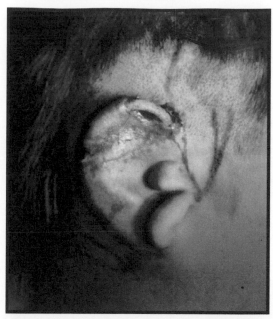

Fig. 19. Example of reconstructed auricle using a PHDPE framework at completion of stage 1, with early complications: exposed PHDPE framework secondary to necrosis of the full-thickness skin grafts.

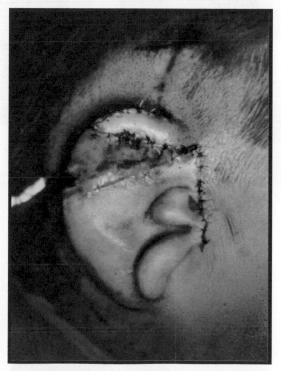

Fig. 20. Reconstruction of auricle using new PHDPE graft and a TPF-free microvascular graft from the contralateral side. Healing pattern is positive due to patient's adherence to good hygiene and avoidance of physical trauma.

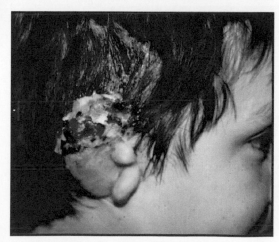

Fig. 18. Infection or compression necrosis of auricular tissue can cause loss of implant.

of a moisturizing ointment, such as bacitracin. Systemic antibiotics are generally not used.

The 10-French suction is removed between 7 and 10 days postoperatively, and the Hemovac is removed between 10 and 14 days postoperatively.

Potential complications and management Infection is a potential complication of any surgery. In alloplastic auricular reconstruction, it can present along a spectrum, from a superficial cellulitis to flap necrosis, and lead to potential loss of the implant. Aside from basic surgical sterility and postoperative wound care, a major factor in preventing implant failure is ensuring that the TPF flap covers the implant in its entirety. Most infections can be managed with the use of oral or intravenous antibiotics, and tissue debridement, if necessary.

Another potential complication is flap ischemia and loss due to compression. Compression can be in the form of trauma, poor flap planning, or from the protective ear cup itself.

Defects smaller than 1 cm can typically be salvaged with either a local advancement flap or additional full-thickness skin grafting. In the rare case of implant loss due to infection or compression necrosis (**Fig. 18**), reconstruction is possible using a new PHDPE graft and a TPF free microvascular flap from the contralateral side (**Figs. 19 and 20**).[24]

RECENT TRENDS AND CONTROVERSIES

A questionnaire-based study indicates that patients in general prefer autologous reconstruction (88%) over osseointegrated implant (11%) when questioned before surgery.[26]

In PHDPE reconstruction, some surgeons have described a 3-stage approach, with an added initial step of skin expander implantation. By generating a larger skin flap, the need for a skin graft is eliminated. Although this adds an extra surgery to the normally 2-staged PHDPE reconstruction, it is

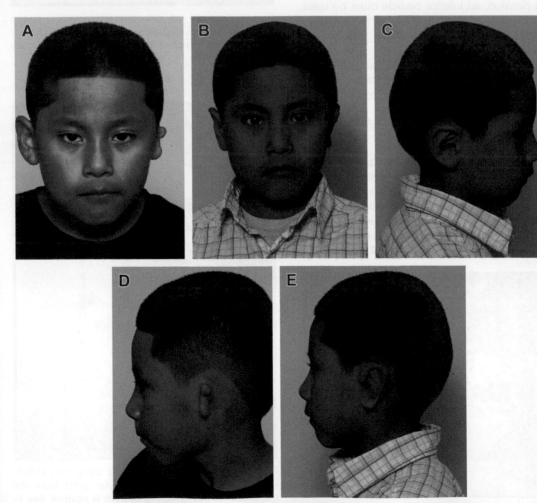

Fig. 21. Left microtia repair with autologous rib in 2 stages, with simultaneous right otoplasty. Preoperative views (*A, D*); postoperative views (*B, C, E*).

thought to create a more stable reconstruction and better skin tone matching.[25]

Future reconstruction will likely involve prefabrication of a biologic framework, derived from tissue engineering, on a scaffold sturdy enough to resist shape distortion from an overlying skin pocket. The source of autogenous cells is controversial, but candidates include stem cells, human chondrocytes, perichondrial cells, and periosteum, none of which are practical options yet.[27]

MEASURING OUTCOMES

There are no standardized objective measures for outcomes in microtia surgery. Investigators generally assess their work subjectively, with attention to shape, anatomic proportions, thickness, and definition (**Fig. 21**).[28]

Surgeons' techniques evolve over time, and continue to modify their framework patterns based on previous experience. Patient satisfaction is ultimately what should be assessed. Ability to wear hearing aids or glasses is an important feature of reconstructive surgery. Patients with a positive impression of their surgery can be seen with shorter haircuts or earrings, indicating some level of overt satisfaction.

SUMMARY

Microtia repair continues to be challenging, given the complex anatomy of the ear and the inherent difficulty in creating an appendage that becomes satisfactorily integrated without complication postimplantation. Although rib reconstruction has been the gold standard, as PHDPE reconstruction becomes more commonplace, there is controversy as to the best option. Given the various options for reconstruction, it is crucial that the surgeon consider the characteristics of the individual patient and family, as well as his or her own comfort level and skill-set, when deciding which of the reconstructive options to pursue. It is only a matter of time before stem cell technology offers a prefabricated ear framework that can be more easily integrated into the patient's body.

SUPPLEMENTARY DATA

Supplementary data related to this article can be found online at http://dx.doi.org/10.1016/j.fsc.2014.07.004.

REFERENCES

1. Romo T III, Reitzen S. Aesthetic microtia reconstruction with Medpor. Facial Plast Surg 2008;24(1):120–8. http://dx.doi.org/10.1055/s-2008-1037453.

2. Quatela VC, Goldman ND. Microtia repair. Facial Plast Surg 1995;11(4):257–73. http://dx.doi.org/10.1055/s-2008-1064542.

3. Converse JM. Reconstruction of the auricle. I. Plast Reconstr Surg Transplant Bull 1958;22(2):150–63.

4. Omori S, Matsumoto K, Nakai H. Follow-up study on reconstruction of microtia with a silicone framework. Plast Reconstr Surg 1974;53(5):555–62.

5. Williams JD, Romo T, Sclafani AP, et al. Porous high-density polyethylene implants in auricular reconstruction. Arch Otolaryngol Head Neck Surg 1997;123(6):578–83.

6. Shanbhag A, Friedman HI, Augustine J, et al. Evaluation of porous polyethylene for external ear reconstruction. Ann Plast Surg 1990;24(1):32–9.

7. Wellisz T. Clinical experience with the Medpor porous polyethylene implant. Aesthetic Plast Surg 1993;17(4):339–44.

8. Wellisz T, Dougherty W, Gross J. Craniofacial applications for the Medpor porous polyethylene flex-block implant. J Craniofac Surg 1992;3(2):101–7.

9. Zim SA. Microtia reconstruction: an update. Curr Opin Otolaryngol Head Neck Surg 2003;11(4):275–81.

10. Brent B. The correction of microtia with autogenous cartilage grafts. 1. The classic deformity. Plast Reconstr Surg 1980;66(1):1–12. http://dx.doi.org/10.1097/00006534-198007000-00001.

11. Brent B. The correction of microtia with autogenous cartilage grafts. 2. Atypical and complex deformities. Plast Reconstr Surg 1980;66(1):13–21. http://dx.doi.org/10.1097/00006534-198007000-00002.

12. Nagata S. Modification of the stages in total reconstruction of the auricle: part I. Grafting the three-dimensional costal cartilage framework for lobule-type microtia. Plast Reconstr Surg 1994;93(2):221–8.

13. Nagata S. Modification of the stages in total reconstruction of the auricle: part II. Grafting the three-dimensional costal cartilage framework for concha-type microtia. Plast Reconstr Surg 1994;93(2):231–8.

14. Nagata S. Modification of the stages in total reconstruction of the auricle: part III. Grafting the three-dimensional costal cartilage framework for small concha-type microtia. Plast Reconstr Surg 1994;93(2):243–8.

15. Murakami CS, Quatela VC, Sie KCY, et al. Microtia reconstruction. In: Cummings otolaryngology—head and neck surgery. 5th edition. St Louis (MO): Mosby; 2010. p. 2741–51.

16. Jahrsdoerfer RA, Kesser BW. Issues on aural atresia for the facial plastic surgeon. Facial Plast Surg 1995;11(4):274–7. http://dx.doi.org/10.1055/s-2008-1064543.

17. Beahm EK, Walton RL. Auricular reconstruction for microtia: part I. Anatomy, embryology, and clinical

evaluation. Plast Reconstr Surg 2002;109(7):2473–82 [quiz following: 2482].

18. Bauer BS. Reconstruction of microtia. Plast Reconstr Surg 2009;124(Suppl):14e–26e. http://dx.doi.org/10.1097/PRS.0b013e3181aa0e79.

19. Brent B. Technical advances in ear reconstruction with autogenous rib cartilage grafts: personal experience with 1200 cases. Plast Reconstr Surg 1999;104(2):319–34.

20. Nagata S. A new method of total reconstruction of the auricle for microtia. Plast Reconstr Surg 1993;92(2):187–201.

21. Tanzer RC. Total reconstruction of the external ear. Plast Reconstr Surg Transplant Bull 1959;23(1):1–15.

22. Ishikura N, Kawakami S, Yoshida J, et al. Vascular supply of the subcutaneous pedicle of Nagata's method in microtia reconstruction. Br J Plast Surg 2004;57(8):780–4. http://dx.doi.org/10.1016/j.bjps.2004.04.004.

23. Nagata S. Modification of the stages in total reconstruction of the auricle: part IV. Ear elevation for the constructed auricle. Plast Reconstr Surg 1994;93(2):254–66 [discussion: 267–8].

24. Romo T III, Fozo MS, Sclafani AP. Microtia reconstruction using a porous polyethylene framework. Facial Plast Surg 2000;16(1):15–22.

25. Yang SL, Zheng JH, Ding Z, et al. Combined fascial flap and expanded skin flap for enveloping Medpor framework in microtia reconstruction. Aesthetic Plast Surg 2008;33(4):518–22. http://dx.doi.org/10.1007/s00266-008-9249-0.

26. Botma M, Aymat A, Gault D, et al. Rib graft reconstruction versus osseointegrated prosthesis for microtia: a significant change in patient preference. Clin Otolaryngol Allied Sci 2001;26(4):274–7.

27. Ciorba A, Martini A. Tissue engineering and cartilage regeneration for auricular reconstruction. Int J Pediatr Otorhinolaryngol 2006;70(9):1507–15. http://dx.doi.org/10.1016/j.ijporl.2006.03.013.

28. Sabbagh W. Early experience in microtia reconstruction: the first 100 cases. Br J Plast Surg 2011;64(4):452–8. http://dx.doi.org/10.1016/j.bjps.2010.07.027.

Soft Tissue Trauma and Scar Revision

Steven R. Mobley, MD*, Phayvanh P. Sjogren, MD

KEYWORDS

- Pediatric facial scar • Scar revision • Pediatric procedural sedation • Topical therapy
- Laser resurfacing • Steroid injection • Tissue expander • Suture material

KEY POINTS

- Scars of the head and neck often have profound physical and psychosocial consequences in children; therefore, treatment should not be delayed in the pediatric population.
- The goal of primary soft tissue trauma of the face is to prevent the need for scar revision by applying proper wound closure techniques.
- The surgeon's armamentarium to improve on the appearance of facial scars should be broad and should generally start from the least to most invasive modalities.
- Treatment planning is an important aspect in children because successful outcomes depend not only on precise surgical technique but also on patient and family cooperation.

INTRODUCTION

Scars of the head and neck region can be physically and psychologically disfiguring. This cannot be emphasized enough in the pediatric population. Wound healing in young children and adolescents is crucial because excessive scarring can lead to low self-esteem and stigmatization.[1] Scars may be the end product of elective or urgent surgery, burns, and trauma. Most superficial facial wounds heal with few long-term sequelae; however, interruption of the reticular dermis likely results in residual scarring.

The ideal scar after complete maturation is narrow, flat, and similar in color to the adjacent skin. Conversely, unfavorable scars are hypertrophic, have wide margins and are misaligned with relaxed skin tension lines.[2] Patients should be made aware that their facial scars cannot be completely eliminated. Nevertheless, a plastic surgeon's armamentarium should include a variety of techniques to minimize initial scar formation and treatments in which to improve on unfavorable scars. The successful application of these techniques requires an understanding of their ideal timing and indications.

MANAGEMENT OF PRIMARY SOFT TISSUE INJURY

The ideal management of facial scars is to prevent the need for scar revision in the first place. This begins with appropriate selection of suture material and meticulous handling of the soft tissue to avoid trauma or closure under tension. Surgeons can achieve this by working in an environment in which they are comfortable. Of equal importance is the ability of patients to tolerate the procedure in an emergency department or outpatient setting. When it comes to treating a pediatric facial lesion,

Disclosure Statement: Dr S.R. Mobley is a national teacher of cosmetic chin implants for Implantech and receives a small remuneration for this annual teaching. Nothing in this work would be related to cosmetic chin implants.
Division of Otolaryngology–Head and Neck Surgery, University of Utah, 50 North Medical Drive, Salt Lake City, UT 84132, USA
* Corresponding author.
E-mail address: Mobley@MobleyMD.com

it may be next to impossible to have a child hold reasonably still to achieve proper repair techniques. Procedural sedation is, therefore, an indispensable tool in this setting.

PROCEDURAL SEDATION

Pediatric procedural sedation refers to the pharmacologic technique of managing a child's pain and anxiety during an uncomfortable procedure.[3] Procedures that are attempted in an uncooperative child often require restraints, which create adverse procedure outcomes and undue stress for patients and families.[4]

All children require a presedation assessment, which includes a focused medical history and physical examination to evaluate for risks of adverse events.[5]

Fasting

The amount of time a child should be fasting before procedural sedation continues to be disputed. Two large prospective trials showed no significant difference in adverse events between fasting and nonfasting children.[6] Several guidelines exist with differing recommendations regarding nothing-by-mouth timing; thus, the risks of immediate sedation must be considered in accordance with the urgency and nature of the procedure.[7] Potential settings for procedural sedation include emergency departments, subspecialty procedure suites, and physician offices. All locations must have age- and site-appropriate medications and supportive equipment readily available.

Sedatives

A review of the emergency medicine literature illustrates that many medications and cocktails are available to provide pain relief, anxiolysis, or both for a child during procedural sedation.

- Etomidate is a rapid-onset sedative with a short duration of action. It maintains hemodynamic and respiratory stability but reduces intracranial pressure.
- Over the years, ketamine has become commonplace in pediatric emergency departments. The agent creates a dissociative state and provides effective sedation and analgesia. Contraindications include sympathomimetic medical conditions, elevated intracranial pressure, coronary heart disease, and a history of psychosis. Ketamine should not be administered to infants 3 months or younger secondary to risk or respiratory compromise.[8]

- Propofol is a rapid-onset, short-acting agent that offers sedation and antiemetic properties. It has no analgesic properties, however, and therefore warrants coadministration of another agent for pain control. The agent is a potent respiratory depressant and a reversal agent does not yet exist. Thus, it is prudent to monitor the respiratory status of patients under sedation with propofol and provide airway intervention if necessary.[9]
- A sedative combination is available that consists of 1:1 intravenous (IV) ketamine and propofol. Ketamine's sympathomimetic properties act to counter the respiratory depression and hypotension seen with propofol whereas the latter counters ketamine's emetogenic properties.[10] Shah and colleagues[11] conducted a randomized trial that suggested greater satisfaction with the sedative combination among patients and providers versus propofol or ketamine alone. Another randomized controlled trial comparing propofol alone with the combined agent found more patient and provider satisfaction but unchanged respiratory depression.[12] Another group found that the propofol and ketamine combination provided more consistent sedation depth than propofol alone.[13]

Administration of Sedation

Intranasal administration of sedative agents offers more rapid onset of action compared with IV or intramuscular administration, with less discomfort.

Intranasal midazolam can provide anxiolysis during simple procedures, including incision and drainage and minor laceration repair.[14]

Inhaled nitrous oxide (N_2O) is another option for pediatric procedural sedation. One prospective randomized study compared inhaled N_2O and IV ketamine during laceration repair in children.[15] The ketamine group had higher initial pain scores and more emesis than the N_2O group; however, results may be biased secondary to IV placement in the ketamine group alone. A large prospective, observational study showed a good safety profile for sedation with N_2O administered at 70% concentration by nasal mask for procedures of fewer than 15 minutes in children.[16]

SUTURE MATERIAL

Traumatic lacerations are among the most common reasons that children are seen in the emergency medical setting. Pediatric wounds must be closed with special attention to avoid excess tension. Skin elasticity is inversely proportional to patient age with a greater tendency to stretch into a wide scar over time. Local muscle tension and lesions over bony prominences as well as edema increase wound tension.[17] Some wounds can be remedied with surgical adhesive tape and tissue glue but others require sutures depending on the location, size, and width of the defect.[18] The use of absorbable suture and tissue adhesives obviates a return to clinic, thereby decreasing costs associated with missed work and school.

Traditional teaching dictates that nonabsorbable sutures be used for approximating the outermost layer of lacerations, especially those under tension. Several studies have challenged this approach, however. In a single-blind, randomized controlled trial comparing outcomes of traumatic pediatric lacerations repaired with absorbable plain gut and nonabsorbable nylon sutures in an emergency department, no difference was found in the rate of dehiscence or infection. Cosmetic results seemed at least as good as in wounds repaired with nonabsorbable nylon sutures.[19] Parell and Becker[17] compared rotational advancement flaps of the head and neck, in which half the wound was closed with 5-0 polypropylene and the other half with 5-0 polyglactin. At the 6-month mark, no difference was noted in scar formation. One study compared facial lacerations closed with rapid-absorbing gut suture, nylon suture, and tissue adhesive octyl cyanoacrylate and no differences in cosmetic outcomes were identifies at 9 and 12 months.[20] Recently, Luck and colleagues[21] compared nylon sutures with fast-absorbing catgut sutures in the repair of pediatric facial lacerations. In contrast to their previous study[22] in which there was no difference in cosmetic outcomes between the 2 groups, physicians found better results at 3 months in the nylon suture group compared with the absorbable group. Caregivers in this study found no difference, however, with respect to the appearance of the scar. A meta-analysis of the pediatric literature suggested that nonabsorbable sutures were not superior to absorbable sutures in the management of wound repair but larger, methodically sound trials are warranted.[23]

Meticulous technique and ideal suture selection are critical in the repair of the pediatric facial lesion. Other factors are beyond a surgeon's control and include the mechanism of injury and position of the wound as well as a patient's overall health, nutrition status, and tendency to form robust scars. Topical therapies have been investigated as potential adjuncts to decrease the severity of scar formation and to optimize wound healing.

TOPICAL THERAPY

Scar prevention begins with the environment in which is it allowed to heal. In a closed wound, re-epithelialization occurs within 24 to 48 hours. The optimal milieu for wound healing is a moist environment because it encourages cell migration and can double the rate of epithelialization.[24] Occlusive or semiocclusive dressings can be used to generate a moist environment and additionally can wick away excess fluid that can macerate surrounding tissue or encourage bacterial growth.[25] Topical therapies for the prevention and minimization of scars remain an area of controversy. To date, no single topical treatment is touted as the ideal agent in the prevention or elimination of hypertrophic scars.

Vitamin E

Vitamin E consists of a group of fat-soluble tocopherol and tocotrienol derivatives with robust antioxidant properties. Vitamin E theoretically modulates scar formation by reduction of inflammation, fibroblast proliferation, and collagen synthesis.[26] A prospective single-blind study compared postoperative twice-daily application of vitamin E to petrolatum in children. Based on assessments by an external surgeon and the caregiver, 96% of the treatment group showed better cosmetic results compared with 76% in the control group.[27] A double-blind controlled study of 15 patients, however, who had undergone skin cancer excision, applied a petroleum-based ointment with and without vitamin E to the wounds twice daily for 4 weeks. In 90% of the cases, topical vitamin E either had no effect on or actually worsened the cosmetic appearance of scars and 33% developed a contact dermatitis.[28] Given the paucity of scientific evidence available and risk of contact dermatitis, the routine use of topical vitamin E is generally not encouraged.

Allium cepa

Onion extract, or Allium cepa, has antiinflammatory, bacteriostatic, and fibrinolytic properties.[29] The topical gel Mederma (Merz Pharmaceuticals, Frankfurt, Germany) contains 10% aqueous A cepa. Use of onion extract has been suggested to be efficacious in reducing various types of scars but such studies lack a proper control arm. A newer formulation of Mederma Advanced Scar Gel contains a higher concentration of onion extract along with a proprietary liposomal skin penetrator system. A clinical trial of this new formulation suggested improved overall appearance, redness, softness, and smoothness of treated lesions, but the control group had no topical treatment at all.[30] Chung and colleagues[31] conducted a randomized, double-blind, split-scar study of 24 patients who showed no scar improvement compared with a petrolatum ointment. Treatment of 17 scars after Mohs surgery had no statistically significant difference in erythema and pruritus after 1 month of thrice-daily applications and had better results with the petrolatum control group, which suggests that scar hydration plays a more important role in wound healing.[32] At this time, there is insufficient evidence to support the routine use of onion extract as a topical therapy.

Silicone

Silicone is a soft, semiocclusive scar cover made of cross-linked polydimethysiloxane polymer with several available formulations.[33] The mechanism of action in scar remodeling has not been well elucidated, although its healing properties are thought to stem from hydration, occlusion,[34] reduced capillary activity, and fibroblast-induced collagen deposition.[35,36] Silicone gel alone compared with silicone cream with occlusive dressing showed a 22% versus 82% decrease in erythema, tenderness, pruritus, and hardness, suggesting that the occlusive factor may be synergistic and that silicone sheeting may be more effective than silicone gel alone.[37] A small study of children with hypertrophic scars treated with silicone sheeting showed that 3 of the 5 treated children showed initial improvements in scar size, thickness, softness, and vascularity[38]; however, adverse side effects included rash and skin breakdown. Silicone gel sheeting has been demonstrated to increase the elasticity of preexisting scars between 1 and 6 months.[39,40] An international advisory panel has supported silicone gel sheeting as a primary option in the treatment of hypertrophic or keloid scars. Silicone gel sheeting, as opposed to silicone gel alone, seems efficacious in improving the appearance of new and preexisting hypertrophic scars.[41]

If Topical Therapies Fail

Despite superb primary repair techniques and the use of topical therapies, the wound may not appear optimal in the eyes of the surgeon or family. It is then time to contemplate more invasive interventions to improve the long-term outcome of the final scar. Intralesional steroid administration is a useful office procedure that can soften and mold either a maturing primary scar or older matured scar into a less visible lesion.

TRIAMCINOLONE INJECTION

Facial plastic surgeons wishing to maximize the management of their patients with facial scars should become comfortable with the use of intralesional scar tissue triamcinolone injections. For the purpose of this discussion, it is difficult to outline an exact formulation because there is great variability in judgment with the application of intralesional steroid injections. Nevertheless, general guidelines can steer a maturing facial plastic surgeon to develop a strong working knowledge on the use of this important office-based clinical intervention.

Indications for steroid injections include

- Persistent tissue edema after scar revision
- As adjunctive treatment of hypertrophic scars and keloids

Hypertropic scars and keloids are typically associated with a facial scar that rises above the natural surface level of the surrounding skin. Medical triamcinolone designed for injections typically comes in 2 standard concentrations. A surgeon starting to gain comfort with this procedure may start with a concentration of 10 mg/mL and should strongly consider diluting this to 2.5 mg/mL until confidence with this intervention is gained. For concentrations of triamcinolone at 2.5 mg/mL, the surgeon may inject 0.05 to 0.1 mL of medication per approximate linear 5 to 8 mm of scar tissue.

A key aspect to keep in mind when mastering this technique is that although it is always possible to bring a patient back for repeated injection sessions, it is impossible to uninject a patient. It is always more prudent to do multiple injections spread out over the course of several weeks or months than to accomplish maximum scar softening or flattening with a single injection. When a surgeon attempts to soften and/or flatten the scar with a single higher concentration injection, there is a risk of overflattening the area. Subcutaneous fat atrophy can additionally lead to a post-treatment divot in the treated area, which can be difficult to permanently reverse although cosmetic fillers can be a temporary remedy.

Timing of Steroid Injections

Injections are typically performed between 2- and 6-week intervals, with 4 weeks the most common time interval. Patients are advised to massage the treated area for approximately 24 hours after injection. The logic is that after the initial injection, the concentration of the antiinflammatory agent is at its highest, and patients should therefore be instructed to perform firm digital massage of the target area to gain maximum softening and flattening benefits.

Lip Scar Injections

Scars in the upper and lower lips are particularly amendable to steroid injection. The senior author has observed that over the course of many years of treating patients with routine lip lacerations, even after proper initial wound management and closure, patients often develop a firm, subcutaneous nodularity in the lip tissue. Typically, patients present with this finding 1 to 2 months after a successful lip laceration repair. Whether this is a result of the effect of the initial laceration on minor salivary gland tissue has not yet been fully elucidated. Patients may describe this phenomenon as a small bump in the affected tissues of the lip. This nodularity can be palpated on physical examination by performing a gloved examination with 1 finger inside the oral cavity to stabilize the tissue and a thumb pressing against the outer skin. These particular lesions respond effectively to triamcinolone injections. Again, this is an area where starting at a concentration of 2.5 mg/mL of triamcinolone is most prudent. As the surgeon develops experience with this technique, the concentration of triamcinolone injections can be increased to 10 mg/mL. The amount injected typically ranges from 0.05 to 0.2 mL during 1 session.

Risks with Intralesional Steroid Injections

Surgeons should always counsel patients on the risks of intralesional steroid injections, which include excessive subcutaneous fat atrophy that can create divots, telangiectasias of the surrounding skin, and thinning of the dermis. In the senior author's experience, the negative side effects of intralesional steroids can be significantly reduced with injections completed at lower concentrations, performed at the appropriate time intervals and with close clinical follow-up.

Analysis of Treatment Options

The initial assessment of any scar in the office setting by a facial plastic surgeon should include analysis of the treatment options applying a reconstructive ladder model, which implies starting with the simplest treatments before seeking more invasive management options. Can the wound be managed simply with topical therapy, such as silicone sheeting? Or would intralesional steroids be more appropriate? More invasive options of a scar revision include laser application, dermabrasion, and surgical intervention.

LASERS

Laser therapy in children poses unique advantages as well as challenges compared with their adult counterparts. Pediatric lesions are often smaller and thinner. With aging, the composition of vascular and pigmented lesions becomes more resistant to laser therapy; therefore, treatment of lesions at an early age allows for enhanced results in fewer sessions. Laser parameters should be adjusted for smaller vessel caliber and the unpredictable nature of scarring in pediatric skin.[42,43]

Laser-tissue interactions are guided by principles of selective photothermolysis, which include adequate fluence to damage the target tissue while minimizing collateral damage to surrounding tissue. A light wavelength is chosen that is selectively absorbed by tissues of interest, and a pulse duration is selected equal to or less than the thermal relaxation time of the target tissue to avoid conduction of thermal energy to surrounding tissues. This is defined as the time required for 90% of the tissue to cool to half of the temperature achieved immediately after laser exposure. The fluence, which is the energy density of the laser in J/cm^2, should be sufficient to heat the target tissue. The choice of light wavelength and laser parameters depends on the scar size, color, texture, and classification.[44]

Laser Selection for Scars and Keloids

The carbon dioxide (CO_2) and erbium:YAG (Er:-YAG) lasers traditionally were used to treat hypertrophic scars and keloids. The pulsed dye laser (PDL) has become the preferred laser for these lesions.[45] The proposed mechanisms of action include selective photothermolysis of vasculature,[46] release of mast cell constituents that alter collagen metabolism,[47] reduction of transforming growth factor β expression, fibroblast proliferation, and collagen type III deposition.[48] The heating action of the PDL is also thought to disrupt disulfide bonds with subsequent realignment of collagen fibers.[49] The PDL has been shown to improve scar size, erythema, pliability, pruritus, and texture; results of treatment on facial scars have been promising.[50,51] Post-treatment purpura is the most encountered adverse side effect and can last for several days. Other postoperative complications include edema, vesiculation, and crusting. Hyperpigmentation has been reported in 1% to 24% of cases,[52,53] and treatment should be resumed only after resolution to ensure extra melanin does not interfere with laser absorption.

Ablative Lasers

Depressed scars are caused by inflammation and collagen destruction with atrophy. The goal of laser treatment of these hypopigmented and fibrotic lesions is to decrease the appearance of scar borders while stimulating collagen deposition in the wound depression. Ablative lasers cause a photothermal effect with subsequent collagen contraction and remodeling that improves textural irregularities.[54] Recontouring of the scar can be achieved with the Er:YAG or CO_2 lasers. Both are preferentially absorbed by intracellular water, but the shorter wavelength of the Er:YAG laser increases its absorption rate by 16-fold.[55] Compared with the CO_2 wavelength, the Er:YAG light is associated with fewer pigmentary changes but may cause pinpoint bleeding due to inferior hemostasis.[56] Side effects include erythema and edema with occasional serous discharge. The erythema typically appears worse in first several days with gradual resolution over the subsequent weeks.[57] Hyperpigmentation, rather than hypopigmentation, is the more common side effect and is usually observed during the first 3 to 4 weeks post-treatment. The high cost and potential side effects may limit the use of ablative lasers in pediatric patients.[58]

Nonablative Lasers

Nonablative lasers selectively target the dermis, thus sparing the epidermis. For this reason, nonablative lasers have a lower side-effect profile, which includes local erythema, edema, and, less frequently, herpes simplex reactivation or vesiculation. The tradeoff of the lower-risk profile is reduced clinical efficacy.[56] Children and their families may find it challenging to comply with the 3 to 5 sessions required each month to achieve clinical results. Visible changes are noticeable within 3 to 6 months.[59,60] The reduced side effects of nonablative lasers may be a better option because pediatric skin has a propensity to remain erythematous longer compared with adult skin, although more investigations in this area are warranted.

Fractional lasers create microcolumns of dermal necrosis surrounded by zones of viable tissue. The intact surrounding tissue acts as a reservoir of healthy epidermal and dermal cells that aid in wound healing.[61] Fractional lasers are available in both nonablative and ablative forms. The nonablative fractional laser (NAFL) preserves the stratum corneum, thereby preserving the epidermal barrier. Superior clinical results can be obtained with greater energy settings and multiple laser passes, but a higher density is more likely associated with erythema, edema, and

hyperpigmentation.[62] Typically, patients require monthly treatments with more appreciable cosmetic results after each successive session.[52]

Ablative Fractional Laser

The ablative fractional laser similarly creates laser microarrays in the skin but does not preserve the stratum corneum.[63] Although there remain areas of viable epidermis to aid in healing, immediate post-treatment results are similar to purely ablative treatment, including severe erythema and serosanguinous drainage due to lack of protective columnar regions.[64] Compared with NAFL, fewer sessions are required because most patients benefit from 1 to 2 treatments every 6 to 12 months.[56] In a prospective study of 24 children with facial scars who underwent fractional CO_2 laser resurfacing, clinical improvement was found excellent in 58% and good in 29% of cases without adverse events.[65]

DERMABRASION

Another option for minimally invasive management of the facial scar is dermabrasion. This technique consists of controlled resurfacing of the superficial skin to smooth surface contour irregularities and to soften the appearance of scars. The skin of the face is unique in its rich vascular and adnexal system that allows blood, oxygen, and macronutrients to be readily available in the wound healing process.[66] The optimal timing of postoperative scar dermabrasion is variable. When the technique was initially described, the ideal timing was suggested to be 4 to 8 weeks postinjury.[67] Before 4 weeks, scars have a propensity to spread due to insufficient tensile strength. Katz and Oca[68] investigated wound healing after dermabrasion with a diamond fraise in a split-scar model. Scars were improved at 4 and 6 weeks; however, a greater number of patients responded at 8 weeks. Other investigators contend that dermabrasion should be performed at 6 to 8 weeks during maximum collagen remodeling.[69] In a study of skin cancer defect reconstruction, investigators suggested that dermabrasion is most useful 6 to 12 weeks after closure during active collagen remodeling.[70] A review of the literature shows that although skin resurfacing has been studied in pediatric burn patients, no investigations have focused on the use of dermabrasion for scar revision in children.

RE-EXCISION AND CLOSURE

When a surgeon has attempted the treatments (described previously) without adequate improvement or concluded that the initial wound has enough characteristics to warrant surgical revision, several options are available.

- Would the scar benefit from simple excision and secondary closure (re-excision with everted closure)?
- Does the scar need to be reoriented, requiring a Z-plasty?
- Would the scar benefit from irregularization techniques as in a W-plasty or GBLC?

The selection process among these differing modalities is discussed.

When contemplating re-excision, a scar typically has a good orientation on the face but is wide, depressed, or excessively elevated. Subcutaneous or surrounding tissue fullness is another reason to consider re-excision. For most facial scars, maturing surgeons may focus more keenly

on the closure technique. With time and experience, however, surgeons learn that when performing re-excision, the initial contact of the scalpel blade with the skin surface can be one of the subtlest yet most important determining factors in creating a more pleasing, hidden facial scar.

There are specific nuances concerning the initial contact of the blade with skin that should be followed.

Re-excision nuances:

- The skin should be marked in place without tension applied.
- The re-excision should be made as small as possible so as not to increase the defect on the patient's face. The re-excision scar is a few millimeters longer in linear length in order to re-encompass the original scar tissue (**Fig. 1**).

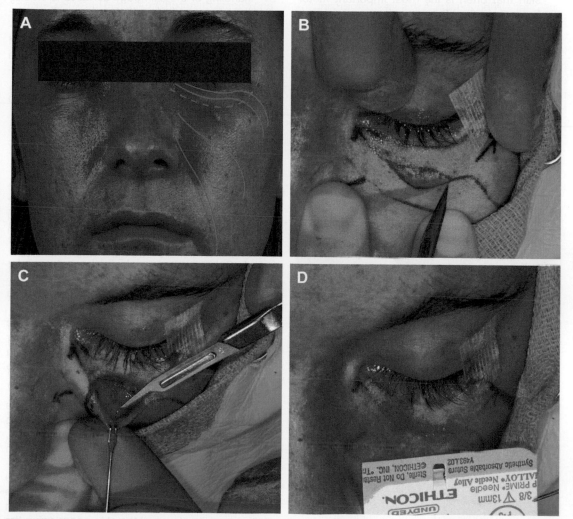

Fig. 1. (*A*) The incision is marked in accordance with relaxed skin tension lines. (*B*) The initial contact of the blade with skin is under extreme 4-point tension, (*C*) followed by sharp tissue undermining (*D*) and final closure of the revised scar.

- On initial execution of the scar, the choice of surgical scalpel is important. For an extremely small scar, the senior author prefers to use a Surgistar 15 degree Microknife (**Fig. 2**). For a majority of facial scars, a 15-blade should be selected, and when the scar is longer in linear length, a 10-blade is adequate. As a general rule, as the linear length of the scar increases, surgeons are better served by using an increasingly larger blade.

- Once an appropriate scalpel has been selected and the scar carefully marked on a patient's face, the initial contact of the blade with the patient's skin should occur under extreme 4-point tension. This extreme 4-point tension allows the best opportunity for the blade to cut cleanly through the skin, and it is this initial contact of the scalpel with the skin that often is the most important factor for an optimized final scar after re-excision.

- A crucial point of the execution of the initial cut is determined by the angle of the surgeon's blade, which should engage the skin at approximately 10° to 15° from a 90° perpendicular line to the surface of the skin. This sets the stage for a favorable bevel to skin edge and contributes significantly to the final re-excised scar. The importance of this subtle angle cannot be emphasized enough. Despite the challenge of maintaining this angle when re-excising tissue under tension, it is critical to do so for optimal results.

- After the initial skin excision, the epithelial elements of the scar should be partially excised, leaving a thin dermal base in the wound bed. A slightly raised scar can typically be treated in the postoperative period with dilute triamcinolone injections. The depressed scar, however, is more challenging to reverse. For this reason, it is better to leave a thin layer of dermis from the original scar in the newly excised tissue bed to provide a collagen matrix on which the new scar forms.

- After the initial incision and excision of the superficial epithelial component of the scar, modest undermining should be performed. At this point of the operation, delicate handling of the skin edge surfaces is crucial. It is recommended that only small single- and double-prong retractors be used to handle the skin edges. Regular forceps should not be used to handle the skin edges because it induces tissue trauma. Tools, such as fine-tooth pick-ups or Adson-Brown forceps, help create more pristine edges for a more elegant final closure.

- After undermining, standard hemostasis is achieved, and attention is next turned to closure.

- The selection of a subcutaneous stitch depends on a surgeon's experience and the specific clinical scenario. The senior author recommends 3 common sutures depending on the amount of tension involved in closure:

  1. Subcutaneous polyglactin sutures for wounds with low tension
  2. Poliglecaprone sutures for wounds with a medium amount of tension
  3. Polydioxanone suture, which can be reserved for wounds closed under higher tension; however, too many sutures with this material in the subcutaneous closure may lead to suture spitting.

A successful subcutaneous closure should be measured by the simple fact that if everything has been appropriately executed to this point, the skin edges should be touching one another in a slightly everted fashion before any superficial sutures are placed. If there is visible dermis after the subcutaneous closure, then there has been some error in execution either in the original incision (failure to properly bevel the skin edges using the angles previously discussed) or during the deep closure technique.

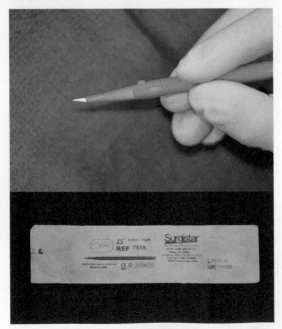

Fig. 2. The Surgistar 15 degree Microknife offers aonctrol and precision for small scars. (*Courtesy of* Surgistar Inc., Vista, CA; with permission.)

- Once a satisfactory deep closure technique has been obtained, the surgeon should then focus on the superficial closure.
- Superficial closure is typically performed with a high-quality monofilament suture, such as polypropylene. Application of either a vertical or horizontal mattress suturing technique achieves everted skin edges that provides for a fine, less visible scar (**Fig. 3**).

Z-PLASTY

For scars that need to be realigned, a Z-plasty is an excellent surgical technique with which every facial plastic surgeon should become familiar. Z-plasties come in various angulations but traditionally have two 60° angles and three limbs of equal length. The 2 flaps are undermined and transposed to theoretically lengthen the scar by 75%; however, the actual length gained is influenced by the elasticity of the surrounding skin. The execution of the Z-plasty should occur using the basic principles outlined for the re-excision procedure in terms of scalpel selection, treatment of the original scar bed, and meticulous handling of the soft tissue.

W-PLASTY

W-plasty can be a useful scar irregularization technique and can be performed as a single or running W. The limbs of each element of the W should be 5 mm or greater. The length of the limb may initially appear large, but as soon as the initial incisions are made, the natural process of scar tissue contracture starts to take place and this length appears short as the case progresses. Surgeons should become comfortable on the various lengths of the limbs based on their own personal experience. It is recommended to avoid limbs less than 5 mm except in the most unique situations. Proper

techniques should be applied when performing the W-plasty, including a good initial skin incision, proper management of the native scar wound bed, and an intact deep layer closure to prevent scar widening postoperatively.

Geometric Broken Line Closure

Geometric broken line closure (GBLC) is another popular and powerful scar irregularization technique. It is based on principles similar to the W-plasty but because the GBLC contains more irregularized components, it is more difficult for the average human eye to follow the scar along the surface of the skin, further camouflaging the original lesion. The design of GBLC consists of random, irregular geometric patterns interlocked with a mirror image pattern on the opposite side of the excision. The limbs here again should be a minimum of 5 mm in linear length and may be longer based on the actual part of the face involved and other elements of the scar being improved. GBLC is classically helpful for scars that occur across the broad surface of the cheeks or the mandibular regions of the face.

TISSUE EXPANSION

Tissue expansion is a powerful technique in the management of problematic facial scars. Key elements are discussed briefly. The decision to use tissue expansion is often appropriate when a surgeon has concluded that there is a paucity of normal tissue to close the defect in question. Facial plastic surgeons can see defects of large sizes on all areas of the face; for example, defects on the forehead after significant skin cancer excision.

Procedural Considerations

- Typically a surgeon wants to stabilize the wound bed at the same time as performing the tissue expansion. A large open wound can be managed with a skin graft or simply by allowing the wound to granulate over the coming weeks during the tissue expansion process.
- A key step is to determine the location of the initial incision for the placement of the tissue expander itself.
- To close the defect, the surgeon must anticipate the subsequent surgical moves ahead of time. The initial skin incision used for the placement of the tissue expander must be complementary to the ultimate planned local flap or adjacent tissue transfer advancement.

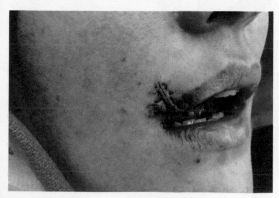

Fig. 3. Demonstration of properly everted skin edges necessary to achieve a less visible scar.

- The effect of the initial skin incision on surrounding neurovascular structures should be considered. For example, forehead expanders must be planned carefully to avoid disruption of the supraorbital nerve.
- Another essential factor to contemplate before surgery is the location of the injection port. The ideal injection port site is in an easily accessible area of low sensitivity, because this area must be frequently penetrated with an injecting needle during the tissue expansion period.

Tissue Expanders

Tissue expanders come in a variety of sizes and shapes and can be obtained through medical distribution companies. Custom tissue expanders can also be obtained, but the senior author prefers prefabricated expanders from one of the national providers. Considerable planning must be dedicated to the base of the expander. Some expanders come with a more stabilized base, and some expand to fill their base as the expander itself enlarges. Based on the amount of donor tissue a surgeon is initially trying to expand, the selection of a stable base or a nonstable base should be considered. If there is a more limited amount of initial skin under which the expander is going to be placed, consideration should be given for a nonstable base type expander. Conversely, if several square centimeters of skin exist under which the expander is going to be placed, then the choice of a stable base tissue expander may be preferable.

Patient Follow-up

Patients undergoing tissue expansion require frequent visits to the office. Therefore,

consideration of follow-up ease must be considered and a unique postoperative plan devised for patients who do not live close to the office. The senior author prefers to see patients every 3 to 5 days for the first few weeks. On the initial visit, the office staff performs the injection. On the second and third visits postoperatively, the office staff can begin to observe the caregiver performing the injection in the office setting. Although there can be variability in different clinical scenarios, it is usually prudent to wait approximately 9 to 10 days postplacement of the expander before beginning the initial injections. Children and parents should be counseled on the physical and emotional challenges during tissue expansion.

Initially the expander is subtle noticeable, and the main concern is simply the discomfort of needle placement into the injection port. As the expanders become larger, however, a period of noticeable physical deformity is inevitable (**Fig. 4**). Therefore, the surgeon should provide emotional support during office visits to help the patient and family tolerate this brief period of deformation, particularly near the end of the tissue expansion process. The office staff also plays a critical role in providing support in the final weeks when significant extra tissue can be created. Tissue expanders provide the ability to repair large surface area defects with adjacent tissue that is similar in color, tone, and texture. In general, the clinical results are overall positive and are well worth the effort.

FREE TISSUE TRANSFER

In rare instances, the pediatric facial defect is so great as to warrant composite soft tissue reconstruction. Indications for microvascular free tissue

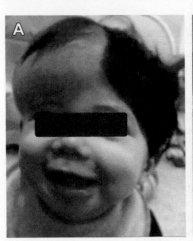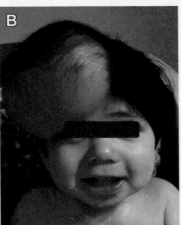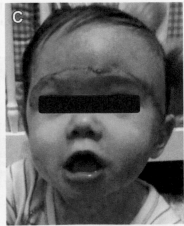

Fig. 4. Application of a tissue expander in a pediatric patient. (*A*) Initial placement of tissue expander in a child's scalp. (*B*) Addition of saline gradually allows the skin to stretch. (*C*) Following repair with the donor tissue. (*Courtesy of* Dr Bruce S. Bauer, Pediatric Plastic and Reconstructive Surgery, North Shore University Health System, Evanston, IL.)

transfer in children differ from in adults and the applications in this age group have not been well established.[71] Although donor site morbidity has been shown to be minor in adults, the ongoing potential for growth at both the donor and reconstructed site in children requires meticulous planning. The application of free flaps requires skill in microvascular surgery, which is arguably the most technically challenging part of the procedure. In younger patients, vasospasm may be decreased due to the underdeveloped muscularis layer in pediatric vessels. Despite the rarity of hypertension, atherosclerosis, and diabetes mellitus in this age group, the risk of thrombosis exists; therefore, postoperative monitoring remains essential.[72,73] Yazar and colleagues[74] demonstrated high flap survival rates in a series of 72 children who underwent head and neck reconstruction with microsurgical free flap transfers. The authors advocate use of the anterolateral thigh perforator flap for intraoral lining, external skin cover, and soft tissue volume reconstruction because it has a generous cutaneous area and adjustable flap thickness. The topic of free tissue transfers in the pediatric population is discussed in more detail in other articles.

SUMMARY

Scars of the head and neck often have profound physical and psychosocial impacts on patients, especially in the pediatric population. Treatment should start early to minimize stigmatization and emotional consequences. A surgeon's armamentarium to improve on the appearance of facial scars should be broad and generally start from the least to most invasive modalities. Treatment planning is an important aspect in children because successful outcomes depend not only on precise surgical technique but also on cooperation and follow-up.

REFERENCES

1. Brown BC, McKenna SP, Siddhi K, et al. The hidden cost of skin scars: quality of life after skin scarring. J Plast Reconstr Aesthet Surg 2008;61: 1049–58.
2. Thomas JR, Prendiville S. Update in scar revision. Facial Plast Surg Clin North Am 2002;10:103.
3. Doyle L, Collotti JE. Pediatric procedural sedation and analgesia. Pediatr Clin North Am 2006;53(2): 279–92.
4. Crock C, Olsson C, Phillips R, et al. General anaesthesia or conscious sedation for painful procedures in childhood cancer: the family's perspective. Arch Dis Child 2003;88:253–7.
5. Bhatt M, Kennedy RM, Osmond MH, et al. Consensus-based recommendations for standardizing terminology and reporting adverse events for emergency department procedural sedation and analgesia in children. Ann Emerg Med 2009; 53(4):426–35.
6. Agrawal D, Manzi SF, Gupta R, et al. Preprocedural fasting state and adverse events in children undergoing procedural sedation and analgesia in a pediatric emergency department. Ann Emerg Med 2003;42:636–46.
7. Green SM, Roback MG, Miner JR, et al. Fasting and emergency department procedural sedation and analgesia: a consensus-based clinical practice advisory. Ann Emerg Med 2007;49(4):454–61.
8. Green SM, Roback MG, Kennedy RM, et al. Clinical practice guideline for emergency department ketamine dissociative sedation: 2011 update. Ann Emerg Med 2011;57(5):449–61.
9. Green SM, Krauss B. Barriers to propofol use in emergency medicine. Ann Emerg Med 2008; 52(4):392–8.
10. Green SM, Andolfatto G, Krauss B. Ketofol for procedural sedation? Pro and con. Ann Emerg Med 2011;57(5):444–8.
11. Shah A, Mosdossy G, McLeod S, et al. A blinded, randomized controlled trial to evaluate ketamine/propofol versus ketamine alone for procedural sedation in children. Ann Emerg Med 2011;57(5): 425–33.
12. David H, Shipp J. A randomized controlled trial of ketamine/propofol versus propofol alone for emergency department procedural sedation. Ann Emerg Med 2011;57(5):435–41.
13. Andolfatto G, Abu-Laban RB, Zed PJ, et al. Ketamine-propofol combination (ketofol) versus propofol alone for emergency department procedural sedation and analgesia: a randomized double-blind trial. Ann Emerg Med 2012;59(6):504–12.
14. Lane RD, Schunk JE. Atomized intranasal midazolam use for minor procedures in the pediatric emergency department. Pediatr Emerg Care 2008; 24(5):300–3.
15. Lee JH, Kim K, Kim TY, et al. A randomized comparison of nitrous oxide versus intravenous ketamine for laceration repair in children. Pediatr Emerg Care 2012;28(12):1297–301.
16. Zier JL, Liu M. Safety of high-concentration nitrous oxide by nasal mask for pediatric procedural sedation: experience with 7802 cases. Pediatr Emerg Care 2011;27(12):1107–12.
17. Parell GJ, Becker GD. Comparison of absorbable with nonabsorbable sutures in closure of facial skin wounds. Arch Facial Plast Surg 2003;5:488–90.
18. Singer AJ, Hollander JE, Quinn JV. Evaluation and management of traumatic lacerations. N Engl J Med 1997;337(16):1142–8.

19. Karounis H, Gouin S, Eisman H, et al. A randomized, controlled trial comparing long-term cosmetic outcomes of traumatic pediatric lacerations repaired with absorbable plain gut versus nonabsorbable nylon sutures. Acad Emerg Med 2004;11(7):730–5.

20. Holger JS, Wandersee SC, Hale DB. Cosmetic outcomes of facial lacerations repaired with tissue-adhesive, absorbable, and nonabsorbable sutures. Am J Emerg Med 2004;22(4):254–7.

21. Luck R, Tredway T, Gerard J, et al. Comparison of cosmetic outcomes of absorbable versus nonabsorbable sutures in pediatric facial lacerations. Pediatr Emerg Care 2013;29(6):691–5.

22. Luck RP, Flood R, Eyal D, et al. Cosmetic outcomes of absorbable versus nonabsorbable sutures in pediatric facial lacerations. Pediatr Emerg Care 2008;24(3):137–42.

23. Al-Abdullah T, Plint AC, Fergusson D. Absorbable versus nonabsorbable sutures in the management of traumatic lacerations and surgical wounds: a meta-analysis. Pediatr Emerg Care 2007;23(5): 339–44.

24. Hom DB, Sun GH, Elluru RG. A contemporary review of wound healing in otolaryngology: current state and future promise. Laryngoscope 2009; 119(11):2099–110.

25. Pitzer GB, Patel KG. Proper care of early wounds to optimize healing and prevent complications. Facial Plast Surg Clin North Am 2011;19(3):491–504.

26. Erlich HP, Tarver H, Hunt TK. Inhibitory effects of vitamin E on collagen synthesis and wound repair. Ann Surg 1972;175(2):235–40.

27. Zampieri N, Suin V, Burro R. A prospective study in children: pre- and post-surgery use of vitamin E in surgical incisions. J Plast Reconstr Aesthet Surg 2009;63(9):1474–8.

28. Baumann LS, Spencer J. The effects of topical vitamin E on the cosmetic appearance of scars. Dermatol Surg 1999;25(4):311–5.

29. Augusti KT. Therapeutic calues of onion (Allium cepa L) and garlic (Allium sativum L). Indian J Exp Biol 1996;34(7):634–40.

30. Draelos ZD. The ability of onion extract gel to improve the cosmetic appearance of postsurgical scars. J Cosmet Dermatol 2008;7(2):101–4.

31. Chung VQ, Kelley L, Marra D, et al. Onion extract gel versus petrolatum emollient on new surgical scars: prospective double-blinded study. Dermatol Surg 2006;32(2):193–7.

32. Jackson BA, Shelton AJ. Pilot study evaluating topical onion extract as treatment for postsurgical scars. Dermatol Surg 1999;25(4):267–9.

33. Zurada JM, Kriegel D, Davis IC. Topical treatments for hypertrophic scars. J Am Acad Dermatol 2006; 55(6):1024–31.

34. Chang CC, Kuo YF, Chiu HC, et al. Hydration, not silicone, modulates the effects of keratinocytes on fibroblasts. J Surg Res 1995;59(6):705–11.

35. Momeni M, Hafezi F, Rahbar H, et al. Effects of silicone gel on burn scars. Burns 2009;35(1):70–4.

36. Quinn KJ, Evans JH, Courtney JM, et al. Non-pressure treatment of hypertrophic scars. Burns Incl Therm Inj 1985;12(2):102–8.

37. Sawada Y, Sone K. Hydration and occlusion treatment for hypertrophic scars and keloids. Br J Plast Surg 1992;45(8):599–603.

38. Gibbons M, Zuker R, Brown M, et al. Experience with silastic gel sheeting in pediatric scarring. J Burn Care Rehabil 1994;15(1):69–73.

39. Ahn ST, Monafo WW, Mustoe TA. Topical silicone gel for the prevention and treatment of hypertrophic scar. Arch Surg 1991;126(4):499–504.

40. Carney SA, Cason CG, Gowar JP, et al. Cica-Care gel sheeting in the management of hypertrophic scarring. Burns 1994;20(2):163–7.

41. Mustoe TA, Cooter RD, Gold MH, et al. International clinical recommendations on scar management. Plast Reconstr Surg 2002;110(2):560–71.

42. Cantatore JL, Kriegel DA. Laser surgery: an approach to the pediatric patient. J Am Acad Dermatol 2004;50(2):165–84.

43. Chapas AM, Geronemus RG. Our approach to pediatric dermatologic laser surgery. Lasers Surg Med 2005;37(4):255–63.

44. Cordisco MR. An update on lasers in children. Curr Opin Pediatr 2009;21(4):499–504.

45. Vrijman C, van Drooge AM, Limpens J, et al. Laser and intense pulsed light therapy for the treatment of hypertrophic scars: a systematic review. Br J Dermatol 2011;165(5):934–42.

46. Reiken SR, Wolfort SF, Berthiaume F, et al. Control of hypertrophic scar growth using selective photothermolysis. Lasers Surg Med 1997;21(1):7–12.

47. Alster TS, Williams CM. Treatment of keloid sternotomy scars with 585 nm flashlamp-pumped pulsed-dye laser. Lancet 1995;345(8959):1198–200.

48. Kuo YR, Jeng SF, Wang FS, et al. Flashlamp pulsed dye laser (PDL) suppression of keloid proliferation through down-regulation of TGF-beta1 expression and extracellular matrix expression. Lasers Surg Med 2004;34(2):104–8.

49. Alster TS, Nanni CA. Pulsed dye laser treatment of hypertrophic burn scars. Plast Reconstr Surg 1998; 102(6):2190–5.

50. Alster TS, McMeekin TO. Improvement of facial acne scars by the 585 nm flashlamp-pumped pulsed dye laser. J Am Acad Dermatol 1996;35(1):79–81.

51. Nouri K, Jimenez GP, Harrison-Balestra C, et al. 585-nm pulsed dye laser in the treatment of surgical scars starting on the suture removal day. Dermatol Surg 2003;29(1):65–73.

52. Manuskiatti W, Wanitphakdeedecha R, Fitzpatrick RE. Effect of pulse width of a 595-nm flashlamp-pumped pulsed dye laser on the treatment response of keloidal and hypertrophic sternotomy scars. Dermatol Surg 2007;33(2):152–61.

53. Fiskerstrand EJ, Svaasand LO, Volden G. Pigmentary changes after pulsed dye laser treatment in 125 northern European patients with port wine stains. Br J Dermatol 1998;138(3):477–9.

54. Fitzpatrick RE, Rostan EF, Marchell N. Collagen tightening induced by carbon dioxide laser versus erbium:YAG laser. Lasers Surg Med 2000;27(5): 395–403.

55. Nelson JS. In this issue. Dermatologic laser surgery. Lasers Surg Med 2000;26(2):105–7.

56. Sobanko JF, Alster TS. Laser treatment for improvement and minimization of facial scars. Facial Plast Surg Clin North Am 2011;19(3):527–42.

57. Alora MB, Anderson RR. Recent developments in cutaneous lasers. Lasers Surg Med 2000;26(2): 108–18.

58. West TB. Laser resurfacing of atrophic scars. Dermatol Clin 1997;15(3):449–57.

59. Tanzi EL, Alster TS. Comparison of a 1450-nm diode laser and a 1320-nm Nd:YAG laser in the treatment of atrophic facial scars: a prospective clinical and histologic study. Dermatol Surg 2004; 30:152–7.

60. Friedman PM, Jih MH, Skover GR, et al. Treatment of atrophic facial acne scars with the 1064-nm Q-switched Nd:YAG laser: six-month follow-up study. Arch Dermatol 2004;140(11):1337–41.

61. Laubach HJ, Tannous Z, Anderson RR, et al. Skin responses to fractional photothermolysis. Lasers Surg Med 2006;38(2):142–9.

62. Manstein D, Zurakowski D, Thongsima S, et al. The effects of multiple passes on the epidermal thermal damage pattern in nonablative fractional resurfacing. Lasers Surg Med 2009;41(2):149–53.

63. Hantash BM, Bedi VP, Kapadia B, et al. In vivo histological evaluation of a novel ablative fractional resurfacing device. Lasers Surg Med 2007;39(2): 96–107.

64. Waibel J, Beer K, Narurkar V, et al. Preliminary observations on fractional ablative resurfacing devices: clinical impressions. J Drugs Dermatol 2009;8(5): 481–5.

65. Lapidoth M, Halachmi S, Cohen S, et al. Fractional CO2 laser in the treatment of facial scars in children. Lasers Med Sci 2014;29(2):855–7.

66. Smith JE. Dermabrasion. Facial Plast Surg 2014; 30(1):35–9.

67. Yarborough JM Jr. Ablation of facial scars by programmed dermabrasion. J Dermatol Surg Oncol 1988;14(3):292–4.

68. Katz BE, Oca AG. A controlled study of the effectiveness of spot dermabrasion ('scarabrasion') on the appearance of surgical scars. J Am Acad Dermatol 1991;24(3):462–6.

69. Oliaei S, Nelson JS, Fitzpatrick R, et al. Use of lasers in acute management of surgical and traumatic incisions on the face. Facial Plast Surg Clin North Am 2011;19(3):543–50.

70. Brenner MJ, Perro CA. Recontouring, resurfacing, and scar revision in skin cancer reconstruction. Facial Plast Surg Clin North Am 2009;17(3):469–87.

71. Arnold DJ, Wax MK. Microvascular Committee of the American Academy of Otolaryngology–Head and Neck Surgery. Pediatric microvascular reconstruction: a report from the Microvascular Committee. Otolaryngol Head Neck Surg 2007; 136(5):848–51.

72. Yücel A, Aydin Y, Yazar S, et al. Elective free-tissue transfer in pediatric patients. J Reconstr Microsurg 2001;17(1):27–36.

73. Parry SW, Toth BA, Elliott LF. Microvascular free-tissue transfer in children. Plast Reconstr Surg 1988;81(6):838–40.

74. Yazar S, Wei FC, Cheng MH, et al. Safety and reliability of microsurgical free tissue transfers in paediatric head and neck reconstruction–a report of 72 cases. J Plast Reconstr Aesthet Surg 2008;61(7):767–71.

Craniofacial Distraction Osteogenesis

Ryan Winters, MD, Sherard A. Tatum, MD*

KEYWORDS

- Distraction osteogenesis • Distraction osseogenesis • Craniofacial surgery • Orthognathic surgery
- Maxillofacial surgery • Pediatric craniomaxillofacial surgery

KEY POINTS

- Distraction osteogenesis has a wide variety of applications in the craniofacial skeleton.
- Greater degrees of skeletal movement can be achieved with distraction osteogenesis compared with conventional techniques.
- The decision to use distraction osteogenesis, conventional osteotomy, or a combination of techniques should be based on individual patient situations.

OVERVIEW

Distraction osteogenesis (DO) is a method of inducing new bone formation within a gap between 2 bony surfaces of an osteotomy via gradual application of an external separating force. Orthopedic surgeons have used this technique for nearly a century to lengthen long bones, and much of the current understanding of the biomechanics involved and progression of the osteoneogenesis has been extrapolated from this literature.[1–3] Initial interest in application of DO to surgical osteotomies in the craniofacial skeleton centered on lengthening the mandible or on repairing segmental mandibular defects. In the early 20th century, European surgeons pioneered mandibular DO in animal models. From the 1970s through the 1990s, various canine models were used to develop techniques to lengthen the mandible via distraction at a surgically created osteotomy.[4] Rosenthal reported the first clinical results of DO of the human mandible in 1927, and since then DO has been applied to an ever-expanding list of locations and clinical scenarios throughout the craniofacial skeleton.[5,6]

The underlying goal of DO, regardless of specific anatomic location, is to lengthen the chosen bone, thereby establishing more normal anatomic size and position relative to surrounding structures. The surgical osteotomy is created (or the distractor can be placed across an existing suture), the distractor device is applied, and a latency period is allowed to elapse before beginning distraction. This latency phase allows initial bone healing to begin at the osteotomy gap via bony callus formation. The bony segments are gradually separated by activating the distractor device over a period of several days. This is the distraction phase, gradually stretching the callus, inducing osteoneogenesis. Once the desired length is achieved, distraction stops, and the soft immature bone now present in the distraction gap mineralizes, eventually resembling mature bone. This newly formed bone is likely never as strong as native bone. The cross-section of the regenerate can only be as big as the cross-section of the bone at the osteotomy and is frequently smaller. This should factor into the planning of the osteotomy location. During this consolidation phase, the distractor device is left in situ to provide rigid fixation

Disclosure: None.
Division of Facial Plastic & Reconstructive Surgery, Department of Otolaryngology & Communication Sciences, SUNY Upstate Medical University, 750 East Adams Street, Syracuse, NY 13202, USA
* Corresponding author.
E-mail address: tatums@upstate.edu

Facial Plast Surg Clin N Am 22 (2014) 653–664
http://dx.doi.org/10.1016/j.fsc.2014.08.003

to the bony segments, facilitating maturation of the bony regenerate and preventing skeletal relapse and pseudoarthrosis.

PREOPERATIVE PLANNING

When considering DO of the craniofacial skeleton, planning begins with a thorough history and physical examination. Particular attention should be given to occlusion, cranial vault shape, and position of the orbits (and globes within them), as well as the overall shape and symmetry of the maxillofacial region. Photographs are taken and placed in the medical record. Cephalograms, both lateral and frontal, are useful in nearly all patients. Pantomograms of the tooth-bearing areas are helpful as well. High-resolution 3D computed tomograms are most useful for analysis and planning although the radiation particularly of children should be considered and minimized. Computer-aided design/computer-aided manufacturing systems are widely available to construct life-size acrylic models or perform virtual surgery for planning purposes. Detailed anatomy, including defect or malposition magnitude and precise location of brain, eye, tooth, and other important structures, are well visualized. An additional advantage is the ability to clearly evaluate surrounding bone stock to ensure adequate amounts are available to generate bone and secure the selected distractor devices. This technology allows planning osteotomy sites, device placement, and final desired position of the distracted bones. Plastic jigs or guides can be constructive for intraoperative guiding of these steps. The distractors in some cases can be custom made or shaped for a specific situation.

Surgical Technique

A detailed discussion of the individual procedures performed for craniomaxillofacial distraction osteogenesis is not the purpose here. Certain important points bear mention. With regard to positioning and prepping, there are 2 points. Regardless of the approach chosen, there is a reasonable chance the aerodigestive tract will be traversed at some point. Therefore, we prefer complete irrigation of the nasal, oral, and pharyngeal cavities with 3% hydrogen peroxide solution, including brushing teeth if present. A second irrigation of the same areas is done with 10% povidone-iodine solution (Betadine, Purdue Pharma, LP, Stamford, CT), and the teeth if present are brushed again. For scalp incisions the hair is washed with Betadine scrub. Then the external field is prepped with the same povidone-iodine solution.

PATIENT POSITIONING

For the majority of craniofacial DO surgeries, the patient is placed supine, with the head of the operating table rotated about 120° away from the anesthesiologist to allow the surgical team maximum access to all sides of the head. For bilateral mandibular distraction, the table usually is not turned. The head of the operating table is extended, and the whole table is placed in reverse Trendelenburg position.

Although we have found this positioning to be amenable to nearly all DO surgeries (including some posterior cranial vault distractions), some authors prefer either the standard prone position or the "sphinx" position, wherein the patient is placed prone with the neck maximally extended and head elevated with the arms placed anteriorly. These positions allow better access to the entire skull and posterior cranium, but special care must be taken to pad the multiple pressure points created along the chin and mandible and especially to secure the endotracheal tube, which can be disastrous if dislodged in this position.[7–9] Air embolism might be more likely with the sphinx position as well, owing to the open circulation of the medullary space and the skull osteotomies being elevated significantly above the heart. In the senior author's practice, the prone position is reserved for cases where successful posterior distraction requires osteotomy to the level of the foramen magnum.

DISTRACTOR SELECTION

The first choice is (semi)internal versus external devices. The prefix "semi-" refers to intraoral devices where all or part of the body of the device is not buried under the tissues but remains contained in the mouth. Otherwise the internal devices are buried, but there is always a partially exposed activator mechanism. The external devices are outside the patient connected to the bone percutaneously.

External Distractors

In the current practice of the senior author (S.A.T.), the majority of DO performed utilizes internal devices; however, some situations exist wherein external devices may be superior. Arguments for internal or external devices exist throughout the literature.[6,10] Internal devices may increase long-term patient compliance because they are less conspicuous and less likely to be dislodged by patient activity. Some authors feel the distraction forces are better transmitted via the direct fixation of the device to bone with screws rather than the more distant percutaneous fixation of external devices. The internal devices require more exposure and dissection to place. Their vector cannot be altered once placed (some designs offer limited adjustability), and perhaps most important, they require a second frequently difficult procedure for removal. Often the distraction process has moved the devices away from the incision used to place them, making their exposure even more difficult.

External devices allow more fine tuning of distraction vectors, better facilitate multivector distraction, and may be used when inadequate bone stock exists for implanted devices to be anchored. There are external scars at every percutaneous entry site and some of these pins and wires migrate through the soft tissue, amplifying the scarring. The halo devices (**Fig. 1**) often require transcutaneous facial attachments, but some are used exclusively with custom intraoral appliances having builtin attachments.[11] They are not at all hidden, and they are more subject to dislodgement by patient activity. If placed away from the typical mandibular osteotomy site, the pins might present less harm to the dentition than the screws of an internal device placed right over the osteotomy. Additionally, their removal is typically a minor procedure, often appropriately done in the office.

In some direct comparative series, these devices were found to be less effective than external, percutaneous systems; however, both DO devices outperformed traditional orthognathic surgery in long-term outcomes.[11,12] The authors prefer to utilize internal distractors whenever possible, with the understanding that removal of these devices is a more significant operation than removal of external distractors. The benefits of improved transmission of distraction force and increased patient comfort and compliance are felt to outweigh these drawbacks.

Mandibular Distraction

For infant distraction when airway compromise persists through nonoperative measures and a tracheotomy is being contemplated, mandibular distraction offers another option. External multivector devices anchored percutaneously with osteotomies performed through intraoral incisions have been traditional. New internal devices are available that are small enough to fit on the bone stock of the neonatal mandible. These are typically placed through retromandibular or submandibular incisions.

In older patients, there is greater variety in distractor type and technique applied. For asymmetry

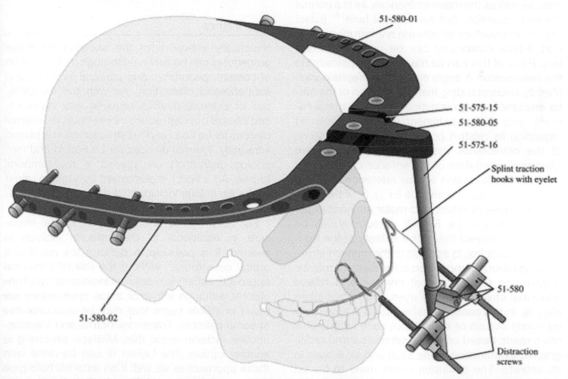

Fig. 1. External midface distractor. (*From* Imola MJ, Tatum SA. Craniofacial distraction osteogenesis. Facial Plast Surg Clin North Am 2002;10:291; with permission.)

problems like craniofacial microsomia, the movements can be very complex and require careful planning. There is often a combination of ramus lengthening, body lengthening, and gonial angle rotation. This type of movement requires external multivector devices. Symmetric mandibular distraction with gonial angle rotation is frequently performed with curvilinear, internal distractor devices placed via intraoral incisions.

Upper and Midface Distraction

Midface distraction can be performed at the Le Fort I, II, or III or monobloc levels. When DO is being entertained for midface hypoplasia, it is essential to consider cranial volume, periorbital aesthetics and function, and occlusal needs separately. Cranial volume and periorbital function and aesthetics include the position of the anterior cranium, the frontoorbital bar, the malar eminence, and the infraorbital rim relative to the globe position. Retro positioning of these structures can result in increases in intracranial and intraorbital pressures damaging both brain and eye function if left untreated.[13] This analysis dictates the specific distraction level necessary to achieve the desired result. If only the lower midface is retruded, a LeFort I advancement may suffice to correct the occlusion. If the forehead and frontoorbital complex, as well as the malar eminences, lie in a normal anatomic position, but the "central face[14]" (nasal and lower maxillary structures) are retruded, a LeFort II-type osteotomy can be used to correct this. Parts of this can be measured empirically via the sella-nasion A angle on a lateral cephalogram (**Fig. 2**), understanding that the position of the malar eminence will go unnoticed with this measurement, and clinical judgment must be employed regarding its relative position. Additionally, some of the craniofacial dysostosis syndromes have abnormal orientation of the anterior cranial fossa rendering sella-nasion a poor reference line. The normal sella-nasion A angle is $81° \pm 3°$. If the nasal complex, inferior orbits, and malar eminences are also retruded, a Le Fort III osteotomy will be required to correct this. If the entirety of the frontoorbital complex, in addition to the midface structures, is retruded, monobloc advancement may be required to restore normal contour and relieve abnormal stresses on the eyes and frontal lobes (**Fig. 3**). In this case, the sella-nasion A angle may be overly obtuse or normal, but such judgment is often made based on an overall clinical and radiographic examination of the skull and skull base in its entirety. The occlusion might need to be set separately from the upper and midface aesthetics with later Le Fort I level or mandibular movement.

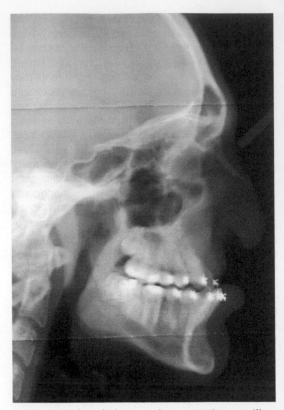

Fig. 2. Lateral cephalogram demonstrating maxillary hypoplasia and resultant midface retrusion.

Approaches

Necessary exposure of the skeleton for these procedures can be achieved through a combination of coronal, periorbital, and intraoral incisions and subperiosteal dissection. As with the mandible, use of external devices requires less exposure, and internal devices require more exposure. Internal devices for Le Fort I and II distraction can be placed intraorally. Internal devices for Le Fort III and monobloc distraction are placed in the temporal fossae. A Le Fort I is performed through an upper vestibular sulcus incision that also provides exposure for intraoral device placement.

For LeFort II advancement, nasoorbital exposure in additional to the intraoral incision is needed. It is possible to perform the nasal and orbital osteotomies without the use of a coronal approach, either via nasal root incision or Lynch incisions, although either of these approaches will result in visible scars that may be unacceptable to some patients. Transconjunctival and transcaruncular incision avoid this. Midface degloving is another option. The LeFort III can be done with these approaches as well if an external halo type distractor is to be used. For a Le Fort III with internal devices or a monobloc distraction with either

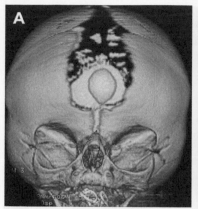
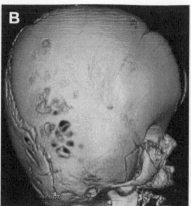
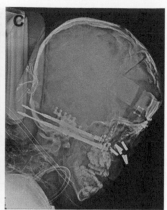

Fig. 3. Preoperative 3-dimensional computed tomograms images of turricephalic patient with concurrent maxillary and frontal cranial retrusion and hypoplasia (*A*, *B*). Immediate postoperative cephalogram showing successful placement of distraction devices for monobloc advancement (*C*). The turricephaly was addressed with subsequent posterior cranial vault remodeling.

an internal or external device, a coronal incision is necessary. A camouflaged sigmoid or saw tooth type of incision is recommended.[15]

Osteotomies and Device Placement

The osteotomies are performed no differently for distraction than for standard skeletal movements, although many surgeons prefer to place the devices and drill the anchoring screw holes before performing osteotomies. The most important point is that the need for complete segment mobility is obvious when the segment is to be moved. However, when it is not to be initially moved but to be moved by distraction, it is a pitfall not to ensure totally the mobility of the segment as well. Distraction will fail if the mobilized segment is not totally mobilized. Another point worth mentioning is sealing of the anterior cranial fossa during a monobloc. When traditional monobloc advancement is done, the cranial cavity is generally sealed with a pericranial flap and fibrin glue. When the osteotomy is done without initial advancement, it should still be sealed at least with glue if not also the flap to separate the sinonasal contents from the dura.

Once complete segment mobilization is assured, the devices are placed. Previously drilled holes or custom drill guides from computer planning determine internal device placement for the desired vector of distraction. Generally, 3 or 4 screws on each side of the osteotomy are required, with care being taken to avoid underlying neurovascular and dental structures. If a halo device is to be used, careful planning of bandeau and craniotomy osteotomies is required to ensure adequate stable skull posterior to these cuts to support the distractor hardware. The devices

should be test activated once placed to ensure proper function.

Cranial Vault Distraction

The use of DO as an alternative to conventional surgery for singlesuture and multisuture craniosynostosis is a recent development and an area of active research. Although they work slightly differently than distractors, springs should be mentioned as a less invasive method for cranial alteration as well. It may be possible to achieve similar results in terms of cranial growth and stability to standard surgical methods using DO or springs with the potential for shorter operative times and fewer complications. Thus far, available data from some centers suggest that there is no difference in terms of outcomes, complications, length of stay, or blood loss.[16,17] Given the rarity of the underlying conditions, it has been proposed a certain learning curve exists, and as surgeons' experience increases, some of these anticipated benefits might be demonstrated (**Fig. 4**).

POSTOPERATIVE CARE

In the authors' practice, all postoperative DO patients are admitted to the step down unit or intensive care unit. Airway monitoring is always a concern, and if a tracheostomy was placed routine care for this is best achieved in an intensive care setting in the acute period. The onset, rate, and rhythm of distraction depend on the patient age and type of distraction performed. Neonatal mandibular distraction routinely commences with a short latency of 24 hours postoperatively and proceeds at 2 to 3 mm/d. Midfacial distraction in

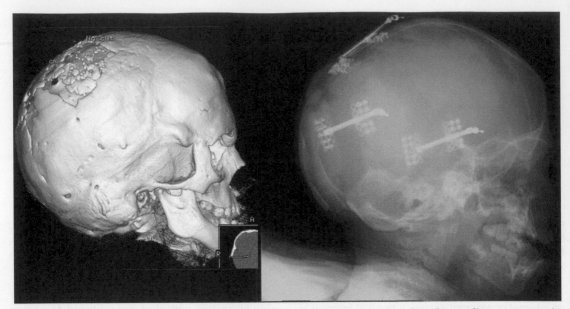

Fig. 4. Preoperative 3-dimensional computed tomograms of posterior cranial vault and immediate postoperative cephalogram showing appropriate positioning of the 3 distractors: One on each lambdoid suture and one at the apex of the lambda.

older patients commences 4 to 5 days postoperatively and proceeds at 1 to 1.5 mm/d.

In mandibular DO patients where airway was a significant concern, the endotracheal tube may be left in place for several days. In midfacial DO patients, the management of the airway is on a case-by-case basis. If tracheostomy was performed prior, things are somewhat simpler. Airway protection in paramount in these children and prolonged intubation in this age group carries a very real risk of acquired subglottic stenosis.

After the latency phase, distraction proceeds at a rate of 1 to 3 mm/d. This is usually performed via twice or thrice daily activation of the device, with the precise number of turns at each session guided by the goal rate and device used. A confirmatory roentgenogram is obtained once distraction is complete to ensure the goal has been reached before removing the activation arms (**Fig. 5**).

FOLLOW-UP CARE

The patient is hospitalized until the functional goals of distraction are met, such as airway expansion, eye protection, and adequate feeding. Older patients with stable airways can be discharged during the distraction. The patients are seen weekly as long as there are no problems during distraction, and more frequently if needed. If applicable, removable activator arms are removed and the consolidation phase proceeds, typically at least

double the length of the distraction phase. Then plans are made for distractor removal at the completion of the consolidation phase.

COMPLICATIONS

As with any operative procedure, complications can occur. DO is generally very well tolerated, and the severity and frequency of complications that may occur is correlated with the extent of the surgery. Fortunately, many of these complications can be avoided with meticulous technique and planning, but early recognition of them when they occur will optimize outcomes for the patient and family.

Relapse

This is the most common complication in any DO procedure, although its frequency is greatly variable depending on the anatomic location of DO performed. For mandibular distraction, incidence of relapse as high as 65% has been reported in some series,[18] whereas relapse rates for Le Fort advancements seem to be lower, 7.3% in some series.[19] For this reason, 10% to 30% overcorrection is typically included in the initial plan. Analysis of true mandibular DO relapse rates may be complicated by the physical limitations of DO in severely micrognathic patients; there may not be sufficient space within the soft tissue envelope to place a distractor of sufficient size to provide optimal distraction. When this occurs, it is

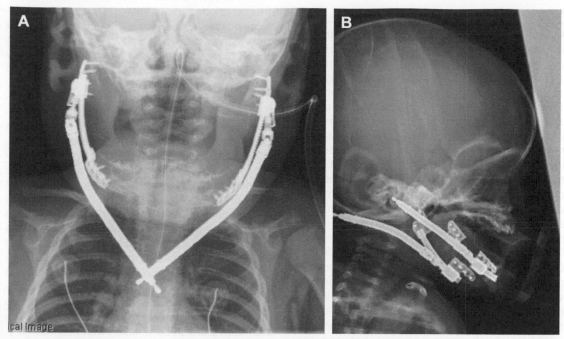

ical Image

Fig. 5. Adequate, symmetric, terminal distraction of both mandibular osteotomies (A). Asymmetric mandibular distraction. Note the difference in the distraction differences in each device (B) despite clinical indication of terminal distractions.

necessary to inform patients of this and to plan for multiple-stage procedures. It is important in any DO surgery to ensure adequate release of surrounding skin and soft tissue elements, because these provide the primary contractile forces that can counteract the desired distraction.

Similarly, it is important to ensure that complete, symmetric distraction is occurring during the distraction phase. In some instances, suboptimal results can be caused by failure of caregivers to recognize premature fusion of the bony segments. Increased resistance to activating the distractors is more common near the end of the distraction phase, where the surrounding soft tissue stretching is at its peak. Optimal distraction rate has been shown to be 1 mm/d, although this is age dependent, yielding the best mix of biomechanical strength and mineralization.[20] Too fast risks a poor quality regenerate. Too slow risks early consolidation, which arrests the process before the goal is reached. Serial radiographs can be used to ensure that distraction is symmetric, and that it is complete before removing the activating arms.

Patients with underlying genetic syndromes may be more prone to complications, and certainly the success of any DO is directly related to the family and social support and involvement of parents and other caregivers during the distraction period. Should relapse occur, it can be managed

conservatively with observation in very mild cases. In cases where the relapse is severe, or when adequate orbital, cranial, or airway expansion is not achieved, repeat distraction or other operative intervention must be undertaken once the consolidation period is complete.

Tooth and Neurovascular Injury

Tooth injury can occur in several settings, although it is much more common in mandibular DO (22.5% in some series of mandibular DO).[18] The most common cause is inadvertent injury to a tooth bud when making the mandibular osteotomy. Preoperative imaging aids in locating tooth buds. Should a tooth bud be encountered, attempts should be made to use a blunt instrument to push the bud into the caudal mandibular segment without violating its capsule. Tooth bud injury can also occur in the maxilla when performing maxillary osteotomies, especially in Le Fort I advancement, so care must be taken to place these cuts superior to the expected location of the tooth roots. Teeth can also be injured during application or subsequent distraction if dental appliances are used to anchor the midface distractor (as with some external devices), and close coordination with dental and orthodontic colleagues is essential for avoiding this problem.

Hypertrophic Scar

As with any cutaneous incision, scar hypertrophy is a possibility regardless of the location. Patients with personal or family history of hypertrophic scarring should be counseled that they might be at increased risk. Maintaining a tension-free closure of all incisions is paramount to avoiding scar widening or hypertrophy, so a layered closure should be employed. Tension-bearing, heavier suture should be used to close deeper layers, with skin sutures providing apposition of the edges in a tension-free manner. Incisions over convex bony prominences or in very mobile areas (scalp incisions and retromandibular incisions, respectively) may be at greater risk of hypertrophy. Master and colleagues[18] in their literature review of complications of mandibular DO noted a 15.6% rate of hypertrophic scar in mandibular DO, even when these principles were adhered to. It is also worth mentioning here that the use of external mandibular distraction devices may predispose some patients to unsightly cheek scars occurring between the proximal and distal percutaneous pins as DO progresses through the distraction phase. This specific situation has largely been avoided with the use of internal distractors.

Nerve Injury

Depending on the approach used for exposure, various nerves are at risk of injury as the distraction devices are placed. For mandibular distraction, the inferior alveolar nerve is at risk from the osteotomy itself, whereas its distal continuation, the mental nerve, may be at risk during intraoral incision. The osteotomy should always be performed carefully to prevent inferior alveolar nerve transection. When making a retromandibular incision, the marginal mandibular branch of the facial nerve is also at risk, so the incision should be placed 1 cm inferior to the inferior border of the angle of the mandible. Blunt dissection should always be performed parallel to the course of the nerve to identify the subperiosteal plane via this approach.

In the coronal approach, the nerves most at risk are the temporal branch of the facial nerve and the supratrochlear and supraorbital nerves. Maintaining a subperiosteal plane will alleviate some of this risk, understanding that the temporalis muscle must be elevated off of the skull and subsequently be resuspended from the temporal line to definitively avoid injury while gaining the wide lateral exposure needed. Maintaining this plane as the surgeon approaches the supraorbital rim will not guarantee safety of the supratrochlear neurovascular bundle, however, so the surgeon must be attuned to position at all times. The majority of patients possess a supraorbital notch through which these nerves pass, although a minority will have a true foramen located more cephalad that may require careful dissection and release to avoid injury.

Elevating in the subperiosteal plane of the anterior maxilla via maxillary gingivobuccal sulcus incision places the infraorbital nerves at risk, so care must be taken to identify these as they exit the infraorbital foramen. In Le Fort osteotomies, the final release of the pterygoids from the maxilla via the transoral osteotomy may place the optic nerve at risk if proper vector and depth of the osteotome is not maintained. Careful orientation of the blade's trajectory parallel to the alignment of the pterygoids and monitoring the depth of penetration can avoid this potentially devastating complication. Last, in monobloc osteotomies, where the frontal aspect of the anterior cranial fossa must be transected to release the frontoorbital bar, the olfactory nerve is at risk because its projections pass through the cribriform plate. In conjunction with neurosurgery, minimal midline elevation of dura off of anterior cranial fossa should be performed, just enough to allow safe retraction of the frontal lobes away from the osteotomy, but disrupting the dural attachments to the cribriform as little as possible.

Infection

Any time the skin or mucosal barriers are surgically disrupted, the potential for infection exists. In the authors' practice, all patients undergoing DO are placed on a 2-week course of postoperative oral antibiotics in addition to topical mupirocin at incision sites for 1 week. Skin flora must be covered, but if intraoral incisions are made, expanded Gram-negative/anaerobic coverage is warranted. Additionally, antibiotics with excellent cerebrospinal fluid penetration are employed during hospitalization if open craniotomy has been performed, with selection and duration guided by our neurosurgical colleagues.

Fortunately, severe infection (osteomyelitis) from the implanted devices is exceedingly rare. Local wound infections occur in less than 10% of patients and are generally successfully managed with intravenous or oral antibiosis.[18] If open craniotomy was performed, there is a risk of meningitis, particularly given the risk of postoperative cerebrospinal fluid leak is significant (up to 20% in some series).[21]

Suboptimal Distraction Vector

This problem can be encountered in one of several scenarios. When single-vector distractors are used, the angle at which they are placed may be asymmetric when 1 side of the face is compared with the other. As a result, differing degrees of projection may result when distraction is completed. In less severe cases, this may be inconsequential; however, problems with occlusion can result if dentition-bearing bone is asymmetrically distracted. This is perhaps more common in the mandible, where rates of approximately 9% have been reported, but can occur in midface distraction as well.[18] The mandible may be more prone to this complication, especially in micrognathic patients, given the relative lack of space and resultant tight contractile forces of the surrounding soft tissue. Serial radiographs should always be employed throughout the distraction phase to ensure symmetric advancement of the distraction segments.

If an asymmetric result is achieved at the end of distraction, management depends on the severity of the resultant malocclusion. Less severe cases may be observed, with definitive management undertaken after permanent teeth have erupted and orthodontic therapy can be instituted. In more severe cases, where the occlusal plane and occlusal relationship is severely abnormal, revision surgery may be required to realign the dental arches.

Device Failure

Although device failure has been reported as high as 7% in some literature reviews, it is important to differentiate "device failure" from "distraction failure."[18] In the former, the device is truly broken or dislodged. Most commonly this manifests as a fracture of the securing plate of the distraction device, or a loosening of the securing screws that results in suboptimal transmission of the distraction forces. Both of these are far less common than "distraction failure," wherein premature bony fusion or inadequate torque is applied to the activators, resulting is a functional device but

poor clinical outcome. Some causes are caretakers activating in the wrong direction and the device itself not holding position after activation. Directionally marked activation tools and ratcheting distractors are measures taken to counteract these problems. Serial radiography is paramount in making this determination, because it allows assessment of the distraction progress as well as the integrity of the devices and their attachments to bone (see **Fig. 5**). If a device is truly broken or malpositioned, reexploration and replacement are warranted.

Mortality

Fortunately, mortality is extremely rare. In the earliest reports of DO, specifically monobloc and frontofacial DO, mortality rates as high as 4.5% were reported by some authors.[21] As overall experience grew, this rate has declined to less than 1%, similar to other intracranial procedures. Even in these early experiences, mortality was seldom a result of the distraction per se, but was associated with the craniotomy and osteotomies required for placement of the DO devices. Despite these encouraging improvements, DO combined with any craniotomy and/or midface osteotomies is major surgery, and patients must be appropriately counseled regarding the risks.

OUTCOMES

When considering outcomes in DO, it is necessary to consider them in the context of the underlying reason for distraction. Outcome measures for mandibular DO are quite different from cranial vault DO.

Mandible Distraction

A major indication for mandibular DO is airway patency, and the possibility of avoiding tracheostomy. Secondary outcomes, often measured

Table 1
Recent series detailing airway outcomes and other complications after mandibular DO

Study	No. of Patients	Avoided Tracheostomy, n (%)	Tooth Injury, n (%)	Malocclusion, n (%)	Nerve Injury, n (%)	Revision Surgery, n (%)
Whittenborn et al,[22] 2004	17	14 (82)	NR	NR	NR	NR
Tiebesar et al,[23] 2010	32	NR	5 (16)	9 (28)	3 (9)	1 (5)
Mudd et al,[24] 2012	24	24 (100)	NR	NR	NR	NR
Murage et al,[25] 2013	50	46 (92)	NR	NR	NR	NR
Senders et al,[26] 2010	11	10 (90)	NR	NR	NR	NR
Hong et al,[27] 2012	10	NR	3 (30)	0 (0)	NR	0 (0)

Abbreviation: NR, not reported.
Data from Refs.[22–27]

Table 2
Reports of outcomes from LeFort and/or monobloc DO

Author	No. of Patients	Mean Distance Advanced (cm)	Resolution of Obstructive Sleep Apnea (% of Affected Patients)	Infection (No. of Patients)	Subsequent Tracheostomy (No. of Patients)	Orbital Volume Change (%)
Fearon,[28] 2001	12	1.9	100	1	1	NR
Chin et al,[29] 1997	9	2	100	1	0	NR
Meling et al,[20] 2006	7	2.3	NR	4	0	NR
Nout et al,[31] 2012	18	1.2	NR	NR	NR	27–28

Abbreviation: NR, not reported.
   Data from Refs.[28–31]

much later in life, involve dental occlusion and projection of the mentum. Outcomes of recent series primarily regarding airway management are detailed in **Table 1**.

Midface Distraction

Indications for DO to advance the midface, with or without concurrent advancement of the orbits or frontal bones, can be grouped into 2 categories: (1) Relief of upper airway obstruction (LeFort II, III, and monobloc) and (2) expansion of orbital and/or cranial vault volume (LeFort III and monobloc). Outcomes for category (1) are often measured by clinical improvements in the airway, either with resolution of obstruction or any obstructive sleep apnea, or successful decannulation or avoidance of tracheostomy. Outcomes for category (2) are often directly measured on lateral cephalogram as distance traveled by the distracted segment. To this regard, an early comparative study of LeFort III DO with conventional LeFort III osteotomy

by Fearon[28] suggests greater advancement is possible with DO than with conventional osteotomy techniques. Outcomes of recent series are detailed in **Table 2**.

Cranial Vault Distraction

The purpose of cranial vault remodeling, whether via DO or traditional osteotomy, is to relieve increased intracranial pressure, ideally while reshaping the skull to a more normal configuration. Outcomes can be measured via formal intracranial pressure measurement with lumbar puncture, but is much more commonly measured by improvement in overt clinical signs and symptoms of increased intracranial pressure (decreased papilledema, mental status improvement, resolution of other neurologic symptoms, etc). Although cranial vault distraction is, comparatively, in its infancy, and therefore long-term data are scarce, **Table 3** summarizes the outcomes of recent studies of cranial vault DO.

Table 3
Recent studies examining volumetric outcomes in posterior vault expansion utilizing DO

Author	No. of Patients	Mean Distraction Distance (cm)	Mean Increase in Volume (%)	Resolution of Increased Intracranial Pressure (%)	Infection (No. of Patients)
Yikontiola et al,[32] 2012	16	2–3 (mean not given)	NR	100	0
Goldstein et al,[33] 2013	22	2.7	21.5	100	NR
Deschamps-Braly et al,[34] 2011	11	NR	6	100	NR

Abbreviation: NR, not reported.
   Data from Refs.[32–34]

SUMMARY

DO may represent the single greatest recent advancement in the field of craniofacial surgery. As experience grows, better data become available regarding the variety of applications of this technology. Although well proven in mandibular and midface disorders, the arrival of new data may yet herald unrecognized advantages of utilizing DO in certain circumstances. Decreased operating times, decreased morbidity and mortality, and better efficacy have all been hypothesized, but emerging data will contain these answers.

REFERENCES

1. Abbott LC. The operative lengthening of the tibia and fibula. J Bone Joint Surg Am 1927;9:128–39.
2. Ilizarov GA. Basic principles of transosseous compression and distraction osteosynthesis. Ortop Travmatol Protez 1971;32:7–9.
3. Hollier LH, Kim JH, Grayson B, et al. Mandibular growth after distraction in patients under 48 months of age. Plast Reconstr Surg 1999;103:1361–70.
4. Costantino PD, Friedman CD, Shindo ML, et al. Experimental mandibular regrowth by distraction osteogenesis. Long term results. Arch Otolaryngol Head Neck Surg 1993;119(5):511–6.
5. McCarthy JG, Schreiber J, Karp N, et al. Lengthening of the human mandible by gradual distraction. Plast Reconstr Surg 1992;89(1):1–10.
6. Imola MJ, Tatum SA III. Craniofacial distraction osteogenesis. Facial Plast Surg Clin North Am 2002; 10:287–301.
7. Lin KY, Ogle RC, Jane J, editors. Craniofacial surgery: science & surgical technique. Philadelphia: WB Saunders Company; 2002.
8. Jimenez DF, Barone CM, Rogers JM. Endoscopic wide vertex craniectomy. In: Jallo GI, Kothbauer KF, Pradilla G, editors. Controversies in pediatric neurosurgery. New York: Thieme Medical Publishers, Inc; 2010. p. 109–20.
9. Davidson EH, Brown D, Shetye PR, et al. The evolution of mandibular distraction: device selection. Plast Reconstr Surg 2010;126(6):2061–70.
10. Meling TR, Tveten S, Due-Tonnessen BJ, et al. Monobloc and midface distraction osteogenesis in pediatric patients with severe syndromal craniosynostosis. Pediatr Neurosurg 2000;33:89–94.
11. Choi HY, Hwang CJ, Kim HJ, et al. Maxillary anterior segmental osteogenesis with 2 different types of distractors. J Craniofac Surg 2012;23:706–11.
12. Baek SH, Lee JK, Lee JH, et al. Comparison of treatment outcome and stability between distraction osteogenesis and LeFort I osteotomy in cleft patients with maxillary hypoplasia. J Craniofac Surg 2007; 18(5):1209–15.
13. Witherow H, Dunaway D, Evans R, et al. Functional outcomes in monobloc advancement by distraction using the rigid external distractor device. Plast Reconstr Surg 2008;121(4):1311–22.
14. Kellman RM. Maxillofacial trauma. In: Cummings W Jr, Haughey BH, Thomas JR, et al, editors. Cumming's otolaryngology – head & neck surgery. 4th edition. St Louis (MO): Mosby; 2005. p. 318–40.
15. Fox AJ, Tatum SA III. The coronal incision: sinusoidal, sawtooth, and postauricular techniques. Arch Facial Plast Surg 2003;5(3):259–62.
16. Taylor JA, Derderian CA, Bartlett SP, et al. Perioperative morbidity in posterior cranial vault expansion: distraction osteogenesis versus conventional osteotomy. Plast Reconstr Surg 2012;129(4):674e–80e.
17. Hopper RA. New trends in cranio-orbital and midface distraction for craniofacial dystosis. Curr Opin Otolaryngol Head Neck Surg 2012;20(4):298–303.
18. Master DL, Hanson PR, Gosain AK. Complications of mandibular distraction osteogenesis. J Craniofac Surg 2010;21(5):1565–70.
19. Greig AV, Davidson EH, Grayson BH, et al. Complications of craniofacial midface distraction: a 10-year review. Plast Reconstr Surg 2012;130(2):371e–2e.
20. Del Santo M, Guerrero CA, Buschang PH, et al. Long-term skeletal and dental effects of mandibular symphyseal distraction osteogenesis. Am J Orthod Dentofacial Orthop 2000;118:485–93.
21. Dunaway DJ, Britto JA, Abela C, et al. Complications of frontofacial advancement. Childs Nerv Syst 2012; 28(9):1571–6.
22. Whittenborn W, Panchal J, Marsh JL, et al. Neonatal distraction surgery for micrognathia reduces obstructive apnea and the need for tracheotomy. J Craniofac Surg 2004;15(4):623–30.
23. Tiebesar RJ, Scott AR, McNamara C, et al. Distraction osteogenesis of the mandible for airway obstruction in children: long-term results. Otolaryngol Head Neck Surg 2010;143:90–6.
24. Mudd PA, Perkins JN, Harwood JE, et al. Early intervention: distraction osteogenesis of the mandible for severe airway obstruction. Otolaryngol Head Neck Surg 2012;146(3):467–72.
25. Murage KP, Tholpady SS, Friel M, et al. Outcomes analysis of mandibular distraction osteogenesis for the treatment of Pierre Robin sequence. Plast Reconstr Surg 2013;132(2):419–21.
26. Senders CW, Kolstad CK, Tollefson TT, et al. Mandibular distraction osteogenesis used to treat upper airway obstruction. Arch Facial Plast Surg 2010;12(1):11–5.
27. Hong P, Graham E, Belyea J, et al. the long-term effects of mandibular osteogenesis on developing deciduous molar teeth. Plast Surg Int 2012;2012:913807.
28. Fearon JA. The LeFort III osteotomy: to distract or not to distract? Plast Reconstr Surg 2001;107(5): 1091–106.

29. Chin M, Toth BA. LeFort III advancement with gradual distraction using internal devices. Plast Reconstr Surg 1997;100(4):819–30.

30. Meling TR, Hans-Erik H, Per S, et al. LeFort III distraction osteogenesis in syndromal craniosynostosis. J Craniofac Surg 2006;17(1):28–39.

31. Nout E, van Bezooijen JS, Koudstaal MJ, et al. Orbital change following LeFort III advancement in syndromic craniosynostosis: quantitative evaluation of orbital volume, infraorbital rim and globe position. J Craniomaxillofac Surg 2012;40(3):223–8.

32. Yikontiola LP, Sandor GK, Salokorpi N, et al. Experience with craniosynostosis treatment using posterior cranial vault distraction osteogenesis. Ann Maxillofac Surg 2012;2(1):4–7.

33. Goldstein JA, Paliga JT, Wink JD, et al. A craniometric analysis of posterior cranial vault distraction osteogenesis. Plast Reconstr Surg 2013;131(6):1367–75.

34. Deschamps-Braly J, Hettinger P, el Amm C, et al. Volumetric analysis of cranial vault distraction for cephalocranial disproportion. Pediatr Neurosurg 2011;47:396–405.

Index

Facial Plast Surg Clin N Am 22 (2014) 665–683
http://dx.doi.org/10.1016/S1064-7406(14)00106-0
1064-7406/14/$ – see front matter © 2014 Elsevier Inc. All rights reserved.

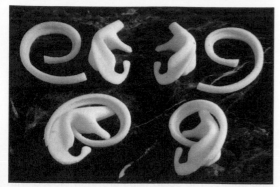

Fig. 12. Porous polyethylene framework. The use of 2 separate elements facilitates shaping for a given patient's ear at the time of surgery and provides additional flexibility and, hence, resistance to trauma.

epinephrine. The full-thickness skin graft donor site, generally harvested from the contralateral postauricular or inguinal region, is also infiltrated with injection preparation at this time.

Raising the TPF flap A #10 scalpel is used to make an incision through the dermal papillae of the hair, but no deeper, so as to not damage the subdermal plexus of the vessels. This reveals the superficial

aspect of the TPF flap. Dissection proceeds anteriorly in the subfollicular plane using a blunt-tipped Stevens tenotomy scissors, elevating 5 cm posterior to the helical rim.

Creating the postauricular sulcus and removal of the cartilage vestige The 0.5% lidocaine in 1:200,000 epinephrine is once again injected, this time into the subcutaneous plane of the auricular vestige, as well as into the subcutaneous plane of the non–hair-bearing skin around the vestige. After several minutes, a Metzenbaum scissor is used to dissect in this subcutaneous plane, in the area inferior to the mastoid. This dissection allows for sufficient contouring of the postauricular sulcus. Once adequate dissection is achieved in this area, the vestige of cartilage is exposed and removed, with bipolar cautery used for hemostasis.

Preparation and placement of the implant The PHDPE implant is composed of 2 separate components: a thin, curled helical rim and a base outlining the shape of the conchal bowl and antihelix (**Fig. 12**). Both of these components are carefully washed in antibiotic solution before a #10 blade is used to size each of the 2 pieces. Once appropriately sized, the helical component is sutured to the base at the helical root and the inferior insertion to the base unit using 3-0 Monocryl sutures.

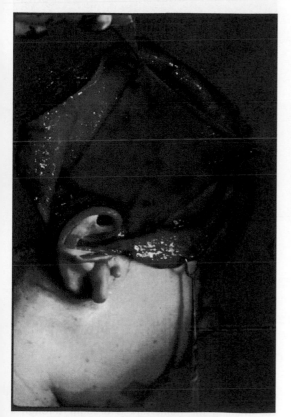

Fig. 13. Harvesting of the temporoparietal facial flap.

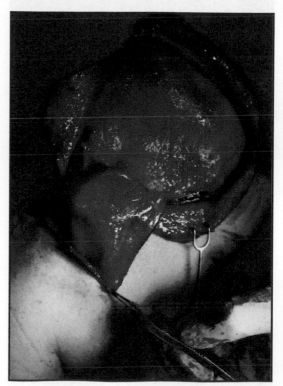

Fig. 14. The TPF is draped over the entire PHDPE framework.

United States Postal Service

Statement of Ownership, Management, and Circulation
(All Periodicals Publications Except Requestor Publications)

1. Publication Title	2. Publication Number	3. Filing Date
Facial Plastic Surgery Clinics of North America	0 1 3 - 1 2 2	9/14/14

4. Issue Frequency	5. Number of Issues Published Annually	6. Annual Subscription Price
Feb, May, Aug, Nov	4	$390.00

7. Complete Mailing Address of Known Office of Publication (Not printer) (Street, city, county, state, and ZIP+4®)

Elsevier Inc.,
360 Park Avenue South
New York, NY 10010-1710

Contact Person
Stephen R. Bushing

Telephone (Include area code)
215-239-3688

8. Complete Mailing Address of Headquarters or General Business Office of Publisher (Not printer)

Elsevier Inc., 360 Park Avenue South, New York, NY 10010-1710

9. Full Names and Complete Mailing Addresses of Publisher, Editor, and Managing Editor (Do not leave blank)
Publisher (Name and complete mailing address)

Linda Belfus, Elsevier Inc., 1600 John F. Kennedy Blvd., Suite 1800, Philadelphia, PA 19103-2899
Editor (Name and complete mailing address)

Joanne Husovski, Elsevier Inc., 1600 John F. Kennedy Blvd., Suite 1800, Philadelphia, PA 19103-2899
Managing Editor (Name and complete mailing address)

Adrianne Brigido, Elsevier Inc., 1600 John F. Kennedy Blvd., Suite 1800, Philadelphia, PA 19103-2899

10. Owner (Do not leave blank. If the publication is owned by a corporation, give the name and address of the corporation immediately followed by the names and addresses of all stockholders owning or holding 1 percent or more of the total amount of stock. If not owned by a corporation, give the names and addresses of the individual owners. If owned by a partnership or other unincorporated firm, give its name and address as well as those of each individual owner. If the publication is published by a nonprofit organization, give its name and address.)

Full Name	Complete Mailing Address
Wholly owned subsidiary of	1600 John F. Kennedy Blvd, Ste. 1800
Reed/Elsevier, US holdings	Philadelphia, PA 19103-2899

11. Known Bondholders, Mortgagees, and Other Security Holders Owning or Holding 1 Percent or More of Total Amount of Bonds, Mortgages, or Other Securities. If none, check box ☐ None

Full Name	Complete Mailing Address
N/A	

12. Tax Status (For completion by nonprofit organizations authorized to mail at nonprofit rates) (Check one)
The purpose, function, and nonprofit status of this organization and the exempt status for federal income tax purposes:
☐ Has Not Changed During Preceding 12 Months
☐ Has Changed During Preceding 12 Months (Publisher must submit explanation of change with this statement)

PS Form 3526, August 2012 (Page 1 of 3 (Instructions Page 3)) PSN 7530-01-000-9931 PRIVACY NOTICE: See our Privacy policy in www.usps.com

---

13. Publication Title	14. Issue Date for Circulation Data Below
Facial Plastic Surgery Clinics of North America	May 2014

15. Extent and Nature of Circulation		Average No. Copies Each Issue During Preceding 12 Months	No. Copies of Single Issue Published Nearest to Filing Date
a. Total Number of Copies (Net press run)		485	507
b. Paid Circulation (By Mail and Outside the Mail)	(1) Mailed Outside-County Paid Subscriptions Stated on PS Form 3541. (Include paid distribution above nominal rate, advertiser's proof copies, and exchange copies)	309	278
	(2) Mailed In-County Paid Subscriptions Stated on PS Form 3541 (Include paid distribution above nominal rate, advertiser's proof copies, and exchange copies)		
	(3) Paid Distribution Outside the Mails Including Sales Through Dealers and Carriers, Street Vendors, Counter Sales, and Other Paid Distribution Outside USPS®	36	35
	(4) Paid Distribution by Other Classes Mailed Through the USPS (e.g. First-Class Mail®)		
c. Total Paid Distribution (Sum of 15b (1), (2), (3), and (4))	▶	345	313
d. Free or Nominal Rate Distribution (By Mail and Outside the Mail)	(1) Free or Nominal Rate Outside-County Copies Included on PS Form 3541	33	44
	(2) Free or Nominal Rate In-County Copies Included on PS Form 3541		
	(3) Free or Nominal Rate Copies Mailed at Other Classes Through the USPS (e.g. First-Class Mail)		
	(4) Free or Nominal Rate Distribution Outside the Mail (Carriers or other means)		
e. Total Free or Nominal Rate Distribution (Sum of 15d (1), (2), (3) and (4))	▶	33	44
f. Total Distribution (Sum of 15c and 15e)	▶	378	357
g. Copies not Distributed (See instructions to publishers #4 (page #3))	▶	107	150
h. Total (Sum of 15f and g)	▶	485	507
i. Percent Paid (15c divided by 15f times 100)	▶	91.27%	87.68%

16. Total circulation includes electronic copies. Report circulation on PS Form 3526-X worksheet.

17. Publication of Statement of Ownership
If the publication is a general publication, publication of this statement is required. Will be printed in the November 2014 issue of this publication.

18. Signature and Title of Editor, Publisher, Business Manager, or Owner	Date
Stephen R. Bushing – Inventory Distribution Coordinator	September 14, 2014

I certify that all information furnished on this form is true and complete. I understand that anyone who furnishes false or misleading information on this form or who omits material or information requested on the form may be subject to criminal sanctions (including fines and imprisonment) and/or civil sanctions (including civil penalties).

PS Form 3526, August 2012 (Page 2 of 3)

Moving?

Make sure your subscription moves with you!

To notify us of your new address, find your **Clinics Account Number** (located on your mailing label above your name), and contact customer service at:

Email: journalscustomerservice-usa@elsevier.com

800-654-2452 (subscribers in the U.S. & Canada)
314-447-8871 (subscribers outside of the U.S. & Canada)

Fax number: 314-447-8029

Elsevier Health Sciences Division
Subscription Customer Service
3251 Riverport Lane
Maryland Heights, MO 63043

*To ensure uninterrupted delivery of your subscription, please notify us at least 4 weeks in advance of move.

Moving?

Make sure your subscription moves with you!

To notify us of your new address, find your Clinics Account Number (located on your mailing label above your name), and contact customer service at:

Email: journalscustomerservice-usa@elsevier.com

800-654-2452 (subscribers in the U.S. & Canada)
314-447-8871 (subscribers outside of the U.S. & Canada)

Fax number: 314-447-8029

Elsevier Health Sciences Division
Subscription Customer Service
3251 Riverport Lane
Maryland Heights, MO 63043

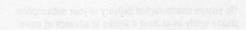

Printed and bound by CPI Group (UK) Ltd, Croydon, CR0 4YY
00/40/2022

81040019-0001

Printed and bound by CPI Group (UK) Ltd, Croydon, CR0 4YY

03/10/2024

01040378-0001